AF335584

Management of
of
Prostate
Cancer

Advances and Controversies

Management of Prostate Cancer

Advances and Controversies

Kenneth B. Cummings M.D.

*Professor and Program Director,
Division of Urology
The Robert Wood Johnson Medical School
University of Medicine and
Dentistry of New Jersey
New Brunswick, NJ, U.S.A.*

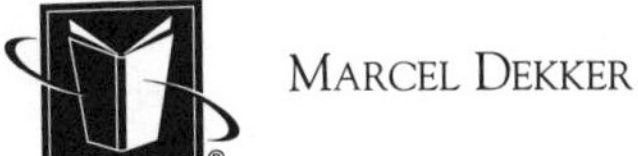

MARCEL DEKKER   NEW YORK

Library of Congress Cataloging-in-Publication Data
A catalog record for this book is available from the Library of Congress.

ISBN: 0-8247-5441-7

This book is printed on acid-free paper.

Headquarters
Marcel Dekker, 270 Madison Avenue, New York, NY 10016, U.S.A.
tel: 212-696-9000; fax: 212-685-4540

Distribution and Customer Service
Marcel Dekker, Cimarron Road, Monticello, New York 12701, U.S.A.
tel: 800-228-1160; fax: 845-796-1772

World Wide Web
http://www.dekker.com

The publisher offers discounts on this book when ordered in bulk quantities. For more information, write to Special Sales/Professional Marketing at the headquarters address above.

Current printing (last digit):

10 9 8 7 6 5 4 3 2 1

PRINTED IN THE UNITED STATES OF AMERICA

Preface

Prostate-Specific Antigen (PSA) testing to detect patients at risk for disease has resulted in increased prostate cancer detection, as well as significant stage migration, with a significant increase in the new cases detected representing patients with localized disease. Additionally, PSA has permitted monitoring of disease progression in treated patients, permitting a greater clarity in efficacy of specific therapeutic interventions.

Associated with the therapeutic advances of the past decade is controversy. The subjects about which uncertainty remain include the best treatment for localized disease and include the comparative efficacy of radical prostatectomy—anatomic radical retropubic prostatectomy (ARRP), radical perineal prostatectomy (RP), laparoscopic radical prostatectomy (LRP), or robot-assisted laparoscopic radical prostatectomy (RARP)—and definitive radiation (three-dimensional conformal radiation, brachytherapy combined modality radiation, or intensity modulated radiation therapy) or Cyroablation. Further, the benefits of postprostatectomy radiation in high-risk, localized disease and its timing (adjuvent or salvage) is not defined. Despite the observation that androgen deprivation (AD) was demonstrated to be of significant clinical benefit for men with advanced prostate cancer over sixty years ago, the timing of AD for PSA progression as the first indication of failure of local treatment remains a major controversy.

The role of "novel therapies" for patients with PSA progression in the absence of imageable metastatic disease may represent an opportunity for experimental therapeutics and "drug discovery." In a disease in which systemic metastasis leads to death from disease, and where no curative therapy has been defined, it is appropriate to examine future perspectives.

Many of the issues of clinical management are contentious and likely are consequent to our inability or unwillingness to subject some of the important clinical questions to well-designed, adequately powered, randomized, and controlled clinical trials.

In the attempt to provide clarity for clinicians, acknowledged leaders in their field and advocates for their therapeutic approach have provided a careful review of their patient selection criteria, staging procedures, therapy, and outcomes. To provide understanding and definition in areas of controversy, a "point–counterpoint" approach has been taken for each presentation with thoughtful critical reflection by acknowledged experts in the field. It is hoped that this volume will be timely, edifying, and of value in aiding clinicians to select an individualized treatment option for the patients for whom they bear "the responsibility of care."

Kenneth B. Cummings, MD
Professor and Program Director,
Division of Urology
The Robert Wood Johnson
Medical School
University of Medicine and
Dentistry of New Jersey,
New Brunswick, NJ, U.S.A.

Contents

Contributors

Sidney C. Abreu, MD Cleveland Clinic Foundation, Cleveland, Ohio, U.S.A.

Neil H. Bander, MD Bernard and Josephine Chaus Professor, Weill Medical College of Cornell University, Attending Surgeon, Brady Urology New York-Presbyterian Hospital-Cornell University Medical Center, New York, NY, U.S.A.

Arie S. Belldegrun, MD Roy and Carol Doumani Chair in Urologic Oncology, Professor of Urology, Chief, Division of Urologic Oncology, David Geffen School of Medicine, University of California School of Medicine, Los Angeles, California, U.S.A.

H. Ballentine Carter, MD Professor of Urology and Oncology, The James Buchanan Brady Urological Institute, The Johns Hopkins Medical Institutions, Baltimore, Maryland, U.S.A.

E. David Crawford, MD Professor of Surgery and Radiation Oncology, University of Colorado Health Sciences Center, Denver, Colorado, U.S.A.

Kenneth B. Cummings, MD Professor and Program Director, Division of Urology, The Robert Wood Johnson Medical School, University of Medicine and Dentistry of New Jersey, New Brunswick, NJ, U.S.A.

Philipp Dahm, MD Assistant Professor Division of Urology, Department of Surgery, Duke University Medical Center, Durham, North Carolina, U.S.A.

Jens Dannull, MD   Assitant Research Professor of Urology, Department of Surgery, Duke University Medical Center, Durham, North Carolina, U.S.A.

Ralph W. de Vere White, MD   Professor and Chairman, Department of Urology, Director UC Davis Cancer Center, University of California Davis, Sacramento, California, U.S.A.

Caner Z. Dinlenc, MD   Department of Urology, Beth Israel Medical Center, New York, NY, U.S.A.

Robert S. DiPaola, MD   Associate Professor of Medicine, The Robert Wood Johnson Medical School, University of Medicine and Dentistry of New Jersey, The Cancer Institute of New Jersey, New Brunswick, NJ, U.S.A.

Michael J. Droller, MD   Katherine and Clifford Goldsmith Professor of Urology, The Mount Sinai Medical Center, New York, NY, U.S.A.

James A. Eastham, MD   Memorial Sloan-Kettering Cancer Center, New York, NY, U.S.A.

Mario A. Eisenberger, MD   R. Dale Hughes Professor of Oncology and Urology, The Johns Hopkins University, Baltimore, MD, U.S.A.

Adrian H. Feng, MD   Resident in Urology, Case Western Reserve University School of Medicine, Cleveland, Ohio, U.S.A.

Molly Gabel, MD   Department of Radiation Oncology, Robert Wood Johnson Medical School, The University of Medicine and Dentistry of New Jersey, The Cancer Institute of New Jersey, New Brunswick, NJ, U.S.A.

Suzanne Generao, MD   Chief Resident in Urology, University of California Davis, Sacramento, California, U.S.A.

Robert P. Gibbons, M.D., Emeritus   Section of Urology and Renal Transplantation, Virginia Mason Clinic, Seattle, WA, U.S.A.

Inderbir S. Gill, MD   Cleveland Clinic Foundation, Cleveland, Ohio, U.S.A.

Jay Y. Gillenwater, MD   Professor of Urology, University of Virginia at the Medical School, Charlottesville, Virginia, U.S.A.

Bertrand Guillonneau, MD   Professor of Urology, Weill Medical College of Cornell University Head, Section of Minimally Invasive Surgery Department of Urology, Memorial Sloan Kettering Cancer Center, Sidney Kimmel Center for Prostate & Urologic Cancer, New York, NY, U.S.A.

Michael J. Harris, MD   Northern Institute of Urology, Traverse City, Michigan, U.S.A.

Ashok K. Hemal, MD   Professor, AIIMS Department of Urology, Vattikuti Urology Institute, Henry Ford Hospital, Detroit, Michigan, U.S.A.

Parvesh Kumar, MD   Professor and Chairman, Department of Radiation Oncology, University of Southern California Keck School of Medicine, Los Angeles, CA, U.S.A.

Daniel W. Lin, MD   Memorial Sloan-Kettering Cancer Center, New York, NY, U.S.A.

Mani Menon, MD   Raj and Padma Vattikuti Distinguished Chair, Director of Vattikuti Urology Institute, Vattikuti Urology Institute, Henry Ford Hospital, Detroit, Michigan, U.S.A.

Edward M. Messing, MD   Professor and Chair Department of Urology, University of Rochester Medical Center, Rochester, NY, U.S.A.

Robert P. Myers, MD   Consultant in Urology, Mayo Clinic, Professor of Urology, Mayo Clinic College of Medicine, Rochester, Minnesota, U.S.A.

Allan J. Pantuck, MD   Assistant Professor of Urology, David Geffen School of Medicine at University of California, Los Angeles, California, U.S.A.

Alan W. Partin, MD   Bernard L. Schwartz Distinguished Professor of Urologic Oncology, The Brady Urological Institute, The Johns Hopkins Medical Institution, Baltimore, MD, U.S.A.

David F. Paulson, MD   Professor of Urologic Surgery, Duke University Medical Center, Durham, North Carolina, U.S.A.

Louis Pisters, MD   Professor of Urology, University of Texas, MD Anderson Cancer Center, Houston, Texas, U.S.A.

Haakon Ragde, MD   The Haakon Ragde Foundation for Advanced Cancer Studies, Seattle, Washington, U.S.A.

Hari Siva Gurunadha Rao Tunuguntla, MD   University of California Davis, Sacramento, California, U.S.A.

Martin I. Resnick, MD   Lester Persky Professor of Urology, Chairman, Department of Urology, Case Western Reserve University School of Medicine, Cleveland, Ohio, U.S.A.

David B. Samadi, MD   Assistant Professor of Urology at Columbia Presbyterian Medical Center, New York, New York, U.S.A.

Peter T. Scardino, MD   Professor and Chairman, Department of Urology, Memorial Sloan-Kettering Cancer Center, New York, NY, U.S.A.

Paul F. Schellhammer, MD   Professor of Urology, Department of Urology, Eastern Virginia Medical School, Norfolk, VA, U.S.A.

Mark Shaves, MD   Assistant Professor, Department of Radiation Oncology, Eastern Virginia Medical School, Norfolk, VA, U.S.A.

Susan F. Slovin, MD, PhD   Genitourinary Oncology Service, Memorial Sloan-Kettering Cancer Center, New York, NY, U.S.A.

Andrew P. Steinberg, MD   Cleveland Clinic Foundation, Cleveland, Ohio, U.S.A.

Richard G. Stock, MD   Professor of Department of Radiation Oncology, Mount Sinai Medical Center, New York, NY, U.S.A.

Nelson N. Stone, MD   Clinical Professor of Urology, Mount Sinai Medical Center, New York, NY, U.S.A.

Donald L. Trump, MD   Professor of Medicine, Senior Vice President for Clinical Research and Chairman of Medicine, Roswell Park Cancer Institute Buffalo, NY, U.S.A.

Johannes Vieweg, MD   Associate Professor of Urology, Department of Surgery, Associate Professor of Immunology, Duke University Medical Center, Durham, North Carolina, U.S.A.

Joseph R. Wagner, MD   Connecticut Surgical Group Hartford Hospital, Hartford, CT, U.S.A.

Amnon Zisman, MD   Assistant Professor of Urology, Assaf-Harofeh Medical Center, Israel

1

Anatomic Radical Prostatectomy in the Management of Localized Prostate Cancer

Daniel W. Lin and James A. Eastham
Department of Urology, Memorial Sloan-Kettering Cancer Center, New York, NY, USA

INTRODUCTION

Prostate cancer remains the most common form of noncutaneous malignancy and the second leading cause of cancer death in American men. It is estimated that more than 198,000 men will be diagnosed with prostate cancer in the United States, and 31,500 will die of this disease [1]. Because prostate cancer incidence increases rapidly with age, the absolute number of diagnosed cases is destined to rise worldwide as life expectancy increases. Indeed, the number of men older than 65 years is likely to double from 1990 to 2020. Prostate cancer will not only cause the death of 3% of all men alive today who are over 50 years old, but will also cause many men to suffer serious complications from local tumor growth or distant metastases, as well as from complications of treatment.

Despite its nearly epidemic proportions, prostate cancer evokes considerable controversy as a result of its unusual biologic features and the lack of firm data regarding the natural history of the disease. Consequently, patients diagnosed with a clinically localized prostate cancer face a daunting variety of treatment choices, including observation (''watchful waiting''), brachytherapy and/or external beam irradiation therapy with or without androgen deprivation therapy, as well as surgery. Because the disease often strikes older men with other co-morbid conditions, the risk to life and health posed by the cancer itself has been difficult to quantify [2–4]. Although preliminary studies [5–6] have supported the use of Prostate-Specific Antigen screening for early detection and treatment and have reported a decrease in disease-specific mortality with aggressive screening, prospective, randomized trials to establish whether early detection (PLCO) or treatment (PIVOT) of localized prostate cancer will decrease the mortality rate from the disease have not yet been completed [7,8]. Until such studies are concluded, patients and their physicians must make the decision whether to treat this aggressively or manage cancer conservatively with the best evidence available today.

For nearly a century, radical prostatectomy has been an effective way to achieve long-term control of clinically localized prostate cancer. The original technique, described by Kuchler in 1858 and developed by Young and, later, by Belt, was performed perineally [9,10]. A retropubic approach for resection of benign adenomas was introduced by Millin in the 1940s. This approach was modified for radical extirpation of the prostate and seminal vesicles and rapidly adopted by urologists [11–14]. Retropubic prostatectomy offers several advantages: the anatomy is more familiar to urologists, there are fewer rectal injuries, a staging pelvic lymphadenectomy can easily be performed, and the wide exposure offers great flexibility to adapt the operation to each individual's anatomy, permitting more consistent preservation of the neurovascular bundles and a lower rate of positive surgical margins. Radical retropubic prostatectomy, therefore, has become our standard procedure for removal of the prostate for treatment of localized prostate cancer.

Since the late 1970s, more accurate definitions of periprostatic anatomy have allowed the development of an operation that is more respectful of the intricate anatomy of the periprostatic tissues [15]. The fine details in surgical technique clearly affect the outcomes after radical retropubic prosatectomy, namely cancer control, as well as recovery of continence and erectile function. Technical refinements have resulted in lower rates of urinary incontinence [16–18] and higher rates of recovery of erectile function [19], less blood loss, fewer transfusions, [20,21] and shorter hospital stays, [22,23] as well as lower rates of positive surgical margins [24–26]. A thorough understanding of periprostatic anatomy, which emphasizes vascular control and meticulous dissection, permits the safe performance of a radical prostatectomy with reduced morbidity.

This chapter describes the rationale for radical retropubic prostatectomy, the preoperative evaluation, and the long-term outcomes, including continence and erectile function. We emphasize key aspects of periprostatic anatomy and surgical technique that allow the procedure to be performed safely with minimal complications.

RATIONALE FOR SURGICAL TREATMENT

Serum PSA, discovered in the late 1970s, has been shown to be effective in the early detection of prostate cancer and is widely considered the most useful tumor marker in oncology [27,28]. Consequently, a dramatic shift in the stage of disease at diagnosis has occurred. Prior to the development of serum PSA testing, only 30% of patients were diagnosed with clinically organ-confined prostate cancer (stage A or B) [29]. Today, 90% of cancers detected in screening trials are clinically confined (stage T1–T2, N0, M0). [30] Accordingly, the incidence of nodal metastases at pelvic lymphadenectomy has declined to 1% to 3% [31]. In 60% of patients with clinically confined prostate cancer, the cancer is completely confined to the prostate pathologically.

Some investigators, however, have questioned the routine use of serum PSA as a screening tool due to the high prevalence of prostate cancer in the aging male. For instance, examination of the prostate gland at autopsy in men 50 years of age or older who had no clinical evidence of cancer identified adenocarcinoma in approximately 30% of cases [32–34]. Yet, the lifetime risk of developing a clinically detected prostate cancer is about 10% [35]. This discrepancy between the high prevalence of prostate cancer found at autopsy and the lower incidence of clinically detected cancer raises the question concerning which prostate cancers might be best managed without immediate treatment. In other words, are cancers detected solely on the basis of an elevated serum PSA level clinically indolent, or are these cancers significant, but identified at an earlier stage?

To examine this question, we compared the pathologic features of impalpable prostate cancers detected by an elevated serum PSA (stage T1c), prostate cancers which were palpable on digital rectal examination (DRE), and prostate cancers found incidentally at cystoprostatectomy for bladder cancer [36]. (Table 1) Prostate cancer was diagnosed in 209 men based solely on an elevated serum PSA. While these tumors were often high grade (55% had a primary or secondary Gleason grade of 4 or 5) and frequently demonstrated extracapsular extension (40%), these tumors had a more favorable profile than a group of 468 men with palpable cancer. Only 25% of clinical stage T1c tumors displayed advanced pathologic features compared to 40% of palpable cancers, while the proportion of indolent tumors was similar (9%) in each group (Table 1) [36]. This distribution of pathologic features contrasts sharply with results from the cystoprostatectomy series in which none had advanced pathologic features and 78% were considered indolent, suggesting that most prostate cancers detected solely on the basis of an elevated serum PSA level are clinically important and are more likely to be cured by radical prostatectomy than palpable tumors.

The natural history of localized prostate cancer has only recently been documented [37–40]. Two large series have been published that document the risk of developing metastases and of death from prostate cancer in men with

TABLE 1 Percentage of Cancers Detected Clinically (Radical Prostatectomy Series) and Incidentally (Cystoprostatectomy Series) that were Indolent, Clinically Important but Curable, and Advanced.* (Modified from Ohori et al., 1994 (137) and reprinted with permission)

		Prognostic category (%)		
Cancer	N	Indolent	Curable	Advanced
Cystoprostatectomy series	90	78	22	0
Radical prostatectomy series	759	10	56	34
Clinical stage T1a, b	73	19	59	22
Palpable tumor	468	9	52	40
Impalpable, elevated PSA level	209	9	66	25
Elevated PSA only, impalpable, nonvisible	110	12	69	19

Abbreviation: PSA, prostate-specific antigen.

* Categories are defined by pathologic criteria. Indolent cancers are <0.5gm and confined to the prostate with no poorly differentiated elements. Advanced cancers are those that are high grade (Gleason sum >6) and extend through the capsule (established extracapsular extension) to the margins of resection, or those that invade the seminal vesicles or metastasize to the pelvic lymph node. Curable cancers are all others in the 2 series.

clinically localized disease managed conservatively. Chodak and associates analyzed the risk of metastases and of death from prostate cancer in a pooled analysis of 828 patients with clinical stage T1-T2 cancers managed conservatively from six medical centers around the world [37]. The risk of metastases at 10 years was 19% for well-differentiated, 42% for moderately differentiated, and 74% for poorly differentiated cancers. (Figure 1) While the confidence intervals were broad beyond 10 years, it was evident that when the primary tumor was not controlled, metastases continued to develop over long periods of time. The cancer-specific mortality rate (13%) at 10 years was identical for well and moderately differentiated tumors, which reflects the inadequacy of a 10-year time interval to assess the full impact of a localized prostate cancer on mortality. Of those patients with poorly differentiated tumors, 66% died of prostate cancer at 10 years.

Albertsen et al. reported the results of a population-based study in Connecticut of 451 men between the ages of 65 and 75 years with clinically localized prostate cancer treated conservatively [38]. The cancer-specific mortality rate at 10 years was 9% for well-differentiated, 24% for moderately differentiated, and 46% for poorly differentiated cancers. When compared to age-matched controls, men with localized prostate cancer (mean age, 70.9 years) lost an estimated 3.8 to 5.2 years of life. While the authors emphasized that men with well-differen-

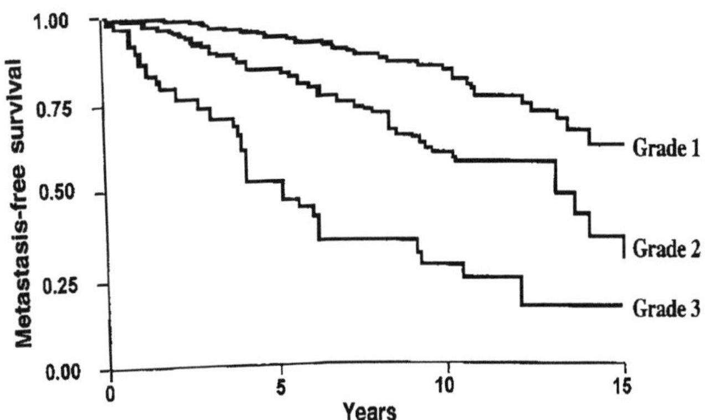

FIGURE 1 Metastasis-Free Survival Among Untreated Patients with Localized Prostate Cancer, According to Tumor Grade. (From Chodak GW, Thisted RA, Gerber GS, et al. Results of conservative management of clinically localized prostate cancer. New Engl J Med 1994; 330:242–248. Reprinted with permission of The New England Journal of Medicine.)

tiated tumors (Gleason sum 2–4) survived as long as age-matched controls, this favorable group comprised only 9% of the patient population. The remaining 91% had a moderately or poorly differentiated tumor and experienced a markedly decreased survival with conservative treatment.

These studies provide strong evidence that clinically localized prostate cancer, while slow growing, can affect patient morbidity and mortality [37–40]. (Table 2) Some prostate cancers progress slowly and present little risk to the overall health of the patient. These cancers almost always fall into the T1a classification or the occasional T1b-T2 cancer that is focal, small, and well differentiated. Expectant management may be a reasonable option for these patients, especially if their life expectancy is less than 10 years. However, most clinically detected prostate cancers are not indolent and pose a significant threat to health and life expectancy and should be treated with the intent to eradicate the primary tumor.

PATIENT SELECTION AND PROGNOSTIC FACTORS

Radical prostatectomy should be reserved for men who are likely to be cured and will live long enough to benefit from the cure. The factors that influence the risk-benefit ratio include the age and health of the patient, the nature of the cancer (the risk of metastasis and death over time if left untreated), the probability that surgery will cure the cancer, and the complications of surgery. Although the efficacy and complication rates of treatment are important factors in the decision-

TABLE 2 Probability of Dying from Prostate Cancer Managed Conservatively According to Biopsy Tumor Grade.

Investigators	N	WellL (2–4)	Mod (5–7)	Poor (8–10)
Chodak et al., 1994[37] (10 years)	828	13	13	34
Albertsen et al., 1995[38] (15 years)	411	9	28	51
Johansson et al., 1997[39] (15 years)	642	6	17	56
Albertsen et al., 1998[40] (15 years)	767	4–7	6–70*	60–87

* Gleason 5= 6–11%; Gleason 6= 18–30%; Gleason 7= 42–70%

analysis model, the dominant features are the metastatic rate of the cancer and the age and life expectancy of the patient [2].

Age and Health

In choosing therapy for an individual patient with clinically localized prostate cancer, the age and general health of the patient remain critically important because of the well-established protracted course of the disease. Mortality from an untreated localized prostate cancer is not likely to occur for 8 to 10 years; yet the risk of death from cancer will continue to increase for at least 15 to 20 years or more. Additionally, the associated morbidity from local progression or metastases can be substantial [39,41–44]. In 1998, the average life expectancy of a 70-year-old man was 12.8 years and for a 75-year-old man it was 10.0 years [45]. Thus, the potential benefits of treatment decrease as a man ages.

Chronological age, however, is only one factor that influences life expectancy. Prostate cancer is frequently diagnosed in older men with associated comorbid conditions. Conversely, some older patients are in excellent health and have a life expectancy greater than the average for their age group. Therefore, an arbitrary age should not be set at which a patient would no longer be considered a surgical candidate. Clinical judgment that thoroughly assesses the life expectancy of the individual patient with prostate cancer will allow the physician to inform the patient fully about the risks and benefits of expectant management, as well as active intervention; in this way, the patient can make a well-informed decision about managing his disease.

Clinical Prognostic Factors

Freedom from progression after radical prostatectomy is associated with several well-established clinical prognostic factors including clinical stage, systematic prostate biopsy information, and serum PSA levels [46–48]. (Table 3 and Figure 2) (Hull GW et al., unpublished data used with permission.) Figure 2 shows the actual nonprogression rates in our series of 1,000 men with clinical stage T1–T2 prostate cancer followed for a mean of 53 months (range, 1 to 170 months) after radical prostatectomy. These survival curves were generated based on preoperative clinical data only. No patient received adjuvant therapy before relapse, and recurrence was defined as a rising PSA level $\geq$ 0.4 ng/mL.

Clinical Stages. In general, as clinical stage increases, so does the risk of disease recurrence [46–48]. (Table 3 and Figure 2) (Hull GW et al., unpublished data used with permission.) Notice, however, that patients with cancers found solely on the basis of an elevated serum PSA level (clinical stage T1c, 328 patients) had an 85% PSA nonprogression rate at 5 years in our series. (Figure 2B) Outcome after radical prostatectomy is influenced by clinical stage, but with the substages considered localized (cT1–T2), it has not proven to be a powerful independent prognostic factor. Between June 1993 and April 1998, we analyzed the progression-free probability after radical prostatectomy for clinically localized prostate cancer in 1,000 consecutive patients. Clinical stage was assigned preoperatively using the 1992 tumor nodal metastasis (TNM) system [49]. Among the clinical T stages, progression rates for T1c and T2a cancers were more favorable than T2b or T2c cancers, while T2b and T2c were similar. In a multivariate analysis of clinical parameters, clinical T stage was an independent predictor of progression, with T1c cancers having a better progression-free survival than T2 cancers. There was no significant difference among the T2 substages in this analysis. (Cagiannos I et al., unpublished data used with permission)

The extent of capsular penetration is an important prognostic feature in patients with clinically localized prostate cancer [50–54]. The role of transrectal ultrasound (TRUS), DRE, and magnetic resonance imaging (MRI) to assess the presence and location of extracapsular extension (ECE) has been reviewed [55,56]. The accuracy of each of these modalities, unfortunately, is limited. The presence of a palpable nodule suggests ECE in 37.4% of patients [49,57], but 18% of patients with no palpable tumor (T1c) have ECE. When the results of DRE and TRUS were combined (if either was positive, the result was considered positive), the results are better, with a positive predictive value of 79% and an overall accuracy of 82% [55]. Endorectal coil MRI may also add to the accuracy of DRE [56,58]. (wei data?)

Seminal vesicle involvement (SVI) is a well-established poor prognostic feature. Patients with SVI not only have an increased incidence of nodal metastasis

TABLE 3 Actuarial (PSA-Based) 5-Year Nonprogression Rates (%) After Radical Prostatectomy for Clinical Stage T1-2NXN0 Prostate Cancer

	Pound et al. (46)	Catalona and Smith (138)	Zincke et al. (48)	Hull et al.[*]
No. patients	1623	925	3170	1000
Clinical Stage				
T1a	100	89[a]		89[a]
T1b	89		85[e]	
T1c	86	99		85
T2a	85	85[b]	81	82
T2b	69		74[f]	67
T2c	63			70
Gleason Score				
2–4	100	91	93[g]	89
5	97		80[h]	84[j]
6		92	89[c]	
7	66		60[i]	60
8–10	41	74		49
Preoperative PSA Level				
0–4	94	95		94
4.1–10.0	82	93		86
10.1–20.0	72	71[d]		65
>20.0	54			41
Pathologic Stage				
Organ/confined	-	91	-	95
Extracapsular extension	-	-	-	76
Seminal vesicle invasion	-	-	-	37
Positive lymph node(s)	-	-	-	18
Surgical Margin				
Negative				81
Positive				36

Abbreviation: PSA, prostate-specific antigen

[*] Hull GW et al., unpublished data used with permission

[a] Includes T1a and T1b [e] Includes T1a, T1b and T1c [i] Includes Gleason score 7 [b] Includes T2a and T2b [f] Includes T2b and T2c [j] Includes Gleason scores 5–6 [c] Includes Gleason scores 5–7 [g] Includes Gleason scores ≤3 [d] Includes PSA > 10 [h] Includes Gleason scores 4–6

A

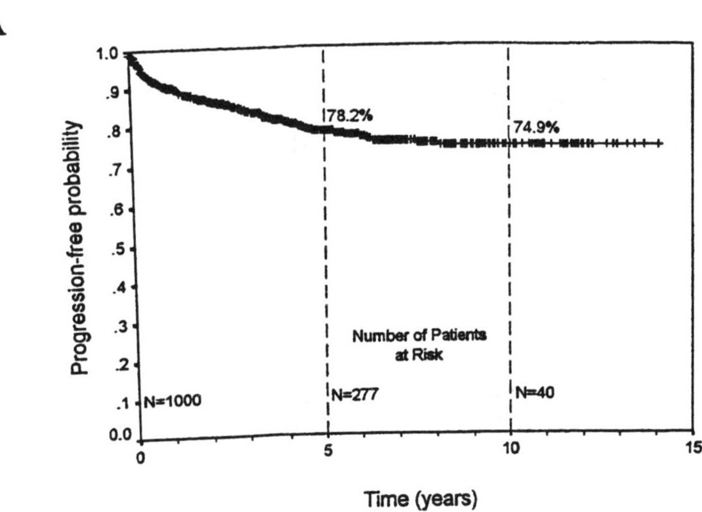

B

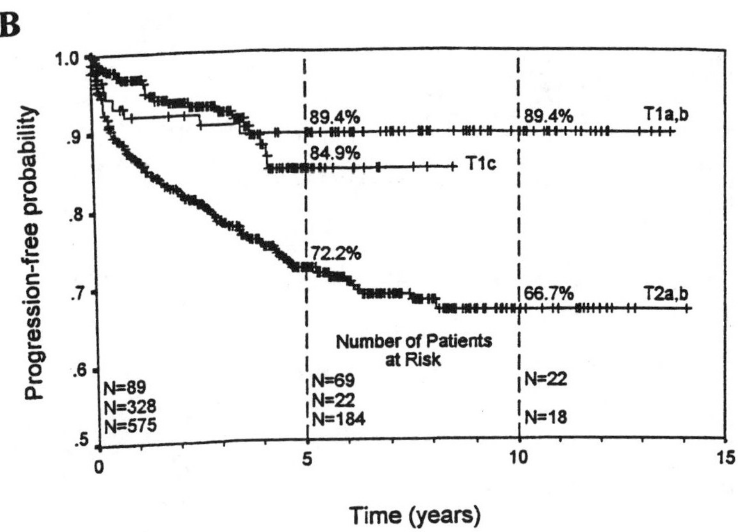

FIGURE 2 ab   Progression-Free Probability for the Overall Population (A) and Based on Clinical Stage (B), Biopsy Gleason Score (BxGS).

C

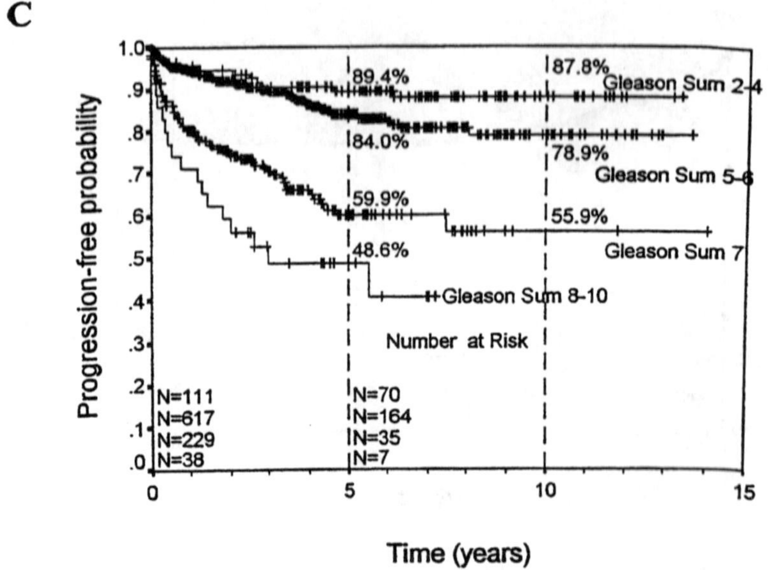

D

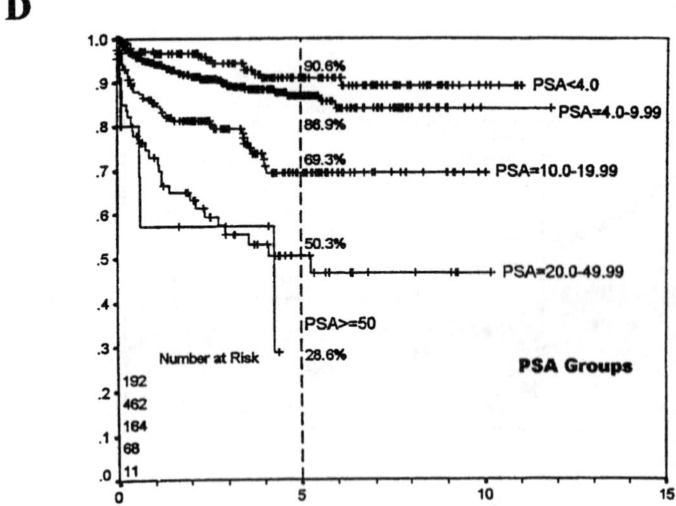

FIGURE 2 cd   (C), and Preoperative Serum Prostate-Specific Antigen (PSA) Level (D). The number of patients is shown on the horizontal axis. (Modified from Hull GW et al., unpublished data and reprinted with permission.)

[59], but also a worse prognosis, even in the absence of lymph node involvement [60,61]. To identify reliable criteria for detecting SVI preoperatively, we compared radical prostatectomy specimens and TRUS [62]. Based on our findings, we developed 3 criteria for SVI: (1) a hypoechoic lesion at the base of the prostate; (2) an "adhesion sign" resulting from loss of the echo reflections from the normal fat plane between the prostate and the seminal vesicle; and (3) "posterior convexity" of the seminal vesicles. These criteria, combined with serum PSA level, allow us to classify patients into those with a low-risk and those with a high-risk of SVI. Sixty-two percent of patients with a PSA > 10 ng/mL and a positive TRUS, had SVI. However, only 3% of patients with a PSA < 10 ng/mL and a negative TRUS had SVI [63]. MRI has proved superior to TRUS in detecting SVI, especially when the image is enhanced by use of an endorectal coil [64,65]. Although SVI may not be an absolute contraindication to radical prostatectomy, its presence has profound implications that could alter treatment recommendations.

Prostate Needle Biopsy Information

While Gleason score is an important prognostic factor, it cannot be used categorically to justify management. PSA nonprogression rates at 5 years following radical prostatectomy according to the biopsy Gleason score are summarized in Table 3 [46–48] (Hull GW et al., unpublished data used with permission.) As the tumor becomes more poorly differentiated, the likelihood of disease recurrence increases. In our own series, a marked decrease was shown in the probability of nonprogression with more poorly differentiated cancers. (Figure 2c; Modified from Hull GW et al., unpublished data used with permission).

We recently conducted a study of 1,039 patients treated with radical prostatectomy for clinically localized prostate cancer to determine if poor results following surgery for high-grade cancers were attributable to the aggressive nature of the cancer itself or to the advanced stage at diagnosis [66]. Poorly differentiated cancer, defined as a Gleason score ≥ 7 in the biopsy specimen, was present in 298 (30%) of 1,003 patients. Cancers detected because of an elevated PSA only (T1c, n = 335) were nearly as likely (24%) to be poorly differentiated as cancers detected by DRE (T2 or T3a, n = 668), of which 32% were poorly differentiated on biopsy. However 49% of the poorly differentiated T1c cancers were confined to the prostate, compared to only 28% of the poorly differentiated cancers detected by DRE (p = 0.001). Additionally, the prognosis for the poorly differentiated T1c cancers was significantly better (5-year freedom from progression, 69% vs. 55%, p = 0.047). Although poorly differentiated tumors frequently extend outside the prostate at the time of diagnosis, a poorly differentiated cancer can be controlled by radical prostatectomy if detected while still organ-confined (5-year freedom from progression was 91%). (Figure 3) Therefore, Gleason grade alone should not be used to exclude a patient with a potentially curable prostate cancer.

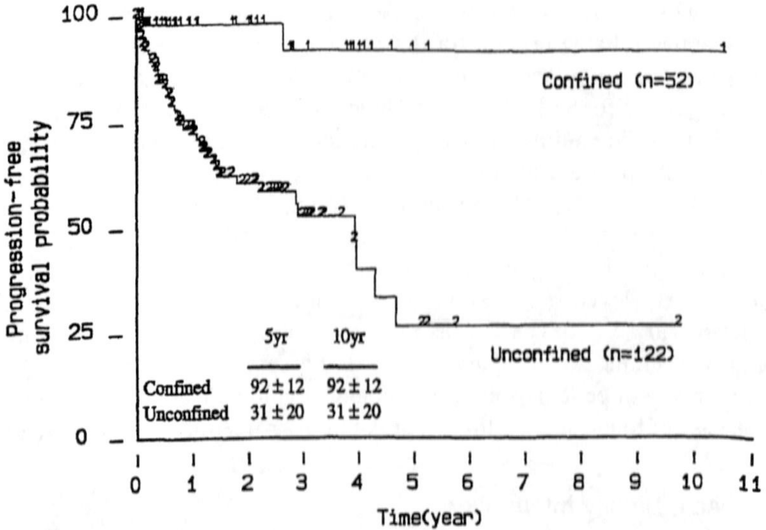

Figure 3 Progression-free rate by pathologic stage (confined versus unconfined) after radical prostatectomy in 174 patients with clinically localized (clinical stage T1–T2 NxMo), poorly differentiated (Gleason score 7–10) cancer on biopsy.

The results of systematic needle biopsy may also indicate areas suspicious for ECE [67]. Information about the location of positive biopsies, the length of cancer in each core, the grade of cancer, and the presence of perineural invasion can help to characterize the location and extent of cancer within the prostate [68–72]. The presence of ECE is not a contraindication to radical prostatectomy, since long-term cancer control is possible in over two-thirds of patients with microscopic ECE. However, knowledge of the presence and location of ECE will allow the surgeon performing radical prostatectomy to modify the operation by performing a wider excision in the involved area so that the tumor can be removed with decreased risk of a positive surgical margin [53,54]. Still, improved imaging studies or other techniques that can detect ECE are urgently needed.

Serum PSA Level

In prostate cancer, the level of serum PSA has been correlated with total tumor volume, clinical and pathological stage, and prognosis [28]. Freedom from PSA progression as a function of preoperative PSA is shown in Table 3 [46–48]. (Hull GW et al., unpublished data used with permission). Preoperative serum PSA levels are also associated with the risk of progression after radical prostatectomy. (Figure 2D) As with clinical stage and biopsy Gleason score, increasing preoperative serum PSA levels are correlated with advanced pathologic stage but with considerable overlap. Higher preoperative serum PSA levels are not always associated with advanced pathologic features, and lower valves do not necessarily suggest organ-confirmed disease. Therefore, the serum PSA level cannot definitively distinguish the stage of the cancer in an individual patient and cannot therefore be used alone as an absolute contraindication to definitive treatment.

Prognostic Models

By combining clinical prognostic factors, risk profiles have been developed to predict the outcome of patients with clinically localized prostate cancer who undergo radical prostatectomy. In 1993, Partin and Walsh first examined the combination of clinical and preoperative pathologic parameters in the prediction of pathological stage [73]. Later, in a multicenter study, Partin and associates examined clinical and pathologic data from 4,133 men who underwent radical prostatectomy at Johns Hopkins Hospital, Baylor College of Medicine, and the University of Michigan School of Medicine [74]. Serum PSA level, TNM clinical stage, and biopsy Gleason score were identified as significant predictors of pathologic stage. Nomograms were developed to predict the probability that a given tumor is a specific pathologic stage (Table 4) [74]. Similarly, Kattan and colleagues combined the serum PSA level, clinical stage, and biopsy Gleason score to develop a nomogram to predict the likelihood of recurrence of disease as detected by serum PSA level after radical prostatectomy [75]. (Figure 4) These prognostic models should enable patients and physicians to make more informed treatment decisions based on the patient's clinical situation.

COMPLICATIONS AND SURGICAL TECHNIQUES TO REDUCE COMPLICATIONS

Early Complications: Hemorrhage, Rectal Injury, and Thromboembolism

Hemorrhage is the most common intraoperative complication during radical retropubic prostatectomy. Historically, radical prostatectomy was accompanied by substantial blood loss and the frequent need for transfusions [15,[76,77]. However, with more accurate descriptions of the dorsal vein complex and periprostatic anatomy and the development of techniques to control the major vessels early in the course of the operation, surgeons can perform the radical retropubic prostatectomy with reduced blood loss [15,[78,79]. The key steps in this surgical procedure are: (a) complete control of the dorsal vein complex and anterior periprostatic veins, (b) identification and control of the small branches from the neurovascular bundles to the prostate posterolaterally, and (c) dissection of the seminal vesicles and vas with control of the many small vessels between the base of the bladder

TABLE 4 Predicted Probability of each Pathologic Stage Based on Preoperative Serum Prostate Specific Antigen (PSA) Level, Clinical Stage, and Gleason Grade in the Biopsy Specimen. Modified with permission, Partin et al (74).

Gleason scores	PSA, 0.0–4.0 ng/mL clinical stage			PSA, 4.1–10.0 ng/mL clinical stage			PSA, 10.1–20.0 ng/mL clinical stage		
	T1c	T2a	T2b	T1c	T2a	T2b	T1c	T2a	T2b
Organ-Confined Disease									
5	81 (76–84)	68 (63–72)	57 (50–62)	71 (67–75)	55 (51–60)	43 (38–49)	60 (54–65)	43 (38–49)	32 (26–37)
6	78 (74–81)	64 (59–68)	52 (46–57)	67 (64–70)	51 (47–54)	38 (34–43)	55 (51–59)	38 (34–43)	26 (23–31)
7	63 (58–68)	47 (41–52)	34 (29–39)	49 (45–54)	33 (29–38)	22 (18–26)	35 (31–40)	22 (18–26)	13 (11–16)
8 to 10	52 (41–62)	36 (27–45)	24 (17–32)	37 (28–46)	23 (16–31)	14 (9–19)	23 (16–32)	14 (9–19)	7 (5–11)
Established Capsular Penetration									
5	18 (15–22)	30 (26–35)	40 (34–46)	27 (23–30)	41 (36–46)	50 (45–55)	35 (30–40)	50 (45–56)	57 (51–63)
6	21 (18–25)	34 (30–38)	43 (38–48)	30 (27–33)	44 (41–48)	52 (48–56)	38 (34–42)	52 (48–57)	57 (51–62)
7	31 (26–36)	45 (40–50)	51 (46–57)	40 (35–44)	52 (48–57)	54 (49–59)	45 (40–50)	55 (50–60)	51 (45–57)
8 to 10	34 (27–44)	47 (38–56)	48 (40–57)	40 (33–49)	49 (42–57)	46 (39–53)	40 (33–49)	46 (38–55)	38 (30–47)
Seminal Vesicle Involvement									
5	1 (1–2)	2 (1–3)	3 (2–4)	2 (1–3)	3 (2–5)	5 (3–8)	3 (2–5)	5 (3–8)	8 (5–11)
6	1 (1–2)	2 (1–3)	3 (2–4)	2 (2–3)	3 (2–4)	5 (4–7)	4 (3–5)	5 (3–7)	7 (5–10)
7	4 (2–7)	6 (4–9)	10 (6–14)	8 (5–11)	10 (8–13)	15 (11–19)	12 (8–16)	14 (10–19)	18 (13–24)
8 to 10	9 (5–16)	12 (7–19)	17 (11–25)	15 (10–22)	19 (13–26)	24 (17–31)	20 (13–28)	22 (15–31)	25 (18–34)
Lymph Node Involvement									
5	0 (0–0)	0 (0–1)	1 (0–2)	0 (0–1)	1 (0–1)	2 (1–3)	1 (0–2)	2 (1–3)	4 (1–7)
6	0 (0–1)	1 (0–1)	2 (1–3)	1 (1–2)	2 (1–3)	4 (3–6)	3 (2–5)	4 (3–6)	10 (7–13)
7	1 (1–3)	2 (1–4)	5 (2–8)	3 (2–5)	4 (3–6)	9 (6–12)	8 (5–11)	9 (6–13)	17 (12–23)
8 to 10	4 (2–7)	5 (2–9)	10 (5–17)	8 (4–12)	9 (5–13)	16 (11–24)	16 (10–24)	17 (11–25)	29 (21–38)

* Numbers represent percent predictive probability (95% confidence interval). Ellipses indicate lack of sufficient data to calculate probability.

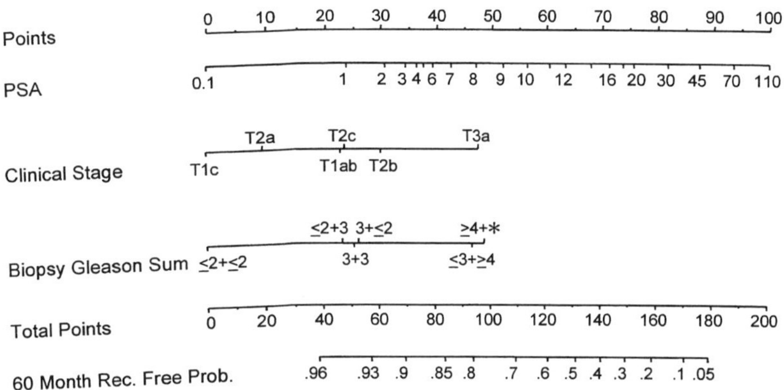

Instructions for Physician: Locate the patient's PSA on the **PSA** axis. Draw a line straight upwards to the **Points** axis to determine how many points towards recurrence the patient receives for his PSA. Repeat this process for the **Clinical Stage** and **Biopsy Gleason Sum** axes, each time drawing straight upward to the **Points** axis. Sum the points achieved for each predictor and locate this sum on the **Total Points** axis. Draw a line straight down to find the patient's probability of remaining recurrence free for 60 months assuming he does not die of another cause first.

Note: This nomogram is not applicable to a man who is not otherwise a candidate for radical prostatectomy. You can use this on only a man who has already selected radical prostatectomy as treatment for his prostate cancer.

Instruction to Patient: "Mr. X, if we had 100 men exactly like you, we would expect between <predicted percentage from nomogram − 10%> and <predicted percentage + 10%> to remain free of their disease at 5 years following radical prostatectomy, and recurrence after 5 years is very rare."   © 1997 Michael W. Kattan and Peter T. Scardino

FIGURE 4 Nomogram that uses preoperative clinical factors (PSA level, biopsy, Gleason grade, and clinical stage) to predict the probability of freedom from progression (defined as a rising serum PSA level or the initiation of any other therapy for prostate cancer). (Modified from Kattan MW, Eastham JA, Stapleton AM, Wheeler TM, Scardino PT. A preoperative nomogram for disease recurrence following radical prostatectomy for prostate cancer. J Natl Cancer Inst 1998; 90(10): 766–71 and reprinted with permission)

and the seminal vesicles [20]. When bleeding is reduced, the surgeon can focus on complete excision of the cancer, selective preservation of the neurovascular bundles responsible for erectile function, and precise construction of the vesicourethral anastomosis.

The estimated blood loss from several large radical prostatectomy series [48,76,80,81] is summarized in Table 5. Over the years, we have modified the operative techniques to significantly reduce blood loss. These techniques, together with a more stringent transfusion policy, have reduced the rate of homologous transfusion to 10% for patients who did not donate autologous blood. Additionally, only 21% of autologous units donated were transfused.

Other intraoperative and perioperative complications occur much less frequently now than in previous decades [42]. Early complication rates from several

TABLE 5 Estimated Blood Loss (EBL) in Patients Undergoing Radical Retropubic Prostatectomy

Series	N	Mean EBL (cc)	Range
Leandri et al (80).	220	300	100–1500
Kavoussi et al (76).	65*	1420	200–2500
	65†	1605	250–3500
Rainwater et al (81).	316	1020	100–4320
Zinke et al (48).	1728	600	–
Baylor	**954**	**800**	**150–5000**

* Hypogastric artery occluded
† Hypogastric artery not occluded

large medical centers are summarized in Table 6 [80,82–84]. Operative mortality, defined as death within 30 days of surgery, occurred in only 11 (0.3%) of 3,834 men. Rectal injury was also uncommon, occurring in less than 1% of patients. Factors that predispose the patient to rectal injury include previous pelvic radiation therapy, rectal surgery, and/or transurethral resection of the prostate [85]. These injuries most often occur during the apical dissection with division of the rectourethralis muscle. If a rectal injury occurs, it should not be repaired until after the prostatectomy has been completed. The injury is closed in two inverted layers, and the anal sphincter is dilated. To reduce the potential of fistula formation, omentum may be placed between the rectum and vesicourethral anastomosis. An opening in the peritoneum is made in the rectovesical cul-de-sac, and the omentum is delivered through the opening [86]. A diverting colostomy is rarely necessary unless the injury is extensive or there is evidence of proctitis from prior radiation treatment.

Deep venous thrombosis and pulmonary embolism occur in approximately 1.1% and 1.3% of patients following radical retropubic prostatectomy, respectively (see Table 6). Considerable controversy exists regarding the role of anticoagulants and sequential pneumatic compression devices in the prevention of these complications. Numerous studies have suggested that sequential pneumatic compression devices are effective in preventing thromboembolic complications. Caprini and colleagues showed that the evidence of deep venous thrombosis detected by figrinogen uptake was decreased from 21% in control patients to 3% in patients wearing sequential pneumatic compression devices [87]. Other studies evaluating urologic patients undergoing pelvic surgery have comfirmed this finding [88,89]. However, a study by Cisek and Walsh reported no difference in the incidence of clinically detected pulmonary emboli or deep venous thrombosis in the thirty-day period following surgery for patients with or without sequential pneumatic compression devices. Thromboembolic complications occurred in 2%

TABLE 6 Perioperative Complications of Radical Retropubic Prostatectomy in Contemporary Series

Complications	Washington University (17) (n=1324)		Mayo Clinic (13) (n=3170)		Ulm (15) (n=418)		Toulose (16) (n=620)		Baylor (n=472)		Overall (n=6004)	
	No	%	No	%	No	%	No	%	No	%	No	%
Rectal Injury	3	0.2	33	1.0	11	2.9	3	0.5	3	0.6	53/6004	0.9
Colostomy	–	–	4	0.1	–	–	–	–	0	0.0	4/3642	0.1
Ureteral Injury	–	–	–	–	1	0.2	0	0.0	1	0.2	2/1510	0.1
Myocardial Infarction	9	0.7	16	0.5	3	0.7	1	0.2	2	0.4	31/6004	0.5
Pulmonary Embolism	22	1.7	58	1.8	6	1.4	5	0.8	5	1.0	96/6004	1.6
Thrombophlebitis/DVT	8	0.6	41	1.3	7	1.7	14	2.3	6	1.3	76/6004	1.3
Sepsis	–	–	–	–	–	–	1	0.2	3	0.6	4/1092	0.4
Wound Infection or Dehiscence	17	1.3	–	–	11	2.6	6	1.0	14	2.9	48/2834	1.7
Lymphocele	–	–	–	–	28	6.7*	14	2.3†	10	2.1*	26/1510	1.7
Prolonged Fluid Leak‡	8	0.6	–	–	–	–	–	–	3	0.6	11/1796	0.6
Premature Catheter Loss	4	0.3	–	–	–	–	–	–	7	1.5	11/1796	0.6
Anostomotic Stricture	–	–	–	–	37	8.6	3	0.5	42	9	82/1510	5.4
Mortality	3	0.2	10	0.3	5	1.2	1	0.2	2	0.4	21/6004	0.3

Note that complications are not mutually exclusive, that is, one patient may have had more than one complication.

* All lymphoceles

† Surgically drained lymphoceles

‡ Urine or lymph

(−) signifies unavailable data

of their patients and most often occurred after discharge from the hospital [90]. As hospital stay after radical prostatectomy continues to decrease, patients should be well informed about the signs and symptoms of deep venous thrombosis and pulmonary embolism to avoid subsequent delays in diagnosis and treatment.

Methods to Reduce Blood Loss

Dorsal Vein Complex Remain

Mobilization of the prosate for adequate dorsal venous complex exposure is first accomplished by incising the endopelvic fascia laterally in the groove between the prostate and the levator ani muscles. This fascial incision is then extended sharply toward the pelvis where the fascia condenses into the puboprostatic ligaments. Blunt dissection using the surgeon's finger will divide the remaining fascia posteriorly and mobilize the prostate from the levator ani muscles. We do not routinely divide the puboprostatic ligaments unless the apex of the prostate is poorly exposed.

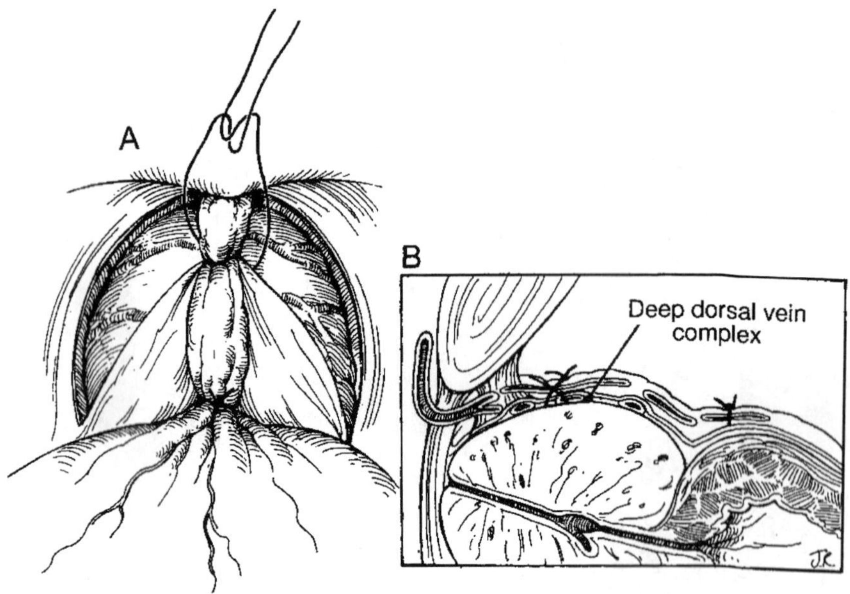

FIGURE 5 The superficial dorsal vein complex is suture ligated at the bladder neck, about 1 cm cephalad to the junction of the prostate and bladder (A and B). A deeper suture is placed around the superficial and deep dorsal vein complex midway toward the apex, extending from one cut edge of endopelvic fascia to the other. These sutures limit back bleeding upon transection of the dorsal vein complex.

To prevent significant back bleeding, the superficial dorsal vein complex is ligated at the bladder neck and the deep dorsal vein complex is suture ligated at the mid prostate. (Figure 5) The first suture marks the site of division of the bladder neck later in the operation. The suture at the level of the mid to apical prostate traverses the anterior surface of the gland from one cut edge of endopelvic fascia to the other. This suture is tied and tagged with a large hemostat. Cephalad traction on this ligature will place tension on the lateral pelvic fascia surrounding the dorsal vein complex, allowing the surgeon to weaken this fascia with blunt finger dissection in the groove between the dorsal vein complex and the urethra just distal to the apex of the prostate [79]. (Figure 6)

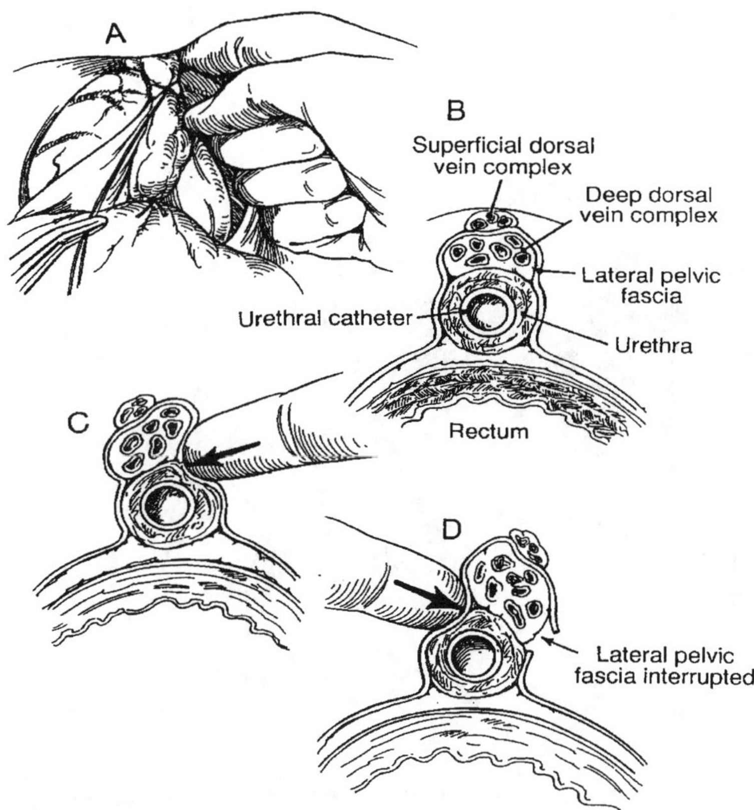

FIGURE 6 Countertraction placed on the hemostatic figure-of-eight suture around the deep dorsal vein complex at midprostate facilitates blunt finger dissection in the plane between the dorsal vein complex and the urethra (A). The lateral pelvic fascia is weakened with finger dissection applied from both sides (C and D).

A right-angle clamp can then be passed through the weakened fascia beneath the entire dorsal vein complex anterior to the urethra. The clamp is used to grasp a 20-gauge stainless steel wire looped on the end. The wire, which is brought beneath the dorsal vein complex (Figure 7), serves as a template so the complex can be transected evenly and sharply with a 15-blade knife. By adjusting the upward tension on the wire and downward traction on the prostate with a sponge stick, the surgeon can divide the dorsal vein complex sufficiently distal to the apex. This maneuver serves to minimize the risk of a positive, apical/anterior surgical margin.

Bleeding from the dorsal vein complex is controlled by suturing the incised edges of the lateral pelvic fascia on either side of the complex, using a continuous 2–0 polyglactin absorbable suture on a CT-2 needle. (Figure 8) Finally, the suture is sewn through the periosteum of the pubis, compressing the superficial veins between the fascia and the pubic bone.

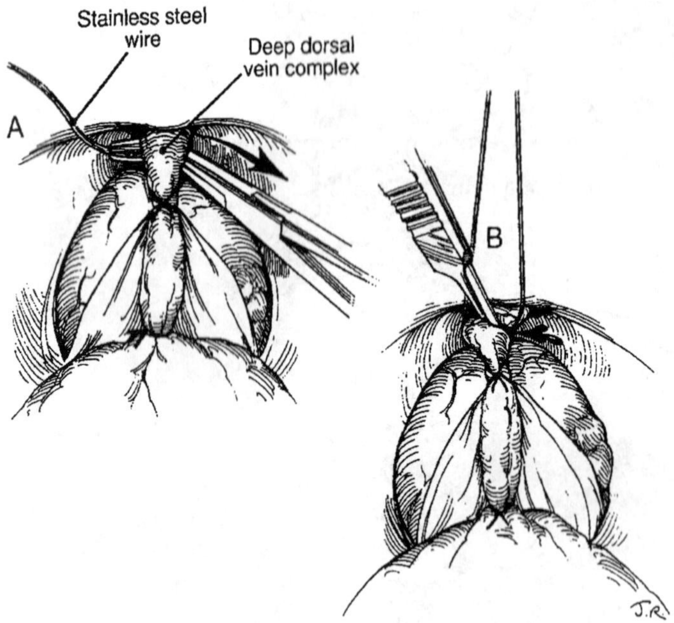

FIGURE 7   A long-nosed right-angled clamp is passed through the weakened fascia between the urethra and dorsal vein complex and grasps a stainless steel wire that is looped on the end (A). The wire serves as a guide to allow a square transection of the dorsal vein complex and its surrounding fascia (B). By this maneuver the dorsal venous complex can be divided close to or far from the apex of the prostate, however the surgeon chooses, with care to avoid a positive surgical margin.

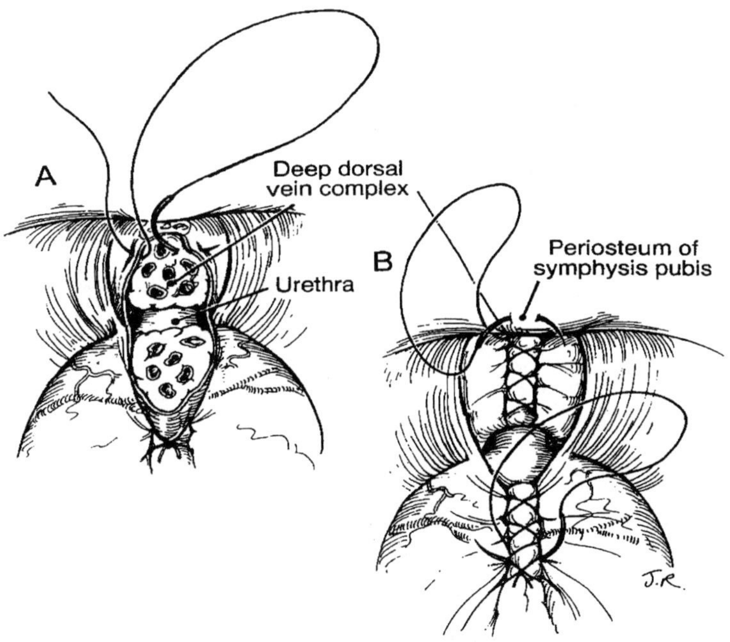

FIGURE 8 Bleeding from the transected dorsal vein complex is controlled by oversewing the cut edges of the lateral pelvic fascia vertically with a continuous suture (A), the last pass of which is brought through the periosteum of the pubis (B) to compress the superficial venous complex above the lateral pelvic fascia and to fix the fascia to the periosteum, simulating the function of the puboprostatic ligaments. Back bleeding from the ventral prostate is controlled with clips or with a continuous hemostatic suture, taking care not to draw the neurovascular bundles medially (B).

Lateral Vascular Pedicles and Seminal Vesicles

The thick lateral vascular pedicle supplying the prostate is encountered toward the base of the prostate. (Figure 9) The lateral vascular pedicles are isolated with a right angle clamp and controlled with clips or ties. (Figure 9A, B) Full division of the lateral pedicle will expose the lateral edge of the seminal vesicle. (Figure 9C)

Control of the bleeding and exposure of the seminal vesicle will be improved if the vascular band of tissue between the bladder and the base of the prostate and seminal vesicles is deliberately isolated, clipped, and divided. (Figure 9C) This assures a wide lateral margin around the base of the prostate. The seminal vesicles can then be bluntly dissected from the bladder base. As the mobilization of the seminal vesicles continues, the vascular pedicle at the tip of

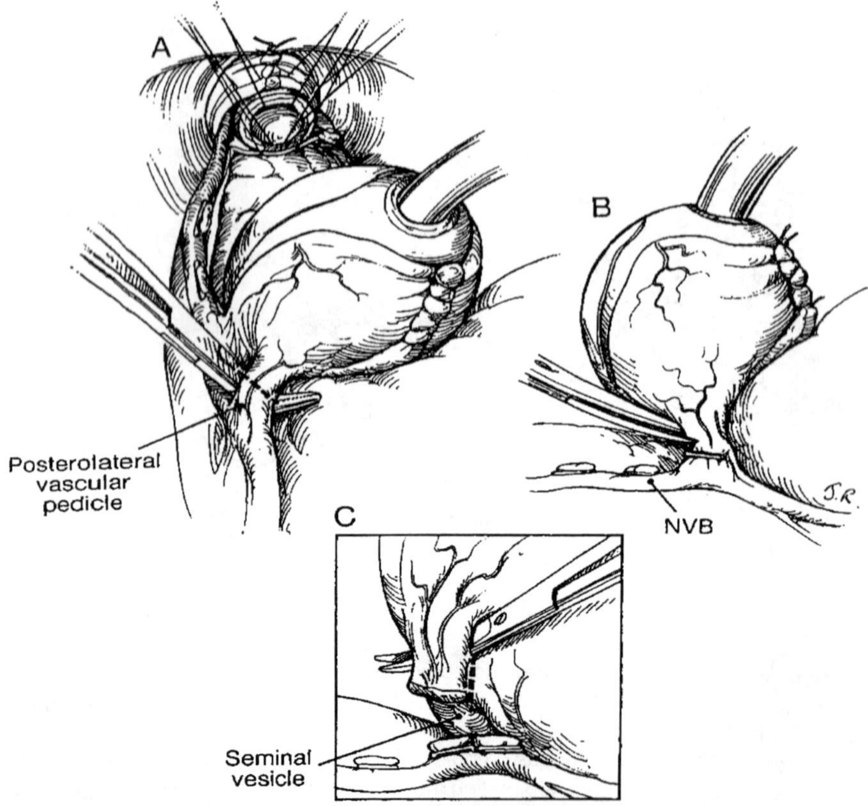

FIGURE 9 Upward traction on the separate catheter placed through the prostate into the bladder allows the lateral vascular pedicles of the prostate to be easily isolated (A), controlled with clips (B), and divided to expose the lateral aspect of the seminal vesicle. Further exposure is gained by division of the vascular bands between the bladder neck and the seminal vesicles and prostate (C).

the seminal vesicles can be exposed, clipped, and divided. (Figure 10) We usually dissect the seminal vesicles from lateral to medial, ending with the identification and division of the ampulla of the vas. Occasionally, this dissection is easier if the vas is divided first. The artery to the vas must be carefully secured. Meticulous control of the small vessels surrounding the seminal vesicles laterally and anteriorly will substantially reduce the overall blood loss during the operation. The seminal vesicles and vas can then be mobilized within their fascia toward the bladder neck.

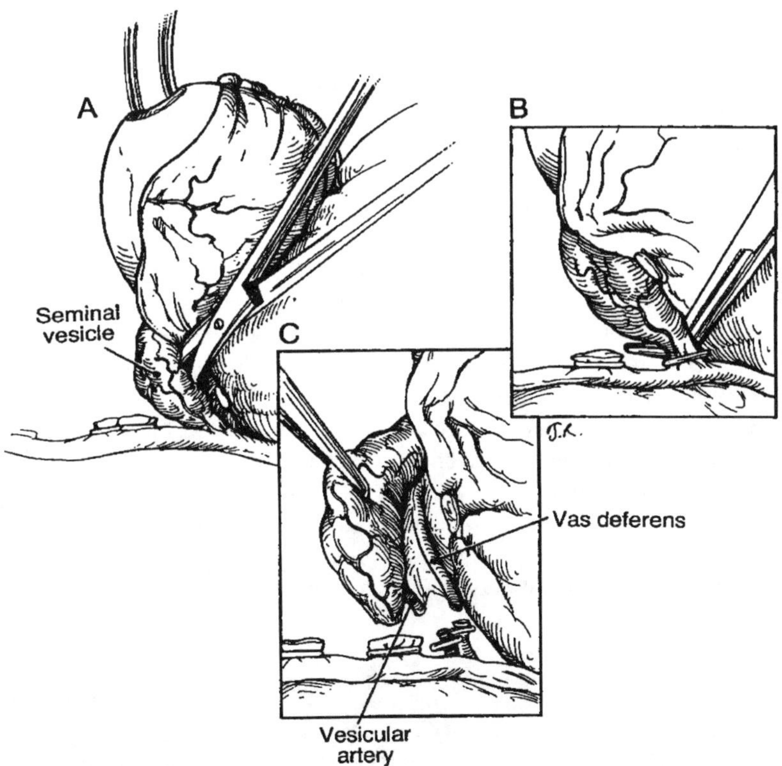

FIGURE 10 The seminal vesicles are typically approached laterally and the plane between the vesicles and the bladder developed with scissors and finger dissection. The major blood supply to the seminal vesicles lies anterior and lateral. When these vessels are clipped and divided close to the wall of the vesicle, it is easier to identify the large artery that enters at the apex of the seminal vesicle. The ampulla of the vas are clipped to include the vasal arteries and then divided.

Late Complications: Bladder Neck Contracture and Incontinence

Bladder neck contractures are usually the result of poor mucosa-to-mucosa apposition at the time of the urethrovesical anastomosis. Careful eversion of the bladder neck mucosa and proper placement of the urethral sutures under direct vision will help reduce the incidence of this complication. Patients with a bladder neck contracture often note a dribbling urinary stream or symptoms of overflow incontinence. Assessment should include a urinary flow rate, determination of postvoid residual urine, and flexible cystoscopy to evaluate the anastomotic site. Severe bladder neck contractures may require cold knife incision and, if recurrent, may require periodic dilatation to maintain an adequate urine flow [91].

Urinary incontinence is still one of the most troubling side effects following radical retropubic prostatectomy. Although an anatomic approach to radical prostatectomy has resulted in a diminished rate of incontinence, incontinence rates vary widely [18–20,48,80,92–97]. (Table 7) The American College of Surgeons surveyed 484 hospitals to examine the status of men who had undergone radical prostatectomy in the United States [95]. Of the 1,796 men who were continent prior to surgery, 330 (19%) wore pads on a daily basis and 3.6% were totally incontinent after surgery. Fowler et al.[93] reported that 31% of a sample population of Medicare patients who responded to a questionnaire reported some degree of wetness. In contrast, most centers with broad expertise in radical prostatectomy report a 5–8% incidence of moderate stress incontinence. (Table 7) These studies are difficult to compare, however, because the definition of continence is not uniform. Importantly, despite the relatively high rates of urinary incontinence reported in population surveys, the majority of these patients were minimally bothered by this complication and were highly satisfied with their treatment [94].

The rate of incontinence, however, is exquisitely sensitive to surgical technique. In 1990, The technique was revised to avoid retraction on the urethra

TABLE 7 Incidence of Incontinence After Radical Prostatectomy (18–20, 48, 80, 92–97)

Series	No. of patients	Incontinence (%)	Definition of incontinence
Interview by treating physician at center of excellence			
Steiner et al., 1991	593	8	Leaks with moderate activity
Leandri et al., 1992	398	5	Leaks with moderate activity
Zincke et al., 1994	1728	5	Requires 3 or more pads per day
Catalona et al., 1999	1325	8	No pads
Geary et al., 1995	458	20	Requires pads
Eastham et al., 1996	581	9	Leaks with moderate activity
Series from patient surveys			
Murphy et al., 1994	1796	19	Requires pads
Litwin et al., 1995	98	25	"Bother" score
Walsh et al., 2000	62	7	Requires pads
Population-based studies using patient surveys			
Fowler et al., 1993	738	31	Pads or clamps
Stanford et al., 2000	1291	8.4	Severe incontinence
		21.6	Requires pads

during the prostatectomy, to place the anastomotic sutures through a small portion of urethra and a larger portion of the lateral pelvic fascia surrounding the oversewn dorsal vein complex, and to form a fully everted (stomatized) bladder neck (see later description and figures). This change resulted in a marked improvement in continence from 82% to 95% at 2 years and decreased the median time to recovery of continence from 5.6 to 1.5 months [16]. (Figure 11) Multivariate analysis has shown that factors independently associated with an increased chance of regaining continence were decreasing age, a modification in the technique of anastomosis, preservation of both neurovascular bundles, and the absence of an anastomotic stricture [16]. (Table 8)

Urodynamic studies of patients who are incontinent following radical prostatectomy have not elucidated a predominant mechanism of incontinence. Most studies have suggested, however, that the functional length of the urethra is the most important factor in post-prostatectomy incontinence [98–101]. (Wei/Coakley

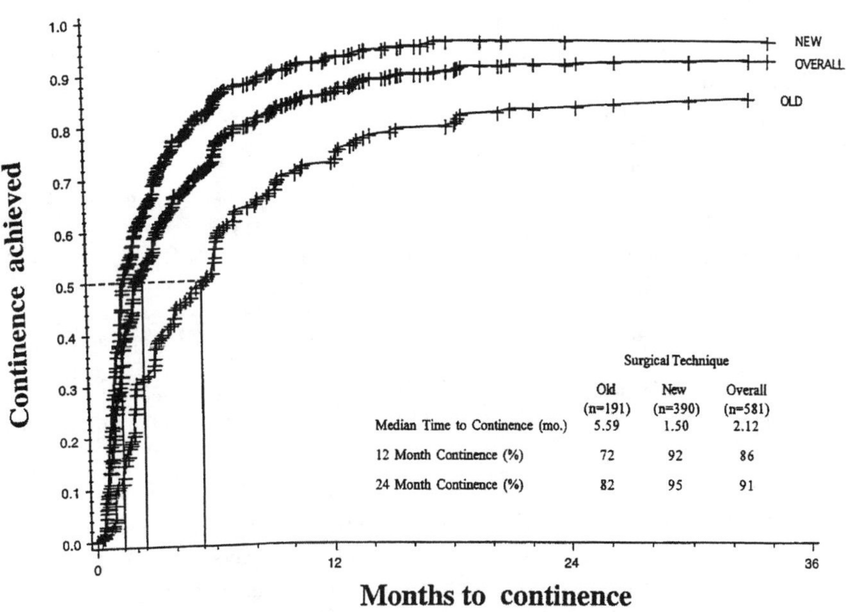

FIGURE 11 Actuarial probability of achieving continence for 581 continent patients who underwent radical prostatectomy for clinically localized (cT1 to T3NXM0) prostate cancer: for the entire group, for the old (191) and the new (390) anastomotic techniques. With the new technique, median time to continence was 1.5 months, and 95% of patients were continent at 24 months. (From: Eastham JA, Goad JR, Rogers E, et al. Risk factors for urinary incontinence after radical prostatectomy. J Urol 1996; 156:1707–1713. Reprinted with permission.)

TABLE 8 Univariate and Multivariate Analysis of the Risk Factors for Incontinence After Radical Prostatectomy

Risk factor	Parameter estimate p value	
	Univariate analysis	Multivariate analysis
Patient weight (continuous)	0.002	Not available
Lower urinary tract symptoms (none versus requiring treatment)		
Obstructive	0.004	0.111
Irritative	0.624	0.186
Prostate size by transrectal ultrasound (continuous)	0.441	0.250
Transurethral resection of prostate (yes or no)	0.001	0.349
Clinical stage (T1a,b/T1c/T2a/T2b/T2c/T3)	0.001	0.158
Tumor palpable at apex	0.289	0.707
Operative blood loss (continuous)	0.016	0.829
Postop, bleeding (presence/absence of clinically significant bleeding)	0.577	0.647
Pathologic stage (confined, ECE versus SVI, +LN)	0.310	0.733
Nerve resection (none versus unilateral versus bilateral)	0.001	0.015
Anastomotic stricture (yes or no)	0.001	0.015
Patient age (continuous)	0.001	0.0001
Anastomotic technique (old or new)	0.001	0.0001

ECE=extracapsular extension; SVI=seminal vesicle involvement; +LN=positive lymph nodes

(From: Eastham JA, Goad JR, Rogers E, et al. Risk factors for urinary incontinence after radical prostatectomy. J Urol 1996; 156:1707–1713. Reprinted with permission.)

data?). We believe a ''hands off'' approach to the external sphincter tissues beyond the apex of the prostate with fixation of the urethra to the lateral pelvic fascia preserves the maximum amount of functional urethral length within the pelvis and contributes significantly to the maintenance of continence following the procedure.

Methods to Reduce Bladder Neck Contracture and Incontinence

Following division of the dorsal venous complex and control of bleeding, the levator ani fibers are bluntly and sharply dissected away from the apex of the prostate, exposing the urethra. It is important to control any operative field bleeding to permit precise division of the anterior urethra. (Figure 12) To secure the cut edge of the urethra, we place the anastomotic sutures at this point rather than attempt to place sutures in the retracted urethral stump later in the procedure. Four 2–0 monocryl absorbable sutures on a UR-6 needle are placed from inside to outside just 3 mm into the urethra then into the hood of the lateral pelvic fascia.

After placement of the four anterior anastomotic sutures, attention is directed to the lateral dissection and the neurovascular bundles (see later discussion). Next, the catheter is withdrawn, exposing the undivided posterior urethra

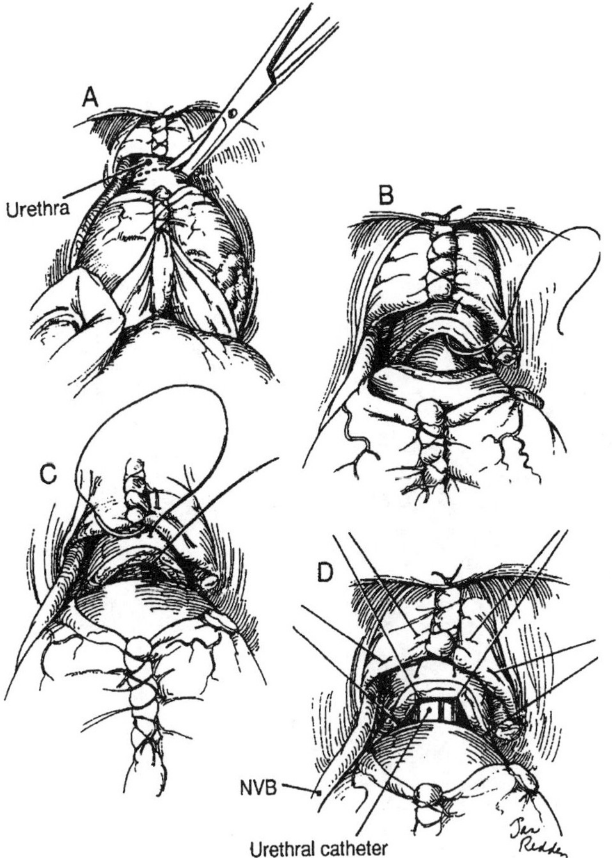

FIGURE 12　Close-up views of urethra at the prostatic apex, illustrating the site of anterior division (A, B) and the placement of the anterior anastomotic sutures beneath the mucosa of the urethra and then separately through the thick layer of lateral pelvic fascia (C, D), which was oversewn to control the dorsal vein complex.

and the firm fibrous layer of Denonvilliers' fascia beneath. (Figure 13A) Two additional posterior sutures are placed through the posterior layer of fascia and through the urethra, from outside to inside, at the 5 and 7 o'clock positions. These two sutures must be well away from the previously mobilized neurovascular bundles. Finally, the rectourethralis muscle is divided and the prostate is dissected away from the rectum beneath Denonvilliers' fascia. (Figure 13B)

Once the bladder neck has been divided and the prostate removed, the bladder neck is reconstructed. The mucosa is everted anteriorly with fine 4–0 absorbable sutures (Figure 14A,B), and the bladder neck is closed posteriorly in a tennis racket fashion with a running 2–0 polyglactin absorbable suture until it is approximately 28 to 32 Fr. in diameter. (Figure 14C) The mucosa must be fully everted 360° around the reconstructed bladder neck. This closure may be reinforced using a running 2–0 polyglactin absorbable suture that reapproximates the lateral vascular pedicles in the midline (Figure 14D,E), securing bleeding from the bed of the seminal vesicles.

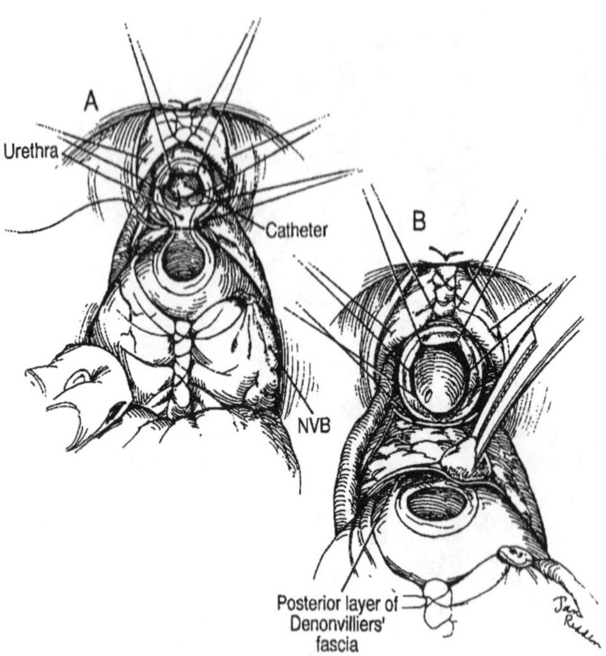

FIGURE 13   After the nerves have been dissected free (or divided), the remaining urethra and posterior layer of Denonvilliers' fascia beneath it are divided (A). Two posterior anastomotic sutures are placed at 5 and 7 o'clock through the fascia and urethra (A). The correct plane of dissection adjacent to the rectum is determined with the aid of a kitner dissector (B).

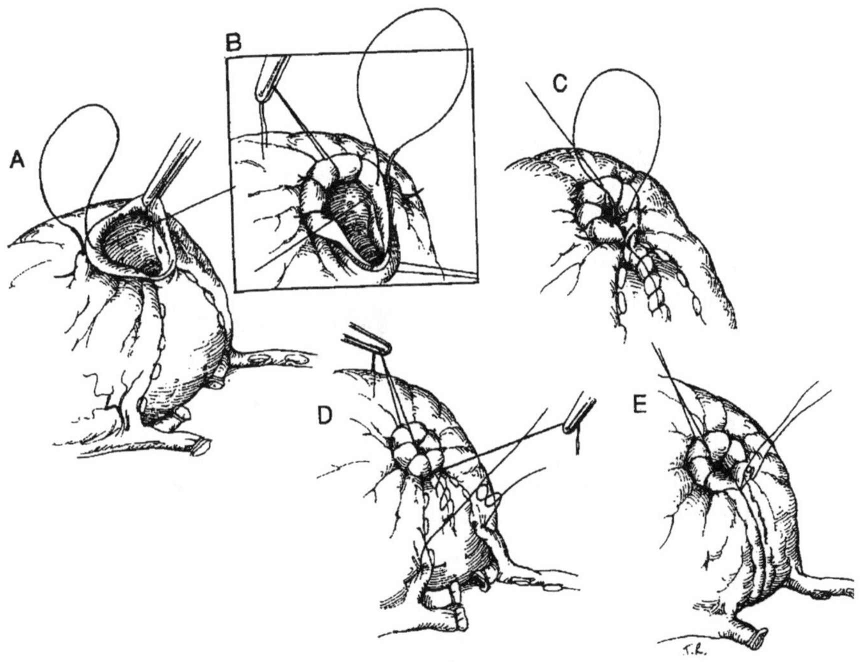

FIGURE 14 The bladder neck is reconstructed by everting the mucosa anteriorly (A and B) and closing the bladder posteriorly with a running suture creating a "tennis-racke" closure (C). The suture closest to the trigone should include muscle but little mucosa to avoid tethering the ureteral orifices. In a separate layer, the lateral vascular pedicles of the bladder are brought together in the midline to reinforce the closure and assure hemostasis (D and E), giving the reconstructed bladder neck a cone shaped.

On completion of the bladder neck reconstruction, the previously placed urethral sutures are placed through the reconstructed bladder neck. (Figure 15) All sutures are placed such that the knots are tied on the outside of the lumen. A Foley catheter (20 Fr., 5 mL balloon) is now passed through the urethra and into the bladder, the balloon inflated with 15 mL sterile water, and the sutures are tied. We often secure the catheter in place with an anchoring suture of No. 2 nylon sewn through the eye of the catheter and passed through the bladder and abdominal wall. This suture is secured to the skin. If the catheter should fall out prematurely, the nylon ligature can be used to guide a new catheter through the vesicourethral anastomosis. If this is not successful, a Coudé cathether can be passed under fluoroscopic control guided by a retrograde urethrogram with the patient in an oblique position. We do not advise cystoscopy for passage of the catheter except as a last resort.

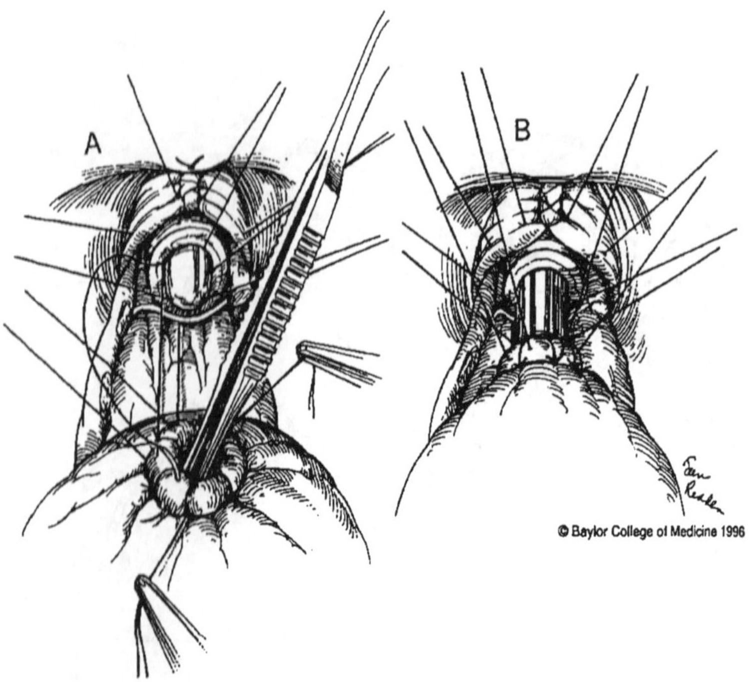

FIGURE 15   The sutures already placed through the urethra are now placed through the bladder neck (A) to provide a mucosa-to-mucosa anastomosis (B).

Late Complications: Positive Surgical Margins and Erectile Dysfunction

Multiple studies have correlated return of erectile function following radical prostatectomy to patient age, pathologic tumor stage, and extent of preservation of the neurovascular bundles [17,80,102,103]. Quinlan and associates [102] demonstrated that recovery of potency was quantitatively related to the preservation of nerves. Approximately 90% of men under 50 years of age were potent if either one or both neurovascular bundles were preserved. For men older than 50, return of potency was more likely if both neurovascular bundles were preserved rather than only one. Catalona and Bigg [54] reported potency in 63% of patients when both nerves were preserved and only 39% when one nerve was spared. Both of these studies also demonstrated a strong correlation of preservation of potency with age and tumor stage.

We recently reviewed our series of 314 previously potent patients treated since 1993 with radical prostatectomy for cT1a-T3a prostate cancer after 1993. Patient age, preoperative potency status, and extent of neurovascular bundle preservation, but not pathological stage, were predictive factors for potency recovery after radical prostatectomy. (Figure 16) At 3 years after the operation, 76% of men younger than age 60 years with full erections preoperatively who had bilateral neurovascular bundle preservation would be expected to regain erections sufficient for intercourse. Compared to the younger men, those 60 to 65 years old were only 56%, and those older than 65 years were 47%, as likely to recover potency. Patients with recently diminished erections were only 63% as likely to

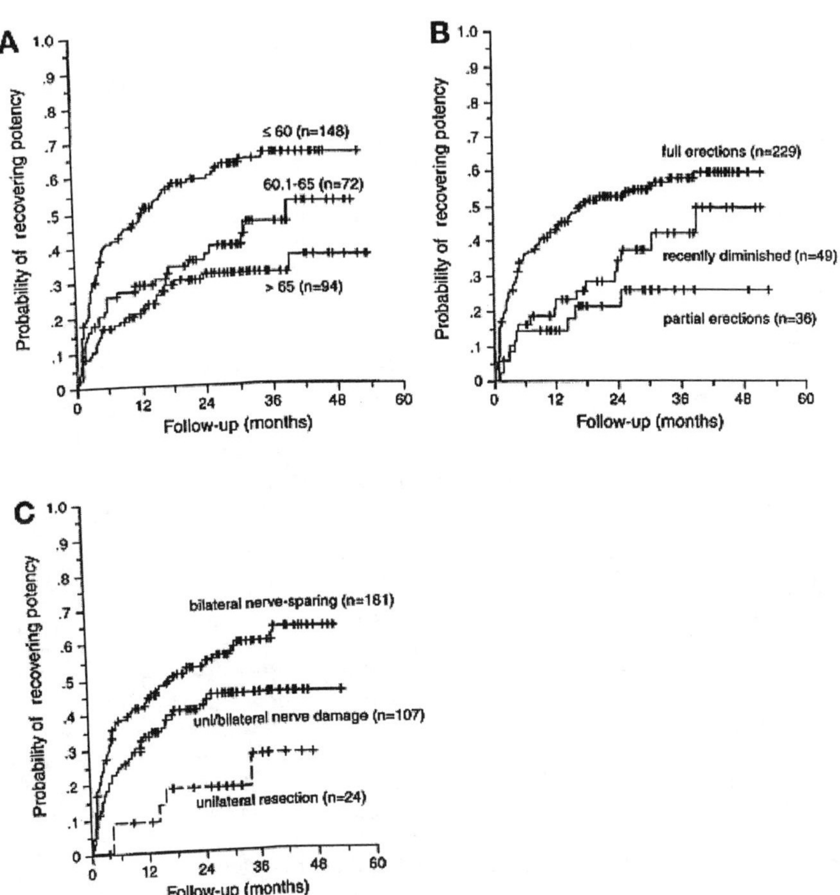

FIGURE 16 Erection recovery according to patient age (*A*), preoperative erectile function (*B*), and extent of preservation of neurovascular bundles (*C*). Two patients undergoing bilateral neurovascular bundle excision were excluded from analysis according to neurovascular bundle status. (From Rabbani F, Stapleton AM, Kattan MW, Wheeler TM, Scardino PT. Factors predicting recovery of erections after radical prostatectomy. J Urol 2000; 164(6): 1929–34. Reprinted with permission.)

recover potency as men with full erections preoperatively, and those with partial erections were only 47% as likely to recover potency. Resection of 1 neurovascular bundle reduced the chance of recovery to approximately 25%, compared to preserving both nerves. We further developed a nomogram that displays these associations derived from a Cox proportional hazards model using only preoperative, or a combination of preoperative and intraoperative, parameters [103] (Table 9)

TABLE 9 Results of Cox Proportional Hazards Analysis for Prediction of Spontaneous Recovery of Erections for 314 Patients Undergoing Radical Prostatectomy Since 1993 for cT1a-T3a Prostate Cancer Based on Preoperative Parameters and the Combination of Preoperative and Intraoperative Parameters.

Probability (%) of recovery of potency by 24 months (36 months)		
PREOPERATIVE PARAMETERS		
Preoperative potency	Age ≤60	Age 60.1–65	Age >65
Full erection	63 (69)	44 (49)	37 (42)
Full erection, recently diminished	48 (54)	31 (36)	26 (30)
Partial erection	35 (40)	22 (25)	18 (21)
PREOPERATIVE AND INTRAOPERATIVE PARAMETERS		
Bilateral nerve-sparing		
Full erection	70 (76)	49 (55)	43 (49)
Full erection, recently diminished	53 (59)	34 (39)	30 (35)
Partial erection	43 (49)	27 (31)	23 (27)
Unilateral or bilateral neurovascular bundle damage		
Full erection	60 (67)	40 (46)	35 (41)
Full erection, recently diminished	44 (50)	28 (32)	24 (28)
Partial erection	35 (40)	21 (25)	18 (21)
Unilateral neurovascular bundle resection		
Full erection	26 (30)	15 (18)	13 (15)
Full erection, recently diminished	17 (20)	10 (12)	8.5 (10)
Partial erection	13 (15)	7.5 (8.8)	6.3 (7.5)

(From: Rabbani F, Stapleton AMF, Kattan MW, Wheelen TM, and Scardino PT: Factors predicting recovery of erections after radical prostatectomy. J Urol 2000; 164(6):1929–34. Reprinted with permission.)

The return of postoperative sexual function following radical retropubic prostatectomy is dependent not only on the preservation of the autonomic innervation to the corpora cavernosa (i.e., the neurovascular bundles), but also on the preservation of the vascular branches to the corpora cavernosa [54]. Accessory arterial branches that supply the corpora have been described [104,105]. When these branches are preserved, a normal arterial inflow to the penis postoperatively will be maintained. Preservation of these branches may enable a patient to remain potent following surgery, or, for a patient who is impotent, adequate arterial inflow will ensure an adequate response to medical treatment.

Complete removal of the cancer (i.e., without positive margins) and preservation of the nerves responsible for erectile function are often competing goals. Cancers most often penetrate the prostatic capsule posterolaterally, directly over the neurovascular bundles [106]. (Figure 17) In several series, attempts to preserve the neurovascular bundles has increased the rate of positive surgical margins posterolaterally [107]. In a review of the literature from centers of excellence, Abbas and Scardino found reported rates of positive margins varied from 14% to 41%, with a mean of 25% [108]. In another review, Weider and Soloway noted the remarkable variation in positive margin rates, varying from 0% to 71% with an overall rate of 28%, in radical retropubic prostatectomy series in which no adjuvant hormonal therapy was used before the operation [25]. Variations in surgical margin rates are related not only to the extent of the cancer and to the processing of the pathology specimen [25,108] but also to the surgical technique. Among 31 urologists who perform radical prostatectomies at Baylor College of Medicine, the rate of positive surgical margins varied from 0 to 76% among patients with ECE. Even among surgeons with ten or more cases, the rate varied from 22% to 45% (Adler et al., unpublished data, 1998).

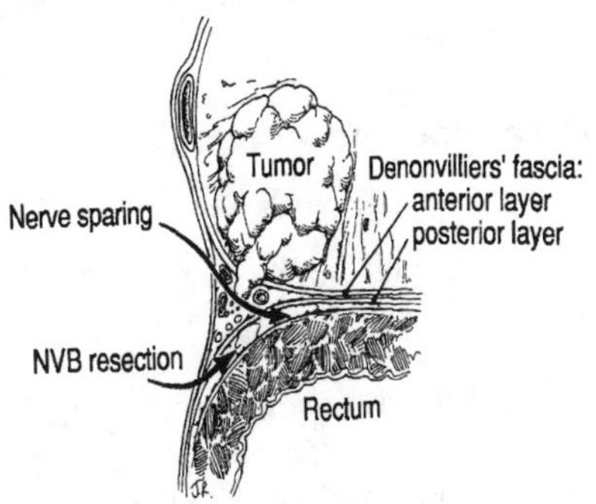

FIGURE 17 The lateral plane of dissection is selected based on preoperative and intraoperative assessment of the extent of the tumor. A wider dissection, i.e., resection of the neurovascular bundle, may be required in an attempt to obtain adequate surgical margins.

TABLE 10 Five-Year Freedom from Progression in Low- and High-Risk Patients with Clinical Stage T1–2 NXM0 Cancers, Comparing Two Surgical Series with Different Rates of Positive Surgical Margins (1987–1993).

	Kupelian et al (109). (N=298)	Baylor. (N=425)
Low risk (Gleason sum <7, PSA <10)		
Patients: N (%)	143 (48%)	140 (33%)
+SM	39%	3.5%
5-year bNED (all patients)	80%	97%
−SM	85%	98%
+SM	63%	80%
High risk (Gleason sum >6 or PSA >10)		
Patients: N (%)	155 (52%)	287 (67%)
+SM	59%	15.3%
5-year bNED (all patients)	37%	71%
−SM	62%	76%
+SM	21%	45%

Positive margins appear to be a strong predictor of long-term cancer control rates for cancers with similar preoperative characteristics (clinical stage, Gleason grade, and PSA). bNED: biochemical no evidence of disease; SM: surgical margin

In multivariate analysis, positive margins confer a greater risk of recurrence [24,109,110]. (Table 10) With deliberate attention to surgical planning and technique, we reduced our rate of positive margins from 24% before 1987 to 8% in 1993 [108]. Consequently, we believe that positive margins are common, that such margins reduce the chances that a cancer will be cured, and that most positive margins can be avoided with careful surgical planning.

Methods to Reduce Positive Surgical Margins and Preserve Erectile Function

Minimizing the rate of positive surgical margins requires careful dissection in four areas: when the dorsal vein complex is divided anteriorly; at the apex; near the neurovascular bundles posterolaterally; and at the bladder neck.

Anterior cancers are difficult to detect preoperatively and difficult to palpate intraoperatively. The dorsal vein complex must be divided sufficiently distal to the anterior prostate to avoid a positive margin. As previously described, adjusting the upward tension of a wire and the downward traction on the prostate will facilitate precise division of the dorsal venous complex and allow a more adequate anterior margin. (see Figure 7B) A lateral approach to the neurovascular bundles allows wide exposure of the apex (Figure 18) so that the apical tissue can be completely

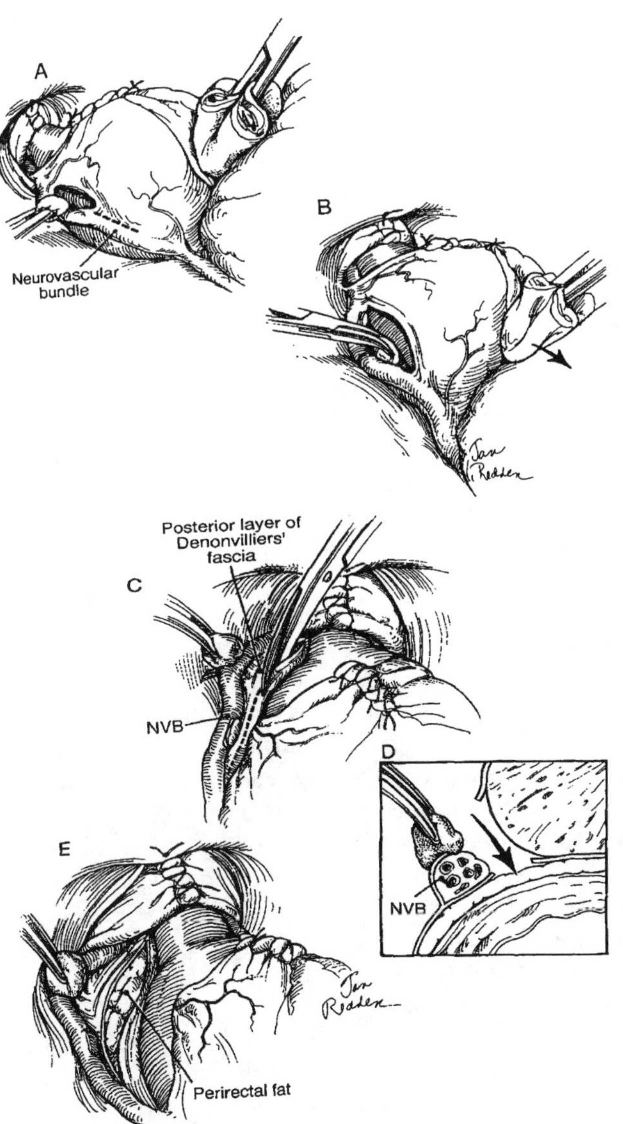

FIGURE 18 Preservation of the left neurovascular bundle. After the dorsal vein complex has been divided, the prostate is rotated to the right, and the levator muscles are bluntly dissected away. The lateral pelvic fascia is then incised in the groove between the prostate and the neurovascular bundle. The neurovascular bundle is most easily dissected away from the apical third of the prostate (A, B). The small branches of the vascular pedicle to the apex must be divided. The posterior layer of Denonvilliers' fascia is then incised, releasing the NVB from the prostate and urethra (C, E) so that the nerves will not be tethered when the urethral anastomotic sutures are tied.

resected. The deep (posterior) layer of Denonvilliers' fascia must be deliberately incised, releasing the neurovascular bundle laterally and allowing a deep plane of dissection along the fat of the anterior rectal wall. The risk of a positive surgical margin will be greatly increased unless this deep layer of fascia is included in the excised specimen. (Figure 18C–E). This apical dissection is performed without a catheter in the prostate to give the prostate more mobility. The lateral pelvic fascia over the neurovascular bundle can be incised more medially or laterally to the nerve, depending on the extent or location of the tumor and whether the nerves are to be preserved. A "peanut" or Kitner dissector is used to gently brush the nerves laterally away from the prostate. Small clips placed parallel to the neurovascular bundle are used to control the small vascular bands that are usually present, particularly near the apex of the prostate. Once the posterior anastomotic sutures are placed (Figure 13), the posterior urethra, together with the firm fibrous layer of Denonvilliers' fascia beneath it, are divided sharply. Finally, the rectourethralis is divided at the apex of the prostate. The prostate is then dissected off the rectum, beneath both layers of Denonvilliers' fascia.

We have been successful in preserving most or all of both neurovascular bundles in the majority of patients using this lateral approach, while still allowing a wider dissection around the apex of the prostate, especially posteriorly. Once the apex is completely mobilized, a second catheter is placed through the urethra to facilitate dissection. (Figure 9) Traction on this catheter allows the remaining neurovascular bundles to be dissected away bluntly. Particular care should be taken near the base of the prostate where the nerves lie in very close apposition to the prostate and seminal vesicles. Dissection too close to the prostate will result in a positive margin in this area, shown to be associated with an increased risk of recurrence. 111 (Table 10)

When resection of one or both neurovascular bundles has been necessary, we have developed, in conjunction with plastic surgeons, a technique for placement of interposition grafts from the sural nerve to one or both neurovascular bundles [112]. (Figure 19) Some patients with bilateral nerve resection and interposition grafts recovered partial spontaneous erections within 8 to 12 months and full erections after 14 months. Of 12 patients followed more than 1 year, 7 have recovered partial or full erections, suggesting that interposition nerve grafts may enhance the recovery of erectile function when the neurovascular bundles are resected. McKeirnan data?

Finally, the bladder neck should be divided well away from the prostate. Tapering the bladder neck into the prostatic urethra does not improve the rate of long-term continence but does increase the rate of positive surgical margins [113]. We do not advocate bladder neck sparing, as the risk of a positive margin at the bladder neck far outweighs the minimal added time and technical ease of bladder neck reconstruction.

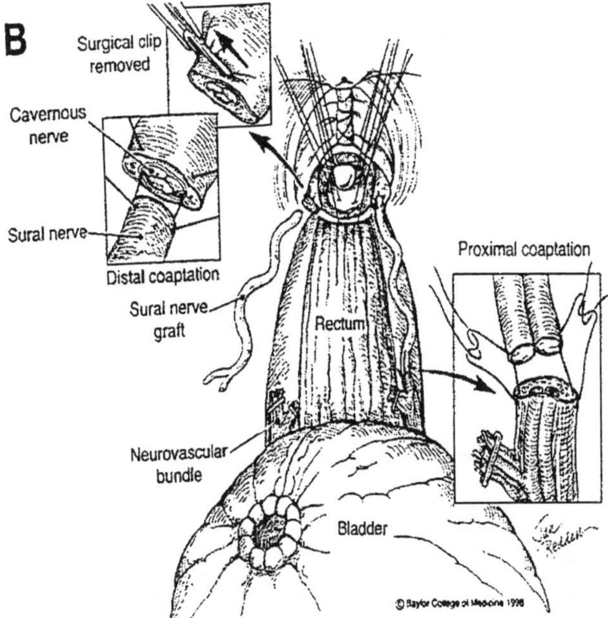

FIGURE 19 Sural nerve grafts can be interposed between severed ends of the cavernous nerves when these nerves must be resected to assure complete excision of the cancer. The nerve graft is reversed and distal branches are coapted to proximal ends of cavernous nerves near the lateral vascular pedicle. Note the surgical clip across the distal end of the severed right neurovascular bundle. (From Kim ED, Scardino PT, Hampel O, Mills N, Wheeler TM, Nath RK. Interposition of sural nerve restores function of cavernous nerves resected during radical prostatectomy. J Urol 1999; 161:188–192. Reprinted with permission.)

CANCER CONTROL AFTER RADICAL RETROPUBIC PROSTATECTOMY

Serum PSA is the most sensitive indicator of disease status after therapy for prostate cancer, and PSA should decline to undetectable levels after radical prostatectomy [114]. Although there are rare reports of disease recurrence following radical prostatectomy in the setting of an undetectable serum PSA level [115–118], a rising PSA is the earliest indicator of persistent or recurrent cancer [114,119–122]. Therefore, treatment outcomes and cancer control should be based primarily on postoperative monitoring of the serum PSA level.

Actuarial nonprogression rates in patients undergoing radical retropubic prostatectomy for clinical stage T1 and T2 prostate cancer have been reported by multiple institutions, revealing approximately 80% nonprogression at 5 years and

TABLE 11 Actuarial 5-Year Progression-Free Probability Rates After Radical Retropubic Prostatectomy, Determined by Prostate-Specific Antigen (PSA), for Clinical Stage T1 and T2 Prostate Cancer.

			PSA Nonprogression (%)	
Group	No. Pts	Years	5 Yr	10 Yr
Pound et al., 1997 (46)	1623[a]	1982–1995	80	68
Trapasso et al., 1994 (123)	425[b]	1987–1992	80	
Zincke et al., 1994 (48)	3170[b]	1966–1991	77	54
Catalona and Smith, 1994 (47)	925[c]	1983–1993	78	–
Hull et al., 2000 **	1000[b]	1983–1998	78	75

** Hull GW et al., unpublished data used with permission
[a] Progression defined as a serum PSA >0.2 ng/mL
[b] Progression defined as a serum PSA >0.4 ng/mL
[c] Progression defined as a serum PSA >0.6 ng/mL

70% at 10 years following prostatectomy [46–48,123]. (Table 11) We recently calculated the risk of recurrence after surgery for a cohort of 1,359 men with clinical stage T1–T2 cancer with "intent to treat" by radical prostatectomy. They have been followed for 1–170 months (mean 44). No patient received adjuvant therapy before relapse. Treatment failure was defined as a serum PSA rising to more than 0.3 ng/mL; clinical, local, or distant recurrence; the initiation of adjuvant treatment; or the abandonment of radical prostatectomy because of positive nodes. Recurrence was documented in 210 (15.5%) patients. Most patients failed during the first year after surgery, and no patient failed after 6 years, suggesting that failure after radical prostatectomy may be largely due to clinical understaging. In the absence of adjuvant treatment, most patients destined to recur do so within 5 years after surgery [124]. (Hull GW et al., unpublished data used with permission)

Pathologic Prognostic Factors

In addition to previously described clinical factors such as preoperative PSA level, biopsy information, and clinical stage, more precise prognostic information can be gained from a detailed analysis of the radical prostatectomy specimen. The single most powerful prognostic factor, considering all clinical and pathologic factors in a multivariate analysis, is the pathologic stage of the cancer [125]. (Figure 20 and Table 3) For patients with prostate cancer pathologically confined to the prostate, 5-year disease-free recurrence determined using the measurement of serum PSA is excellent (>90%). The prognosis is particularly poor when the cancer involves the seminal vesicles or pelvic lymph nodes. Notice, however, that microscopic extracapsular extension is much more favorable. In our series,

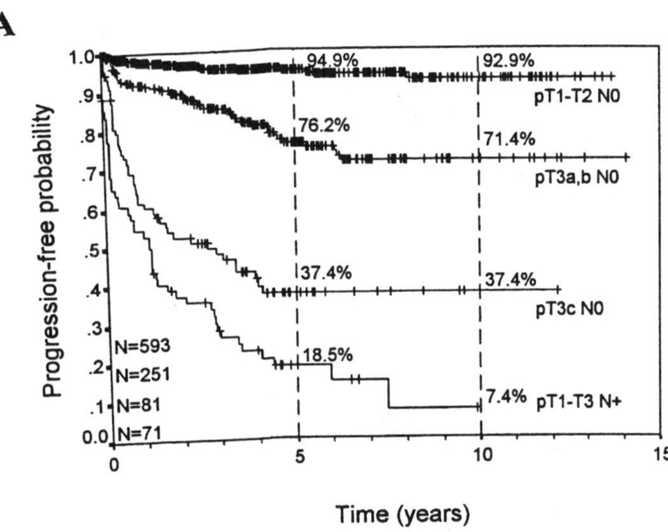

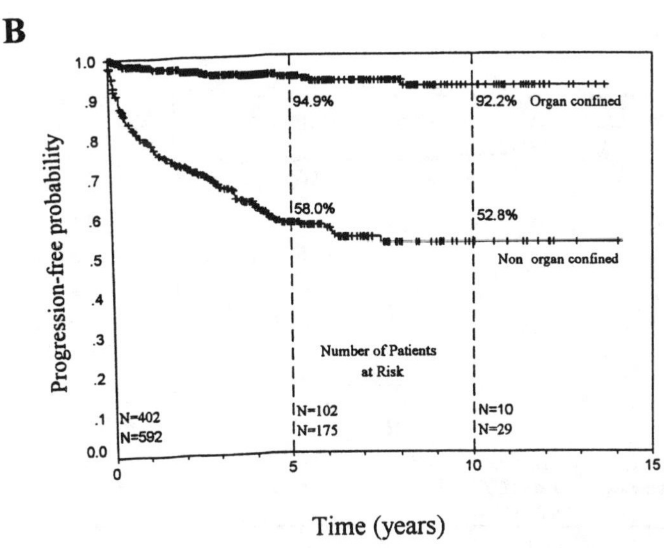

FIGURE 20 Progression-free probability curves based on the pathologic stage (**A**), whether or not the tumor is organ-confined (**B**), the surgical margin status.

C

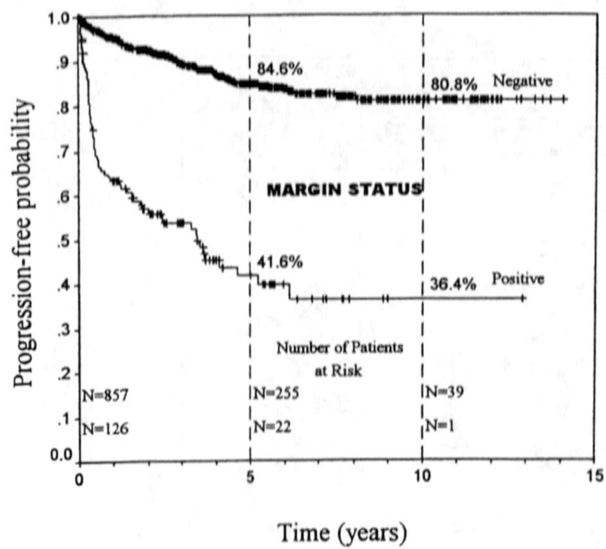

D

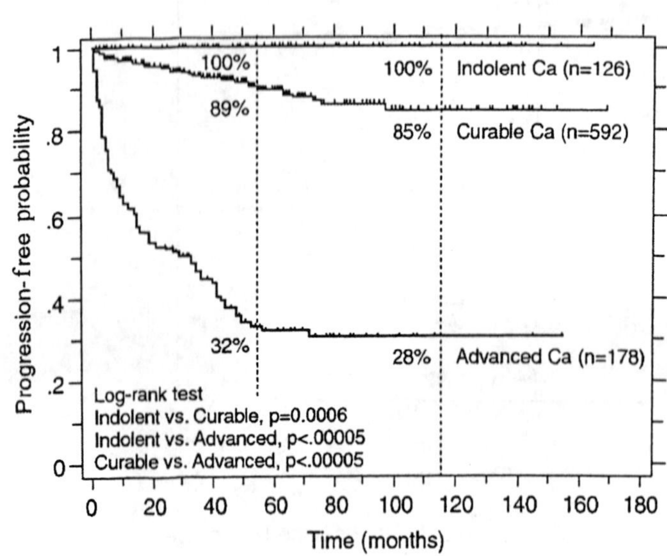

FIGURE 20   (CONT) (**C**), and the prognostic group (**D**). Abbreviations: ECE, extracapsular extension; SVI, seminal vesicle invasion; LN, positive lymph nodes; RRPGS, radical retropubic prostatectomy Gleason score. (Modified from Hull GW et al., unpublished data and reprinted with permission)

76% of such patients are free of disease at 5 years (Table 3). The impact of positive surgical margins in the prostatectomy specimen is summarized in Figure 20C and Table 3. The 5-year nonprogression rate among patients in our series with a positive surgical margin was 41.6% as compared to 84.6% in those patients with a negative margin.

Depending on the pathologic features of the tumor in the radical prostatectomy specimen, patients can be classified as having an indolent, curable, or advanced prostate cancer (see Table 1 for definitions). By assigning patients to one of these three prognostic groups, one can assess the overall risk of progression. (Figure 20D) This classification has implications for therapeutic decision making, such that indolent cancers, if recognized preoperatively, might be treated conservatively—except perhaps in young men—whereas advanced cancers would be excellent candidates for adjuvant therapy. In our series of 896 patients, 126 (14%) were considered to have indolent cancers, and none progressed. Five hundred ninety-two patients had tumors with pathologic features consistent with a clinically important but curable cancer. This group also fared well with a nonprogression rate of 85% at 5 years. Patients whose tumors had advanced pathologic features (n = 178, 20%) did poorly, with only 28% disease free at 5 years. (Hull GW et al., unpublished data used with permission)

In a multivariate analysis of clinical and pathological prognostic factors, Gleason grade in the radical prostatectomy specimen, surgical margin status, and pathologic stage were the dominant factors. (Table 12) (Hull GW et al., unpublished data used with permission) Several other indices have been developed that improve the ability to describe the biologic potential of a given tumor. Some have considered tumor volume an important prognostic [126], but others have found no independent prognostic role for tumor volume [49]. Note that preoperative PSA, PSA density, biopsy Gleason sum, clinical stage, or any other clinical factor did not add significant prognostic information to the information already gain from a thorough pathologic examination of the prostatectomy specimen. Other parameters that have been reported to predict outcomes include a proliferative index measured by Ki67 [127], p53 [128,129], E-cadherin [130], microvessel density , KAI1 expression [131], and measures of relative nuclear roundness [132]. None, however, should be considered a necessary part of the evaluation of a patient with localized disease at this time.

RATIONALE FOR SELECTING RADICAL PROSTATECTOMY AS THE TREATMENT OF CHOICE FOR CLINICALLY LOCALIZED PROSTATE CANCER

While randomized prospective clinical trials comparing different forms of therapy are lacking, biochemical outcome after radical prostatectomy, external beam radiation therapy, and/or interstitial radiation therapy for localized prostate have

TABLE 12 Multivariate Analysis of Risk of Progression Based on Preoperative Clinical Parameters Alone and on Clinical and Pathologic Parameters Combined

Variable	Relative risk (95% CI)	P Value
Preoperative Clinical Parameters		
Clinical stage		.0071
T1a,b versus T1c		NS (.60)
T1c versus T2a		NS (.10)
T1c versus T2b	2.47 (1.52–4.03)	.0003
T1c versus T2c	1.91 (1.06–3.42)	.0304
Biopsy Gleason sum†		<.0001
2–4 versus 5–6		NS (.15)
5–6 versus 7	2.60 (1.75–3.87)	<.0001
5–6 versus 8–10	3.21 (1.72–5.97)	.0002
Log_2 (preoperative PSA)	1.80‡ (1.44–2.24)	<.0001
Clinical and Pathologic Parameters		
Clinical stage		NS (.15)
Biopsy Gleason sum		NS (.12)
Log_2 preoperative PSA		NS (.52)
Gleason sum in prostatectomy specimen		.0008
2–4 versus 5–6		NS (.97)
5–6 versus 7	2.48 (1.34–4.58)	.0038
5–6 versus 8–10	4.55 (2.19–9.42)	<.0001
Extracapsular extension		.0019
Focal versus none	2.17 (1.20–3.92)	.011
Established versus none	2.72 (1.56–4.74)	.0004
Focal versus established		NS (.13)
Surgical margins		
Positive versus negative	4.37 (2.90–6.58)	<.0001
Seminal vesicle involvement		
Present versus absent	2.61 (1.70–4.01)	<.0001
Lymph node metastases		
Present versus absent	3.31 (2.11–5.20)	<.0001

Abbreviations: CI, confidence interval; NS, not statistically significant (p>.05).

‡ Each doubling of the preoperative PSA level (one unit increase in log_2 preoperative PSA level) resulted in an increased relative risk of progression of 1.80.

(Hull GW et al., unpublished data used with permission)

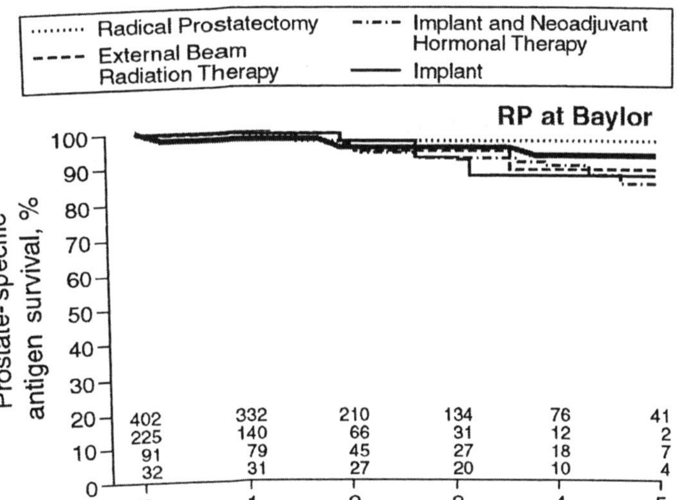

Low Risk Patients Stratified by Modality

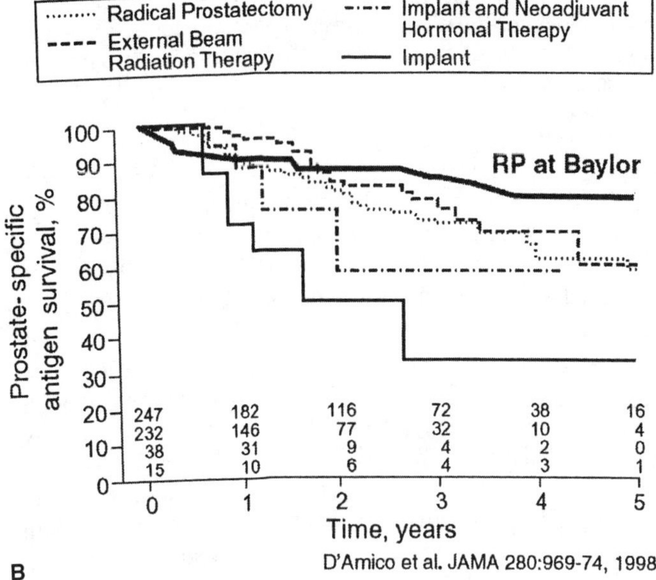

Intermediate Risk Patients Stratified by Modality

FIGURE 21 PSA progression-free survival for low-risk (A), intermediate-risk (B), and high-risk.

High Risk Patients Stratified by Modality

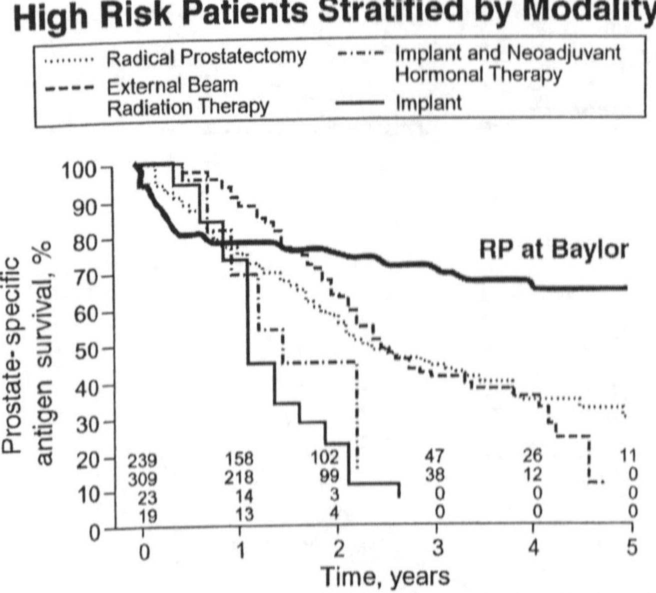

FIGURE 21 (CONT) (C) patients, modified from(136) with permission. The additional line "RP at Baylor" indicates the results of radical prostatectomy in a separate group of 1,000 patients (Hull GW et al., unpublished data used with permission) not reported in D'Amico et al [134].

recently been compared in multiple studies [133,134]. Reasonable comparisons can be made among different forms of local therapy when outcomes are reported in risk-stratified patients. Polascik et al [133]. compared biochemical progression rates in 76 men who underwent radical prostatectomy between 1988 and 1990 to 122 men treated with I-125 brachytherapy without adjuvant treatment. The groups were carefully matched for Gleason score, serum PSA level, and clinical stage. The definition of biochemical failure was defined as a serum PSA level greater than 0.2 ng/ml and greater than 0.5 ng/ml for surgically and radiation managed patients, respectively. The 7-year acturial PSA progression-free survival following radical prostatectomy was 98% (95%, confidence interval [CI] 86% to 99%) compared to 79% (95%, CI not published) for men treated with I-125 brachytherapy. While the authors acknowledge that such comparisons have limitations, they conclude that such data provide a better comparison of biochemical progression than previously reported studies and emphasize the need for caution in interpreting the relative efficacy of brachytherapy in controlling localized prostate cancer [135].

D'Amico et al [134]. examined 1,872 men treated between January 1989 and October 1997 with radical prostatectomy (n = 888), interstitial radiation therapy (n = 218), or external beam radiation therapy (n = 766). Patients were assigned to 1 of 3 risk groups: low-risk (stage T1c, T2a, and serum PSA level ≤10 ng/ml and Gleason score ≤6); intermediate-risk (stage T2b or Gleason score 7 or serum PSA level >10 but <20 ng/ml), or high-risk (stage T2c or serum PSA level ≥20 ng/ml or Gleason score ≥8). A difference was not seen in the 5-year probability of freedom from progression for low-risk cancers treated with radical prostatectomy, three-dimensional (3-D) conformal radiotherapy, and radioactive seed implants with or without neoadjuvant hormonel therapy [134,136] (Figure 21; Hull GW et al., unpublished data used with permission). However, implants were significantly less effective for intermediate- and high-risk cancers, and implants plus hormonel therapy were less effective for high-risk cancers [134,136] (Figure 21) (Hull GW et al., unpublished data used with permission)

Comparing our own series of 1,000 men undergoing radical prostatectomy for clinically localized prostate cancer (Hull GW et al., unpublished data used with permission) with those published by D'Amico et al [134]., similar results are seen regardless of treatment modality for low-risk patients. For intermediate- and high-risk groups, patients in our series had significantly better 5-year cancer control rates. Again, despite the ease of risk group categorization, each group contains a heterogenous population of cancers. This may account for the differences seen in Figure 21, although surgical technique may also play a significant role.

CONCLUSIONS

Prostate cancer poses a great challenge to both physicians and to society due to its remarkable prevalence and heterogenous behavior. Indeed, most prostate cancer is clinically silent, and some patients live out their lives with a prostate cancer that remains stable for decades without treatment. In other cases, the cancer grows aggressively, responds poorly to therapy, and causes death within a few years. The median loss-of-life expectancy for men diagnosed with prostate cancer has been estimated as 9 years. Although major advances have been made in the past 2 decades in the treatment of prostate cancer, further progress will require a more accurate characterization of primary tumors; in this way, treatment—whether conservative or aggressive, surgery or radiation—will be tailored to the individual patient. In particular, imaging studies must be improved if we are to have better, noninvasive ways to identify the presence of a cancer and to define its volume, location, and extent. Additionally, substantial progress against this disease will require major discoveries in our understanding of the etiology of prostate cancer, more accurate ways to assess the biological potential of the tumor, the development of effective chemopreventive agents, and more effective systemic agents to treat metastatic cancer.

Assessing the benefits of active treatment with radical prostatectomy versus conservative management depends on accurate estimations of the life expectancy (age and health) of the patient, the risk that the patient's cancer will metastasize each year if left untreated (indicated most accurately by the grade and PSA level), the probability that surgical excision will eradicate the cancer and prevent metastases, and the frequency, intensity, and bother of complications from the surgical procedure and the cancer itself. Decision analysis models give us a tool to quantitate the degree of benefit (or harm) and will become more useful as the quality and consistency of information about each of these factors improves. The experience with radical prostatectomy reported in the past 5 years clearly documents that this operation effectively eradicates the cancer in a large portion of patients. Preliminary, albeit uncontrolled, comparisons with other treatment modalities support the superb, long-term efficacy of radical prostatectomy, particularly in intermediate- and high-risk patients. Lastly, the operation is generally accompanied by low morbidity and mortality, but recovery of continence and potency are remarkably sensitive to fine details in surgical technique. It remains a challenge to the finest skills of modern surgeons to perform radical prostatectomy without blood transfusions, with complete removal of the cancer and negative surgical margins in all patients, and with preservation of continence and erectile function in those patients continent and potent before the operation.

REFERENCES

1. Greenlee RT, Hill-Harmon MB, Murray T, Thun M. Cancer Statistics, 2001. CA Cancer J Clin 2001; 51(1):15–36.
2. Beck JR, Kattan MW, Miles BJ. A critique of the decision analysis for clinically localized prostate cancer [see comments]. J Urol 1994; 152(5 Pt 2):1894–1899.
3. Fleming C, Wasson JH, Albertsen PC, Barry MJ, Wennberg JE. A decision analysis of alternative treatment strategies for clinically localized prostate cancer. Prostate Patient Outcomes Research Team [see comments]. JAMA 1993; 269(20): 2650–2658.
4. Kattan MW, Miles BJ, Beck JR, Scardino PT. A reexamination of the decision analysis for clinically localized prostate cancer: Age and grade comparisons (abstract #646). J Urol 1995; 153:390A.
5. Bartsch G, Horninger W, Klocker H, Oberaigner W, Severi G, Robertson C, et al. Decrease in prostate cancer mortality following introduction of prostate specific antigen (PSA) screening in the Federal State of Tyrol. J Urol 2000; 163(4 [suppl]): 387a.
6. Labrie F, Candas B, Dupont A, Cusan L, Gomez JL, Suburu RE, et al. Screening decreases prostate cancer death: first analysis of the 1988 Quebec prospective randomized controlled trial. Prostate 1999; 38(2):83–91.
7. Gohagan JK, Prorok PC, Kramer BS, Cornett JE. Prostate cancer screening in the prostate, lung, colorectal and ovarian cancer screening trial of the National Cancer Institute [see comments]. J Urol 1994; 152(5 Pt 2):1905–1909.

8. Wilt TJ, Brawer MK. The prostate cancer intervention versus observation trial (PIVOT). Oncology (Huntingt) 1997; 11(8):1133–1139 discussion 1139–1140, 1143.

9. Young HH. the early diagnosis and radical cure of carcinoma of the prostate: a study of 40 cases and presentation of a radical operation which was carried out in four cases. John Hopkins Hosp Bull 1905; 16:315–321.

10. Belt E, CEE, Surber AC. A new anatomic approach in perineal prosatatectomy. J Urol 1939; 41:482–497.

11. Kuchler H. Uber prostatavergrosserungh. Deutsch Klin 1866; 18:458.

12. Millin T. Retropubic Urinary Surgery: Baltimore: Williams & Wilkins, 1947.

13. Ansell JS. Radical transvesical prostatectomy: preliminary report on an approach to surgical excision of localized prostate malignancy. J Urol 1959; 82:373.

14. Campbell EW. Total prostatectomy with preliminary ligation of the vascular pedicles. J Urol 1959; 81:464.

15. Reiner WG, Walsh PC. An anatomical approach to the surgical management of the dorsal vein and Santorini's plexus during radical retropubic surgery. J Urol 1979; 121(2):198–200.

16. Eastham JA, Kattan MW, Rogers E, Goad JR, Ohori M, Boone TB, et al. Risk factors for urinary incontinence after radical prostatectomy [see comments]. J Urol 1996; 156(5):1707–1713.

17. Catalona WJ. Surgical management of prostate cancer: contemporary results with anatomic radical prostatectomy. Cancer 1995; 75:1903–1906.

18. Steiner MS, Morton RA, Walsh PC. Impact of anatomical radical prostatectomy on urinary continence. J Urol 1991; 145(3):512–514.

19. Walsh PC. Technique of vesicourethral anastomosis may influence recovery of sexual function following radical prostatectomy. Atlas Urol Clin North Am 1994; 2:59–64.

20. Goad J, Scardino PT. Modifications in the technique of radical retropubic prostatectomy to minimize blood loss. Atlas Urol Clin North Am 1994; 2(2):65–80.

21. Goad JR, Eastham JA, Fitzgerald KB, Kattan MW, Collini MP, Yawn DH, et al. Radical retropubic prostatectomy: limited benefit of autologous blood donation. J Urol 1995; 154(6):2103–2129.

22. Smith JA, Bray WL, Koch NO. Cost efficient management of the patient with localized prostate cancer. AUA Update Series 1997; 16:122–131.

23. Leibman BD, Dillioglugil O, Abbas F, Tanli S, Kattan MW, Scardino PT. Impact of a clinical pathway for radical retropubic prostatectomy. Urology 1998; 52(1): 94–99.

24. Ohori M, Wheeler TM, Kattan MW, Goto Y, Scardino PT. Prognostic significance of positive surgical margins in radical prostatectomy specimens. J Urol 1995; 154(5):1818–1824.

25. Wieder JA, Soloway MS. Incidence, etiology, location, prevention and treatment of positive surgical margins after radical prostatectomy for prostate cancer. J Urol 1998; 160(2):299–315.

26. Klein EA, Kupelian PA, Tuason L, Levin HS. Initial dissection of the lateral fascia reduces the positive margin rate in radical prostatectomy. Urology 1998; 51(5): 766–773.

27. Catalona WJ, Smith DS, Ratliff TL, Dodds KM, Coplen DE, Yuan JJ, et al. Measurement of prostate-specific antigen in serum as a screening test for prostate cancer. N Engl J Med 1991; 324(17):1156–1161.

28. Oesterling JE. Prostate specific antigen: a critical assessment of the most useful tumor marker for adenocarcinoma of the prostate. J Urol 1991; 145(5):907–923.

29. Schmidt JD, Mettlin CJ, Natarajan N, Peace BB, Beart RW, Winchester DP, et al. Trends in patterns of care for prostatic cancer, 1974–1983: results of surveys by the American College of Surgeons. J Urol 1986; 136(2):416–421.

30. Smith DS, Catalona WJ, Herschman JD. Longitudinal screening for prostate cancer with prostate-specific antigen [see comments]. Jama 1996; 276(16):1309–1315.

31. Soh S, Kattan MW, Berkman S, Wheeler TM, Scardino PT. Has there been a recent shift in the pathological features and prognosis of patients treated with radical prostatectomy? [see comments]. J Urol 1997; 157(6):2212–2218.

32. Franks LM. Latent carcinoma of the prostate. J Pathol Bact 1954; 68:603–616.

33. McNeal JE. Origin and development of carcinoma in the prostate. Cancer 1969; 23(1):24–34.

34. Sakr WA, Grignon DJ, Crissman JD, et al. High grade prostatic intraepithelial neoplasia (HGPIN) and prostatic adenocarcinoma between the ages of 20–69; An autopsy study of 249 cases. In Vivo 1994; 8(3):439–443.

35. Seidman H, Mushinski MH, Gelb SK, Silverberg E. Probabilities of eventually developing or dying of cancer—United States, 1985. CA Cancer J Clin 1985; 35(1): 36–56.

36. Ohori M, Wheeler TM, Dunn JK, Stamey TA, Scardino PT. The pathological features and prognosis of prostate cancer detectable with current diagnostic tests. J Urol 1994; 152(5 Pt 2):1714–1720.

37. Chodak GW, Thisted RA, Gerber GS, Johansson JE, Adolfsson J, Jones GW, et al. Results of conservative management of clinically localized prostate cancer [see comments]. N Engl J Med 1994; 330(4):242–248.

38. Albertsen PC, Fryback DG, Storer BE, Kolon TF, Fine J. Long-term survival among men with conservatively treated localized prostate cancer [see comments]. JAMA 1995; 274(8):626–631.

39. Albertsen PC, Hanley JA, Gleason DF, Barry MJ. Competing risk analysis of men aged 55 to 74 years at diagnosis managed conservatively for clinically localized prostate cancer [see comments]. JAMA 1998; 280(11):975–980.

40. Johansson JE, Holmbeg L, Johansson S, Bergstrom R, Adami HO. Fifteen-year survival in prostate cancer. A prospective, population-based study in Sweden [see comments] [published erratum appears in JAMA 1997 Jul 16;278(3):206]. JAMA 1997; 277(6):467–471.

41. Aus G, Hugosson J, Norlen L. Long-term survival and mortality in prostate cancer treated with noncurative intent [see comments]. J Urol 1995; 154(2 Pt 1):460–465.

42. Dillioglugil O, Leibman BD, Leibman NS, Kattan MW, Rosas AL, Scardino PT. Risk factors for complications and morbidity after radical retropubic prostatectomy. J Urol 1997; 157(5):1760–1767.

43. Chodak GW. The role of watchful waiting in the management of localized prostate cancer [see comments]. J Urol 1994; 152(5 Pt 2):1766–1768.

44. Brasso K, Friis S, Juel K, Jorgensen T, Iversen P. The need for hospital care of patients with clinically localized prostate cancer managed by noncurative intent: a population based registry study. J Urol 2000; 163(4):1150–1154.

45. Martin JA, Smith BL, TJM, Ventura SJ. Births and deaths: Preliminary data for 1998. Natl Vital Stat Rep 1999; 47(25):1–45.

46. Pound CR, Partin AW, Epstein JI, Walsh PC. Prostate-specific antigen after anatomic radical retropubic prostatectomy. Patterns of recurrence and cancer control. Urol Clin North Am 1997; 24(2):395–406.

47. Catalona WJ, Smith DS. 5-year tumor recurrence rates after anatomical radical retropubic prostatectomy for prostate cancer. J Urol 1994; 152(5Pt2):1837–1842.

48. Zincke H, Oesterling JE, Blute ML, Bergstralh EJ, Myers RP, Barrett DM. Long-term (15 years) results after radical prostatectomy for clinically localized (stage T2c or lower) prostate cancer [see comments]. J Urol 1994; 152(5 Pt 2):1850–1857.

49. Ohori M, Wheeler TM, Scardino PT. The New American Joint Committee on Cancer and International Union Against Cancer TNM classification of prostate cancer. Clinicopathologic correlations. Cancer 1994; 74(1):104–114.

50. Wheeler TM. Anatomic considerations in carcinoma of the prostate. Urol Clin North Am 1989; 16(4):623–634.

51. McNeal JE, Bostwick DG, Kindrachuk RA, Redwine EA, Freiha FS, Stamey TA. Patterns of progression in prostate cancer. Lancet 1986; 1(8472):60–63.

52. Byar DP, Mostofi FK. Carcinoma of the prostate: prognostic evaluation of certain pathologic features in 208 radical prostatectomies. Examined by the step-section technique. Cancer 1972; 30(1):5–13.

53. Scardino PT, Cantini M, Wheeler TM. Radical prostatectomy: assessment of morbidity and pathologic findings. J Urol 1987; 137:192A.

54. Catalona WJ, Bigg SW. Nerve-sparing radical prostatectomy: evaluation of results after 250 patients. J Urol 1990; 143(3):538–543; discussion 544.

55. Ohori M, Egawa S, Shinohara K, Wheeler TM, Scardino PT. Detection of microscopic extracapsular extension prior to radical prostatectomy for clinically localized prostate cancer. Br J Urol 1994; 74(1):72–79.

56. D'Amico AV, Whittington R, Schnall M, Malkowicz SB, Tomaszewski JE, Schultz D, et al. The impact of the inclusion of endorectal coil magnetic resonance imaging in a multivariate analysis to predict clinically unsuspected extraprostatic cancer. Cancer 1995; 75(9):2368–2372.

57. Wheeler TM, Dillioglugil O, Kattan MW, Arakawa A, Soh S, Suyama K, et al. Clinical and pathological significance of the level and extent of capsular invasion in clinical stage T1–2 prostate cancer. Hum Pathol 1998; 29(8):856–862.

58. D'Amico AV, Whittington R, Malkowicz SB, Schultz D, Schnall M, Tomaszewski JE, et al. Critical analysis of the ability of the endorectal coil magnetic resonance imaging scan to predict pathologic stage, margin status, and postoperative prostate-specific antigen failure in patients with clinically organ-confined prostate cancer. J Clin Oncol 1996; 14(6):1770–1777.

59. Middleton RG, Smith JA, Melzer RB, Hamilton PE. Patient survival and local recurrence rate following radical prostatectomy for prostatic carcinoma. J Urol 1986; 136(2):422–424.

60. Epstein JI, Carmichael M, Walsh PC. Adenocarcinoma of the prostate invading the seminal vesicle: definition and relation of tumor volume, grade and margins of resection to prognosis. J Urol 1993; 149(5):1040–1045.

61. Ohori M, Scardino PT, Lapin SL, Seale-Hawkins C, Link J, Wheeler TM. The mechanisms and prognostic significance of seminal vesicle involvement by prostate cancer. Am J Surg Pathol 1993; 17(12):1252–1261.

62. Ohori M, Shinohara K, Wheeler TM, Aihara M, Wessels EC, Carter SS, et al. Ultrasonic detection of non-palpable seminal vesicle invasion: a clinicopathological study. Br J Urol 1993; 72(5 Pt 2):799–808.

63. Terris MK, McNeal JE, Freiha FS, Stamey TA. Efficacy of transrectal ultrasound-guided seminal vesicle biopsies in the detection of seminal vesicle invasion by prostate cancer. J Urol 1993; 149(5):1035–1039.

64. D'Amico AV, Schnall M, Whittington R, Malkowicz SB, Schultz D, Tomaszewski JE, et al. Endorectal coil magnetic resonance imaging identifies locally advanced prostate cancer in select patients with clinically localized disease. Urology 1998; 51(3):449–454.

65. Rorvik J, Halvorsen OJ, Albrektsen G, Ersland L, Daehlin L, Haukaas S. MRI with an endorectal coil for staging of clinically localised prostate cancer prior to radical prostatectomy. Eur Radiol 1999; 9(1):29–34.

66. Balaji KC, Wheeler TM, Scardino PT. Poorly differentiated prostate cancers (PCa) detected by PSA are more likely to be organ confined than those detected by digital rectal examination. Proc Am Soc Clin Oncol 1999; 18:318a.

67. Epstein JI, Walsh PC, Brendler CB. Radical prostatectomy for impalpable prostate cancer: the Johns Hopkins experience with tumors found on transurethral resection (stages T1A and T1B) and on needle biopsy (stage T1C). J Urol 1994; 152(5 Pt 2):1721–1729.

68. Stamey TA. Making the most out of six systematic sextant biopsies. Urology 1995; 45(1):2–12.

69. Scardino PT, Shinohara K, Wheeler TM, Carter SS. Staging of prostate cancer. Value of ultrasonography. Urol Clin North Am 1989; 16(4):713–734.

70. Goto Y, Ohori M, Arakawa A, Kattan MW, Wheeler TM, Scardino PT. Distinguishing clinically important from unimportant prostate cancers before treatment: Value of systematic biopsies. J Urol 1996; 156(3):1059–1063.

71. Bastacky SI, Walsh PC, Epstein JI. Relationship between perineural tumor invasion on needle biopsy and radical prostatectomy capsular penetration in clinical stage B adenocarcinoma of the prostate. Am J Surg Pathol 1993; 17(4):336–341.

72. Ravery V, Chastang C, Toublanc M-, Gibod L, Delmas V. Percentage of cancer on biopsy cores accurately predicts extracapsular extension and biochemical relapse after radical prostatectomy for T1–T2 prostate cancer. Eur Urol 2000; 37(4): 449–455.

73. Partin AW, Yoo J, Carter HB, Pearson JD, Chan DW, Epstein JI, et al. The use of prostate specific antigen, clinical stage and Gleason score to predict pathological stage in men with localized prostate cancer. J Urol 1993; 150(1):110–114.

74. Partin AW, Kattan MW, Subong EN, Walsh PC, Wojno KJ, Oesterling JE, et al. Combination of prostate-specific antigen, clinical stage, and Gleason score to pre-

dict pathological stage of localized prostate cancer. A multi-institutional update [see comments] [published erratum appears in JAMA 1997 Jul 9;278(2):118]. JAMA 1997; 277(18):1445–1451.

75. Kattan MW, Eastham JA, Stapleton AM, Wheeler TM, Scardino PT. A preoperative nomogram for disease recurrence following radical prostatectomy for prostate cancer. J Natl Cancer Inst 1998; 90(10):766–771.

76. Kavoussi LR, Meyers JA, Catalona WJ. Effect of temporary occlusion of the hypogastric arteries on blood loss during radical retropubic prostatectomy. J Urol 1991; 146(2):362–365.

77. Peters CA, Walsh PC. Blood transfusions and anesthetic practices in radical retropubic prostatectomy. J Urol 1985; 134(1):81–83.

78. Myers RP. Improving the exposure of the prostate in radical retropubic prostatectomy: longitudinal bunching of the deep venous plexus. J Urol 1989; 142(5): 1282–1284.

79. Hrebinko RL', Donnell WF. Control of the deep dorsal venous complex in radical retropubic prostatectomy. J Urol 1993; 149(4):799–800; discussion 800–801.

80. Leandri P, Rossignol G, Gautier JR, Ramon J. Radical retropubic prostatectomy: morbidity and quality of life. Experience with 620 consecutive cases. J Urol 1992; 147(3 Pt 2):883–887.

81. Rainwater LM, Segura JW. Technical consideration in radical retropubic prostatectomy: blood loss after ligation of dorsal venous complex. J Urol 1990; 143(6): 1163–1165.

82. Andriole GL, Smith DS, Rao G, Goodnough L, Catalona WJ. Early complications of contemporary anatomical radical retropubic prostatectomy. J Urol 1994; 152(5 Pt 2):1858–1860.

83. Lerner SE, Blute ML, Lieber MM, Zincke H. Morbidity of contemporary radical retropublic prostatectomy for localized prostate cancer. Oncology (Huntingt) 1995; 9(5):379–382; discussion 382, 385–386, 389.

84. Hautmann RE, Sauter TW, Wenderoth UK. Radical retropublic prostatectomy: morbidity and urinary continence in 418 consecutive cases. Urology 1994; 43(2 Suppl): 47–51.

85. McLaren RH, Barrett DM, Zincke H. Rectal injury occurring at radical retropubic prostatectomy for prostate cancer: etiology and treatment. Urology 1993; 42(4): 401–405.

86. Borland RN, Walsh PC. The management of rectal injury during radical retropubic prostatectomy. J Urol 1992; 147(3 Pt 2):905–907.

87. Caprini JA, Chucker JL, Zuckerman L, Vagher JP, Franck CA, Cullen JE. Thrombosis prophylaxis using external compression. Surg Gynecol Obstet 1983; 156(5): 599–604.

88. Coe NP, Collins RE, Klein LA, Bettmann MA, Skillman JJ, Shapiro RM, et al. Prevention of deep vein thrombosis in urological patients: a controlled, randomized trial of low-dose heparin and external pneumatic compression boots. Surgery 1978; 83(2):230–234.

89. Hansberry KL, Thompson IM, Bauman J, Deppe S, Rodriguez FR. A prospective comparison of thromboembolic stockings, external sequential pneumatic compres-

sion stockings and heparin sodium/dihydroergotamine mesylate for the prevention of thromboembolic complications in urological surgery. J Urol 1991; 145(6): 1205–1208.

90. Cisek LJ, Walsh PC. Thromboembolic complications following radical retropublic prostatectomy. Influence of external sequential pneumatic compression devices. Urology 1993; 42(4):406–408.

91. Surya BV, Provet J, Johanson KE, Brown J. Anastomotic strictures following radical prostatectomy: risk factors and management. J Urol 1990; 143(4):755–758.

92. Geary ES, Dendinger TE, Freiha FS, Stamey TA. Incontinence and vesical neck strictures following radical retropubic prostatectomy. Urology 1995; 45(6): 1000–1006.

93. Fowler FJ, Barry MJ, Lu-Yao G, Roman A, Wasson J, Wennberg JE. Patient-reported complications and follow-up treatment after radical prostatectomy. The National Medicare Experience: 1988–1990 (Updated June 1993). Urology 1993; 42(6):622–629.

94. Litwin MS, Hays RD, Fink A, Ganz PA, Leake B, Leach GE, et al. Quality-of-life outcomes in men treated for localized prostate cancer [see comments]. JAMA 1995; 273(2):129–135.

95. Murphy GP, Mettlin C, Menck H, Winchester DP, Davidson AM. National patterns of prostate cancer treatment by radical prostatectomy: results of a survey by the American College of Surgeons Commission on Cancer [see comments]. J Urol 1994; 152(5 Pt 2):1817–1819.

96. Walsh PC. Radical prostatectomy for localized prostate cancer provides durable cancer control with excellent quality of life: a structured debate. J Urol 2000; 163(6): 1802–1807.

97. Stanford JL, Feng Z, Hamilton AS, Gilliland FD, Stephenson RA, Eley JW, et al. Urinary and sexual function after radical prostatectomy for clinically localized prostate cancer: The Prostate Cancer Outcomes Study [In Process Citation]. JAMA 2000; 283(3):354–360.

98. Presti JC, Schmidt RA, Narayan PA, Carroll PR, Tanagho EA. Pathophysiology of urinary incontinence after radical prostatectomy. J Urol 1990; 143(5):975–978.

99. Hutch JA, Fisher R. Continence after radical prostatectomy. Br J Urol 1968; 40(1): 62–67.

100. Rudy DC, Woodside JR, Crawford ED. Urodynamic evaluation of incontinence in patients undergoing modified Campbell radical retropublic prostatectomy: a prospective study. J Urol 1984; 132(4):708–712.

101. O'Donnell PD, Finan BF. Continence following nerve sparing radical prostatectomy [discussion: 1229]. J Urol 1989; 142(5):1227–1228.

102. Quinlan DM, Epstein JI, Carter BS, Walsh PC. Sexual function following radical prostatectomy: influence of preservation of neurovascular bundles. J Urol 1991; 145(5):998–1002.

103. Rabbani F, Stapleton AM, Kattan MW, Wheeler TM, Scardino PT. Factors predicting recovery of erections after radical prostatectomy. J Urol 2000; 164(6): 1929–1934.

104. Bahnson RR, Catalona WJ. Papaverine testing of impotent patients following nerve-sparing radical prostatectomy. J Urol 1988; 139(4):773–774.

105. Breza J, Aboseif SR, Orvis BR, Lue TF, Tanagho EA. Detailed anatomy of penile neurovascular structures: surgical significance. J Urol 1989; 141(2):437–443.

106. Rosen MA, Goldstone L, Lapin S, Wheeler T, Scardino PT. Frequency and location of extracapsular extension and positive surgical margins in radical prostatectomy specimens. J Urol 1992; 148(2 Pt 1):331–337.

107. Killeen KP, Libertino JA, Sughayer MA, Lee AK, Watkins E. Pathologic review of consecutive radical prostatectomy specimens. Nerve sparing versus nonnerve sparing. Urology 1991; 38(3):212–215.

108. Abbas F, Scardino PT. Why neoadjuvant androgen deprivation prior to radical prostatectomy is unnecessary. Urol Clin North Am 1996; 23(4):587–604.

109. Kupelian P, Katcher J, Levin H, Zippe C, Suh J, Macklis R, et al. External beam radiotherapy versus radical prostatectomy for clinical stage T1–2 prostate cancer: therapeutic implications of stratification by pretreatment PSA levels and biopsy Gleason scores. Cancer J Sci Am 1997; 3(2):78–87.

110. Epstein JI. Incidence and significance of positive margins in radical prostatectomy specimens. Urol Clin North Am 1996; 23(4):651–663.

111. Blute ML, Bostwick DG, Bergstralh EJ, Slezak JM, Martin SK, Amling CL, et al. Anatomic site-specific positive margins in organ-confined prostate cancer and its impact on outcome after radical prostatectomy. Urology 1997; 50(5):733–739.

112. Kim ED, Scardino PT, Hampel O, Mills NL, Wheeler TM, Nath RK. Interposition of sural nerve restores function of cavernous nerves resected during radical prostatectomy. J Urol 1999; 161(1):188–192.

113. Licht MR, Klein EA, Tuason L, Levin H. Impact of bladder neck preservation during radical prostatectomy on continence and cancer control. Urology 1994; 44(6):883–887.

114. Oesterling JE, Chan DW, Epstein JI, Kimball AW, Bruzek DJ, Rock RC, et al. Prostate specific antigen in the preoperative and postoperative evaluation of localized prostatic cancer treated with radical prostatectomy. J Urol 1988; 139(4): 766–772.

115. Goldrath DE, Messing EM. Prostate specific antigen: not detectable despite tumor progression after radical prostatectomy. J Urol 1989; 142(4):1082–1084.

116. Takayama TK, Krieger JN, True LD, Lange PH. Recurrent prostate cancer despite undetectable prostate specific antigen. J Urol 1992; 148(5):1541–1542.

117. Leibman BD, Dillioglugil O, Wheeler TM, Scardino PT. Distant metastasis after radical prostatectomy in patients without an elevated serum prostate specific antigen level. Cancer 1995; 76(12):2530–2534.

118. Oefelein MG, Smith N, Carter M, Dalton D, Schaeffer A. The incidence of prostate cancer progression with undetectable serum prostate specific antigen in a series of 394 radical prostatectomies. J Urol 1995; 154(6):2128–2131.

119. Lightner DJ, Lange PH, Reddy PK, Moore L. Prostate specific antigen and local recurrence after radical prostatectomy. J Urol 1990; 144(4):921–926.

120. Stein A, deKernion JB, Dorey F. Prostatic specific antigen related to clinical status 1 to 14 years after radical retropubic prostatectomy. Br J Urol 1991; 67(6):626–631.

121. Morton RA, Steiner MS, Walsh PC. Cancer control following anatomical radical prostatectomy: an interim report. J Urol 1991; 145(6):1197–200.

122. Partin AW, Pound CR, Clemens JQ, Epstein JI, Walsh PC. Serum PSA after anatomic radical prostatectomy. The Johns Hopkins experience after 10 years. Urol Clin North Am 1993; 20(4):713–725.

123. Trapasso JG, deKernion JB, Smith RB, Dorey F. The incidence and significance of detectable levels of serum prostate specific antigen after radical prostatectomy [see comments]. J Urol 1994; 152(5 Pt 2):1821–1825.

124. Dillioglugil O, Leibman BD, Kattan MW, Seale-Hawkins C, Wheeler TM, Scardino PT. Hazard rates for progression after radical prostatectomy for clinically localized prostate cancer. Urology 1997; 50(1):93–99.

125. Epstein JI, Pizov G, Walsh PC. Correlation of pathologic findings with progression after radical retropubic prostatectomy. Cancer 1993; 71(11):3582–3593.

126. McNeal JE, Villers AA, Redwine EA, Freiha FS, Stamey TA. Histologic differentiation, cancer volume, and pelvic lymph node metastasis in adenocarcinoma of the prostate. Cancer 1990; 66(6):1225–1233.

127. Bubendorf L, Tapia C, Gasser TC, Casella R, Grunder B, Moch H, et al. Ki67 labeling index in core needle biopsies independently predicts tumor-specific survival in prostate cancer. Hum Pathol 1998; 29(9):949–954.

128. Massenkeil G, Oberhuber H, Hailemariam S, et al. P53 mutations and loss of heterozygosity on chromosomes 8p, 16q, 17p, and 18q are confined to advanced prostate cancer. Anticancer Res 1994; 14(6B):2785–2790.

129. Mottaz AE, Markwalder R, Fey MF, et al. Abnormal p53 expression is rare in clinically localized human prostate cancer: Comparison between immunohistochemical and molecular detection of p53 mutations. Prostate 1997; 31(4):209–215.

130. Umbas R, Isaacs WB, Bringuier PP, et al. Decreased-E-cadherin expression is associated with poor prognosis in patients with prostate cancer. Cancer Res 1994; 54(14):3929–3933.

131. Ueda T, Ichikawa T, Tamaru J, et al. Expression of the KAII protein in benign prostatic hyperplasia and prostate cancer. Am J Pathol 1996; 149(5):1435–1440.

132. Mohler JL, Metts JC, Zhang XZ, Maygarden SJ. Nuclear morphometry in automatic biopsy and radical prostatectomy specimens of prostatic carcinoma. A comparison. Anal Quant Cytol Histol 1994; 16(6):415–420.

133. Polascik TJ, Pound CR, DeWeese TL, Walsh PC. Comparison of radical prostatectomy and iodine 125 interstitial radiotherapy for the treatment of clinically localized prostate cancer: a 7-year biochemical (PSA) progression analysis [see comments]. Urology 1998; 51(6):884–889; discussion 889–890.

134. D'Amico AV, Whittington R, Malkowicz SB, Schultz D, Blank K, Broderick GA, et al. Biochemical outcome after radical prostatectomy, external beam radiation therapy, or interstitial radiation therapy for clinically localized prostate cancer [see comments]. JAMA 1998; 280(11):969–974.

135. Labrie F, Cusan L, Gomez JL, Diamond P, Suburu R, Lemay M, et al. Neoadjuvant hormonal therapy: the Canadian experience. Urology 1997; 49(3A Suppl):56–64.

136. Witjes WP, Schulman CC, Debruyne FM. Preliminary results of a prospective randomized study comparing radical prostatectomy versus radical prostatectomy associated with neoadjuvant hormonal combination therapy in T2–3 N0 M0 prostatic carcinoma. The European Study Group on Neoadjuvant Treatment of Prostate Cancer. Urology 1997; 49(3A Suppl):65–69.

137. Ohori M, Wheeler TM, Dunn JK, Stamey TA, Scardino PT. The pathological features and prognosis of prostate cancer detectable with current diagnostic tests [see comments]. J Urol 1994; 152(5 Pt 2):1714–1720.

138. Catalona WJ, Smith DS. 5-year tumor recurrence rates after anatomical radical retropubic prostatectomy for prostate cancer [see comments]. J Urol 1994; 152(5 Pt 2):1837–1842.

EDITORIAL COMMENTARY

Robert P. Myers

Consultant in Urology, Mayo Clinic, Professor of Urology, Mayo Clinic College of Medicine, Rochester, Minnesota, USA

The preceding chapter details excellent surgical techniques applied to radical retropubic prostatectomy. In a recent study, the importance of technique was highlighted by the finding that, in multivariate analysis, the occurrence of positive surgical margins was surgeon-dependent [1]. By analogy, the outcomes of pad-free urinary control and resumed erectile function are also surgeon-dependent. The onus, then, is on urologic surgeons to improve their technique, which, if done poorly, can subsequently wreak havoc in the lives of their patients.

Knowing how to use instruments for proper dissection is paramount. However, nothing is of greater importance to a surgeon than an acute understanding of the variable anatomy of the prostate, its fascial enclosures, surrounding vessels, and the variations encountered from case-to-case at the prostate apex and at the junction of the prostate with the bladder neck [2].

Important variables for radical prostatectomy include size of the prostate, configuration of the apex, and the presence or absence of benign prostatic hyperplasia. Prostates of varying apical configuration are shown in Figure 1. The presence of BPH specifically affects the anteroposterior angulation of the prostatic urethra at the veru (verumontanum, seminal colliculus), placement of the veru with respect to the apex of the prostate, the presence or absence of prostate overlap of the sphincteric (membranous) urethra, the size of the anterior commissure, and placement of the neurovascular bundles. Furthermore, BPH affects the detrusor apron [3], which obscures the anterior surface of the prostate as it forms a pubovesical complex [4], including the dorsal veins of the penis at the penile hilus [5]. The detrusor apron is an extension, over the anterior surface of the prostate, of outer longitudinal detrusor muscle beyond or distal to where the bladder forms a neck with the internal urethral meatus.

It is surgically advantageous to bring the detrusor apron and associated vascular plexus together in the midline with suture material, as demonstrated by the authors in their Figures 5 through 8, and herein in Figures 2A and 2B. In addition to achieving hemostasis [6], this bunching together of tissue improves visualization of the lateral surfaces of the prostate before the critical apical dissec-

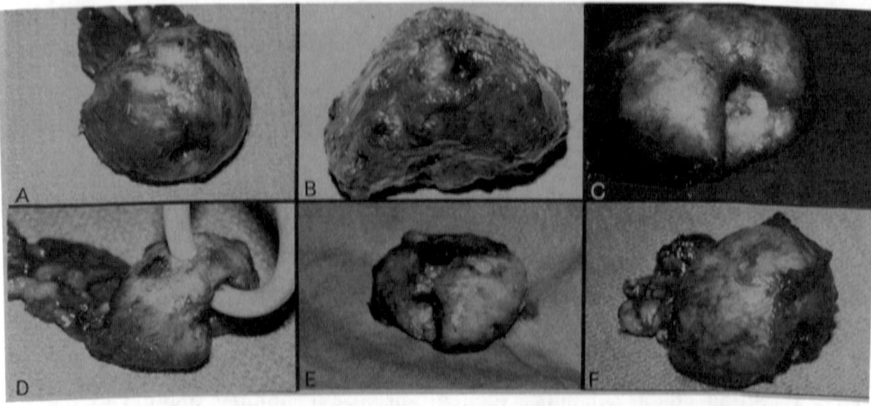

FIGURE 1   Six gross radical prostatectomy specimens, each of different size and apical configuration. Urethral opening at each prostate apex is clearly seen in the midline or to lower left of each specimen. (From Myers [2]. With permission from the American Urological Association.)

tion. Adequate exposure of the lateral surfaces is necessary for proper release of the neurovascular bundles. This bunching maneuver also facilitates access to the neurovascular bundles where they angle sharply at the prostatourethral junction [7]. If the superficial layer of periprostatic fascia is opened first early and linearly along the prostatourethral junction to a point just anterior to the nerve bundle, then there is no substantial risk to the nerve bundle from maneuvers used to control the dorsal vein complex; for example, see the vertical continuous oversewing of the complex seen in the authors' Figure 8B.

BPH affects the size of the anterior commissure, the bridge of prostate tissue anterior to the urethra: the more BPH, the larger the commissure. The larger the commissure, the longer the distance from the bladder neck to the prostatourethral junction. Surgeons should expect variations in this element of prostate anatomy as dissection is carried distally. In the absence of BPH, the anterior commissure (isthmus of the prostate) may be nothing more than a tiny band of tissue. With advanced BPH, the anterior commissure may be enormous [8]. Depending on the size of the commissure, the surgeon will encounter a varying-length avascular plane along the commissure from the point where the bladder attachment ends and the prostatourethral junction begins [3]. As the dissection proceeds distally along the avascular plane segment of the commissure, the surgeon may encounter what seems to be an acute cliff-like drop-off to the prostatourethral junction. The cliff is just one of the problem apices that urologic surgeons encounter. The cliff often overlaps the urethra at the prostatourethral junction. Vertical transection of the urethra commensurate with the end of the

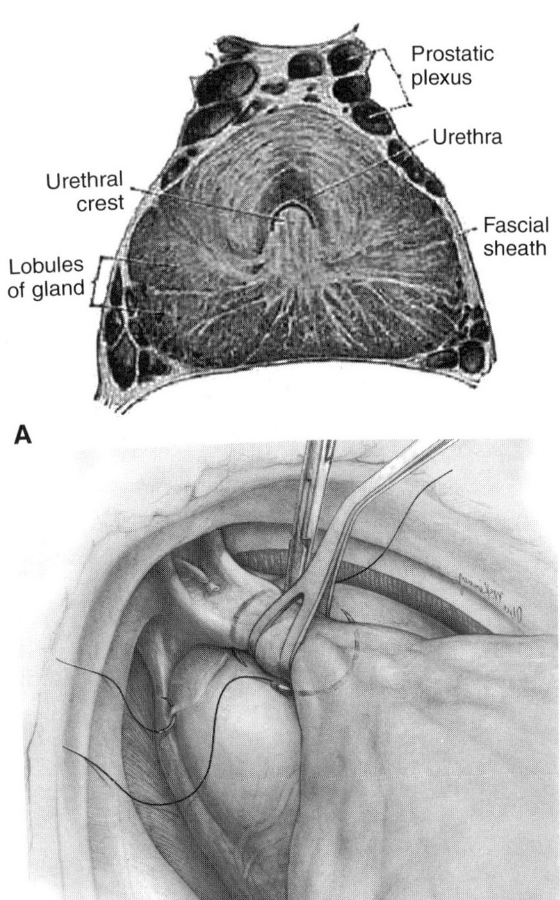

FIGURE 2 **A**: Typical vascular plexus distribution in axial section through the prostate. Major plexus is anterior; minor plexuses accompany posterolateral neurovascular bundles. (From Martin CP. Urogenital system. In: Brash JC, ed. Cunningham's Textbook of Anatomy. 9th ed. London: Oxford University Press, 1953: 727. By permission of the publisher.) **B**: Use of modified Babcock forceps to grasp detrusor apron with its associated major, vascular plexus. (From Myers [6]. With permission from Mayo Foundation for Medical Education and Research.)

cliff will result in transection of the urethra distal to the prostatourethral junction, and the residual urethral stump will be too short for postoperative recovery of urinary control.

Significant overlap of the sphincter by prostate does not occur in most cases because most patients do well with urethral transection at the apex or 1 to 2 mm distal to the apex. Up to 80% certainly can be expected to be pad-free [9]. The remaining 20% have less-than-perfect control and may have what can be called, as mentioned earlier, a "problem apex." This means finding a significant overlap of the sphincter by prostate or a sphincteric (membranous) urethra that is critically short at the beginning. Overlap can be identified intraoperatively but also by preoperative T2-weighted magnetic resonance imaging [10,11], and a short urethra can be identified with preoperative retrograde urethrography [8]. Overlap may be anterior, posterior, unilateral, bilateral, or circumferential. For standard radical prostatectomy that involves leaving several millimeters of urethra, sacrifice of a possibly significant portion of the sphincteric tissue is readily identified in coronal whole-mount histologic section [12], as shown in Figure 3.

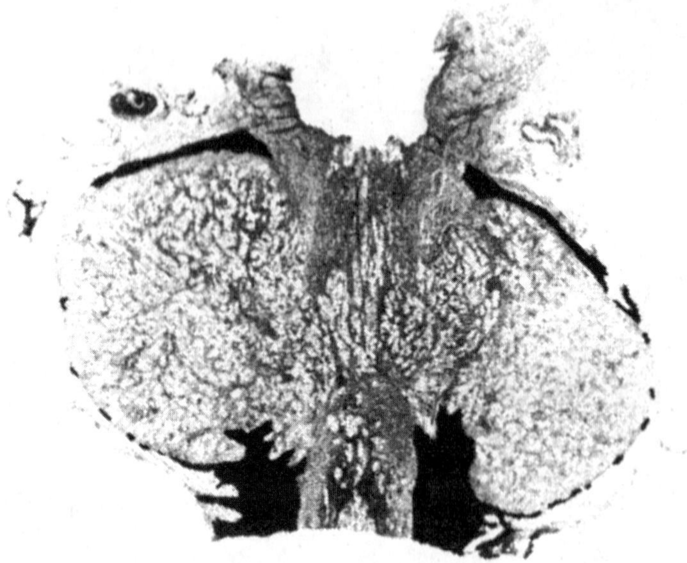

FIGURE 3 Prostate in coronal section with point of transection of urethra and sphincter as performed in "standard" radical prostatectomy sacrifices significant portion of critical smooth muscle and elastic tissue as well as striated muscle of distal continence mechanism. (Black & white rendition of phosphotungstic acid-hematoxylin section.) (From Blacklock [12]. With permission from William Heinemann Medical Books.)

The fact that overlap of the sphincter by the prostate may exist is an important consideration for anyone doing the apical dissection. The overlap involves the inframontanal prostatic urethra, which should be no more than 1 cm in length. The distance from the distal aspect of the veru to the posterior apex will vary from 0 to 1 cm. In such "problem apex" cases, it may be helpful to retract the prostate parenchyma gently before urethral transection in order to gain the required suitable residual functional urethral length [8]. A recent nonrandomized study of apical prostate dissection to preserve the intraprostatic portion of the urethral stump resulted in statistically improved urinary continence rates when compared with flush transection of the urethra at the prostate apex [13]. The authors wrote of a "long intraprostatic urethral stump," but the necessary intraprostatic urethral portion comprises a relatively short component (no more than 1 cm) of most urethral stumps, including their membranous urethral portions. In patients undergoing the intraprostatic urethral stump salvage, the authors reported that the rate of positive apical margins actually decreased, which is surprising. This may reflect stage migration and better selection of patients in their second series.

REFERENCES

1. Eastham JA, Kattan MW, Gerigk C, Scardino PT. Surgeon is an independent risk factor for positive surgical margins (+SM) at the time of radical prostatectomy (RP) (abstract). J Urol 2002; 167(Suppl:):233.
2. Myers RP. Practical pelvic anatomy pertinent to radical retropubic prostatectomy. AUA Update Series 1994; 13(Lesson 4):26–32.
3. Myers RP. Detrusor apron, associated vascular plexus, and avascular plane: relevance to radical retropubic prostatectomy—anatomic and surgical commentary. Urology 2002; 59:472–479.
4. Cummings KB, Pantuck AJ, Glazier DB. Nerve-sparing radical retropubic prostatectomy: refining the anatomic approach (abstract). J Urol 2001; 165(Suppl:):181.
5. Devine CJ, Angermeier KW. Anatomy of the penis and male perineum: Part I. AUA Update Series 1994; 13:9–16.
6. Myers RP. The surgical management of prostate cancer: radical retropubic and radical perineal prostatectomy. In: Lepor H, Ed. Prostatic Diseases. Philadelphia: WB Saunders Company, 2000:410–443.
7. Walsh PC. Anatomic radical retropubic prostatectomy. In: Walsh PC, Retik AB, Vaughan ED, Wein AJ, Kavoussi LR, Novick AC, Partin AW, Peters CA, Eds. Campbell's urology. 8th ed. Vol. 4. Philadelphia: Saunders, 2002:3107–3129.
8. Myers RP. Male urethral sphincteric anatomy and radical prostatectomy. Urol Clin North Am 1991; 18:211–227.
9. Stamey TA. Prostate cancer: who should be treated?. Monogr Urol 1995; 16:3–16.
10. Myers RP, Cahill DR, Devine RM, King BF. Anatomy of radical prostatectomy as defined by magnetic resonance imaging. J Urol 1998; 159:2148–2158.

11. Myers RP. Practical surgical anatomy for radical prostatectomy. Urol Clin North Am 2001; 28:473–490.

12. Blacklock NJ. Surgical anatomy of the prostate. In: Williams DI, Chisholm GD, Eds. Scientific foundations of urology. Vol. 2. London: William Heinemann Medical Books, 1976:113–125.

13. Randenborgh HV, Paul R, Breul J, Hartung R. Improved urinary continence in radical retropubic prostatectomy after preparation of a long intraprostatic urethral stump—results of a questionnaire in 575 consecutive cases (abstract). J Urol 2002; 167(Suppl:):357.

EDITORIAL COMMENTARY

Alan W. Partin

Bernard L. Schwartz Distinguished Professor of Urologic Oncology, The Brady Urological Institute, The Johns Hopkins Medical Institution, Baltimore, MD, USA

Two decades following the first description by Patrick C. Walsh, M.D. of the anatomical radical retropubic prostatectomy for the management of localized prostate cancer, radical retropubic removal of the prostate for treatment of clinical localized prostate cancer remains the number one choice of definitive local therapy elected by patients newly diagnosed with prostate cancer. The introduction of other local treatment modalities such as brachytherapy, cryosurgery, and laparoscopic radical retropubic prostatectomy have enhanced the armamentarium for treatment of localized prostate cancer, which, prior to these new methods, was limited to external beam radiation therapy and radical surgery. However, modifications to the selection of patients and the surgical approach to localized prostate cancer, brought about through decades of careful research and attention to this important operation, have not only decreased the morbidity associated with this treatment method but also greatly enhanced long-term cure rates and potential mortality rates for prostate cancer. This chapter represents an excellent discussion of the anatomic radical retropubic prostatectomy. Drs. Lin, Eastham, and Scardino have carefully outlined the rationale for use of this operation in treating men with localized prostate cancer, important factors regarding patient selection and prognosis prediction, complications related to the technique, description of the surgical procedure, and a careful elucidation of cancer control following radical retropubic prostatectomy. The authors conclude this chapter with a rationale for selecting radical prostatectomy as the treatment of choice for clinically localized prostate cancer.

Of equal importance in determining the rationale for coupling the procedure to the patient is rational approach to the selection of the candidate for that procedure. These authors have carefully outlined the important features in rational patient selection for radical retropubic prostatectomy. These factors include: age, curability, comorbidities, and stage and grade of the prostate cancer; all are important when considering whether an individual patient is a good candidate for this type of treatment for localized prostate cancer. While age, in and of itself, is not an absolute criteria for selecting an ideal candidate for radical retropubic prostatectomy, life expectancy is. If a patient is not likely to benefit from a cure from prostate cancer, with respect to his potential life expectancy, then an alternate, potentially less morbid, form of therapy should be chosen. The recommended cut-off age for potential candidates for radical retropubic prostatectomy ranges between 65 and 75 years of age. This cut-off age is often altered as time passes based on the ever increasing life expectancy of the male population. While no specific recommendations regarding an age cut-off exist, one should take into account the patient's life expectancy when determining whether or not they are an ideal candidate for a radical retropubic prostatectomy. The authors carefully discuss this topic in this chapter. Clinical and pathological factors, such as the grade of the tumor and the stage of the disease (both clinically and pathologically), must also be taken into account when determining whether or not a patient is an ideal candidate for a radical retorpubic prostatectomy. Additionally, a factor such as the number of prostate needle biopsies involved with the cancer, as well as the grade and degree to which these biopsy materials are involved, coupled with serum PSA level, have been used in the past to develop nomograms and models for predicting the likelihood of cure when a patient is confronted with the decision as to whether or not they are a candidate for a radical retropubic prostatectomy. The authors have carefully outlined how these factors can be used in making this important determination.

In summary, this chapter represents an excellent review of the implementation, surgical utilization, and outcomes regarding the anatomical retropubic prostatectomy for localized prostate cancer. Careful attention to the selection of the patients for this procedure is imperative to help ensure an optimal outcome.

EDITORIAL OVERVIEW

Kenneth B. Cummings

Anatomic radical retropubic prostatectomy (RRP) two decades after Dr. Patrick C. Walsh's description remains the undisputed favorite treatment for localized prostate cancer. The occurrence of positive surgical margins as shown by Scardino is surgeon dependent [1] as is, by analogy, the incidence of incontinence and erectile dysfunction. The RRP affords the opportunity to simultaneously examine the pelvic lymph nodes, in contrast to radical perineal prostatectomy or radiation therapy. This having been stated, positive lymph nodes in contemporary series in a prostate-specific antigen era have precipitously dropped as a function of patient selection.

Refinements to the initially described operation continue as attention has been directed to the anatomy of the prostate, to which Myers has been a significant contributor [2–5], and alterations in surgical technique [6].

Refinement in patient selection led by the contributions by Partin has included consideration of clinical and pathologic factors [7,8] to predict the likelihood of freedom from disease.

In a disease where ''disease-specific survival'' is the end-point, surgical extirpation offers unparalleled 15- to 20-year survival data.

REFERENCES

1. Easthan JA, Kattan MW, Gerigk C, Scardino PT. Surgeon is an independent risk factor for positive surgical margins (+SM) at the time of radical prostatectomy (RP) (abstract). J Urol 2002; 167(Suppl:):233.
2. Myers RP. Practical pelvic anatomy pertinent to radical retropubic prostatectomy. AUA Update Series 1994; 13(Lesson 4):26–32.
3. Myers RP. Detrusor apron, associated vascular plexus, and avascular plan: relevance to radical retropubic prostatectomy—anatomic and surgical commentary. Urology 2002; 59:472–479.
4. Myers RP, Cahill RP, Devine RM, King BF. Anatomy of radical prostatectomy as defined by magnetic resonance imaging. J Urol 1998; 159:2148–2158.
5. Myers RP. Male urethral sphincteric anatomy and radical prostatectomy. Urol Clin North Am 1991; 18:211–227.
6. Cummings KB, Pantuck AJ, Glazier DB. Nerve-sparing radical retropubic prostatectomy: refining the anatomic approach (abstract). J Urol 181; 165(Suppl:).
7. Partin AW, Yoo J, Carter HB, Pearson JD, Chan DW, Epstein JI, Walsh, PC. The use of prostate-specific antigen, clinical stage and Gleason score to predict pathological stage in men with localized prostate cancer. J Urol 1993; 150(1):110–114.
8. Kattan MW, Easthan JA, Stapleton AM, Wheeler TM, Scardino PT. A preoperative nomogram for disease recurrence following radical prostatectomy for prostate cancer. J Natl Cancer Inst 1998; 90(10):766–771.

2

Radical Perineal Prostatectomy in the Management of Localized Prostate Cancer

Adrian H. Feng and Martin I. Resnick

Case Western Reserve University School of Medicine, Cleveland, Ohio, USA

I. INTRODUCTION

Prostate cancer is the most common noncutaneous malignancy and the second leading cause of cancer death in American men behind lung cancer. A combination of factors has resulted in an increase in prostate cancer detection or incidence since the 1980s (figure 1). Among these factors are longer life expectancy, a growing section of the male population over the age of 50, refinements in transrectal ultrasound guided prostate biopsy techniques, increases in the frequency of transurethral resections of prostate (TURP) performed in the 1980s, the maturation of prostate-specific antigen (PSA) as a screening adjunct to digital rectal examination (DRE), and an increased awareness of the cancer [1]. These factors have lead to an overall shift toward detecting prostate cancer at earlier stages than in the past. The resulting increase in the number of organ-confined cancers has promoted interest in different ways of treatment. Radical perineal prostatectomy has been and still is a proven technique of oncological therapy for patients with prostate cancer.

II. HISTORY OF THE PERINEAL PROSTATECTOMY

Perineal prostatectomy for cancer was first performed in a mostly blunt fashion by Christian Albert Theodor Billroth in 1867 [2]. Detailed anatomic dissection

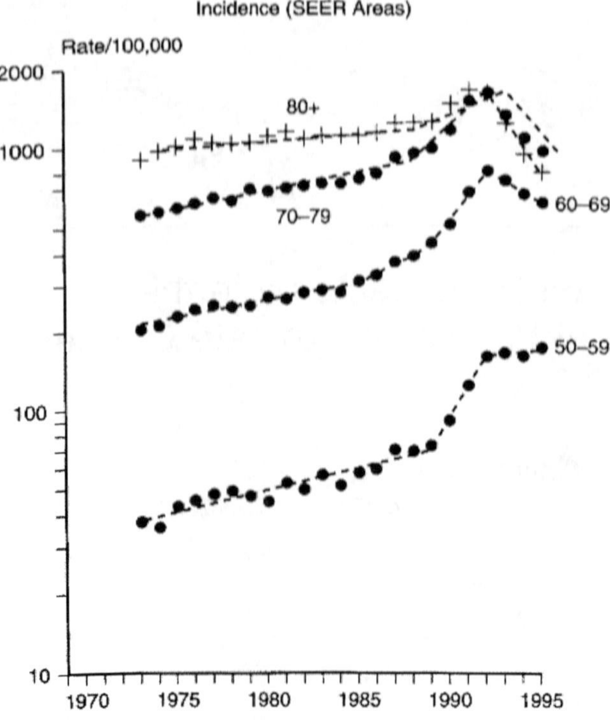

FIGURE 1   Surveillance, Epidemiology, and End Results (SEER) chart of prostate cancer incidence by age. Note the increase in prostate cancer incidence through 1992, followed by a progressive decline in incidence in all age groups except the group 50 to 59 years of age. These findings are consistent with a screening effect. (From Reiter RE, deKernion JB [55], used with permission)

(Zuckerkandl, 1889) and use of a perineal traction system (Proust and Albarran, 1901) led to improvements in exposure (figure 2). George Goodfellow, a urologist and gunfighter from Arizona, is credited as having performed the first radical perineal prostatectomy in the United States [3]. Hugh Hampton Young, however, in 1905, is credited with improving the surgical technique of the operation and developing innovative instrumentation for performing the surgery [4]. Based on his work, technical advances for allowing visualized performance of the vesicourethral anastomosis and improved hemostasis were developed. The procedure became important in the management of patients with adenocarcinoma of the prostate. In 1939, Elmer Belt described a modification of the procedure, thereby introducing subsphincteric dissection as a route toward the prostate (figure 3). Many surgeons subsequently adopted this approach over the following decades

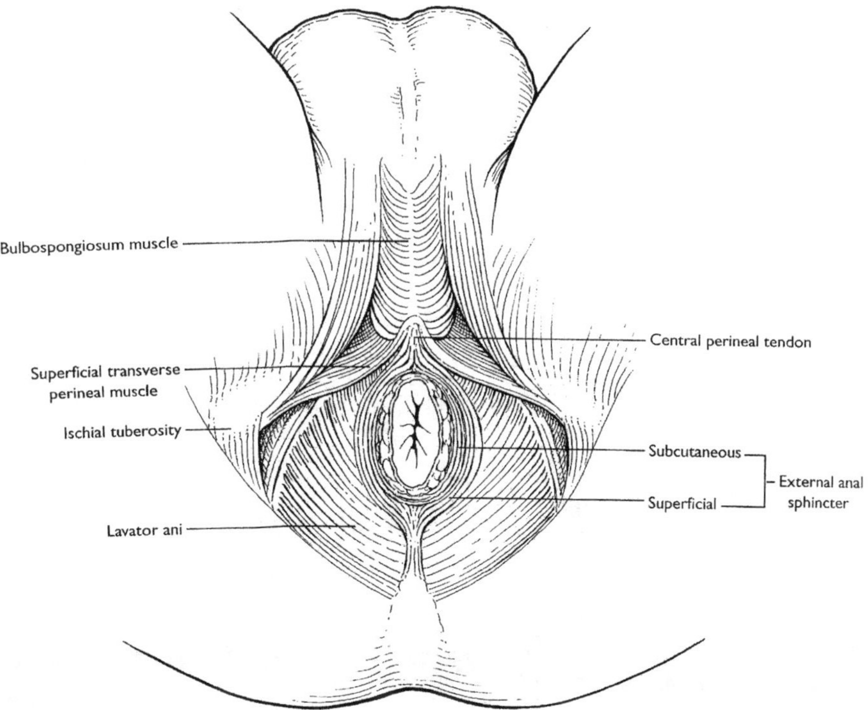

FIGURE 2 Anatomy of the pelvic musculature. (From Haas CA and Resnick MI [56], used with permission)

[5–6]. Radical perineal prostatectomy enjoyed popularity among urologists trained prior to the mid 1970s, and, up until the late 1970s, the procedure had become the preferred surgical approach for treatment of patients with localized prostate cancer.

As understanding of the importance of pelvic lymphadenectomy for disease staging developed, perineal prostatectomy was gradually replaced by the retropubic prostatectomy, which allowed for staging pelvic lymphadenectomy and radical prostatectomy through the same incision and anesthetic. Patrick Walsh's advances in the anatomical knowledge of the cavernous nerves responsible for erections, control of the dorsal venous complex, and of Santorini's plexus, as well as his refined understanding of anatomical and functional relationships, resulted in decreased surgical blood loss, decreased incontinence rates, and decreased impotency rates [7–9]. These factors have currently made the retropubic approach the most popular way of prostatic extirpation for localized carcinoma of the prostate among urologists today.

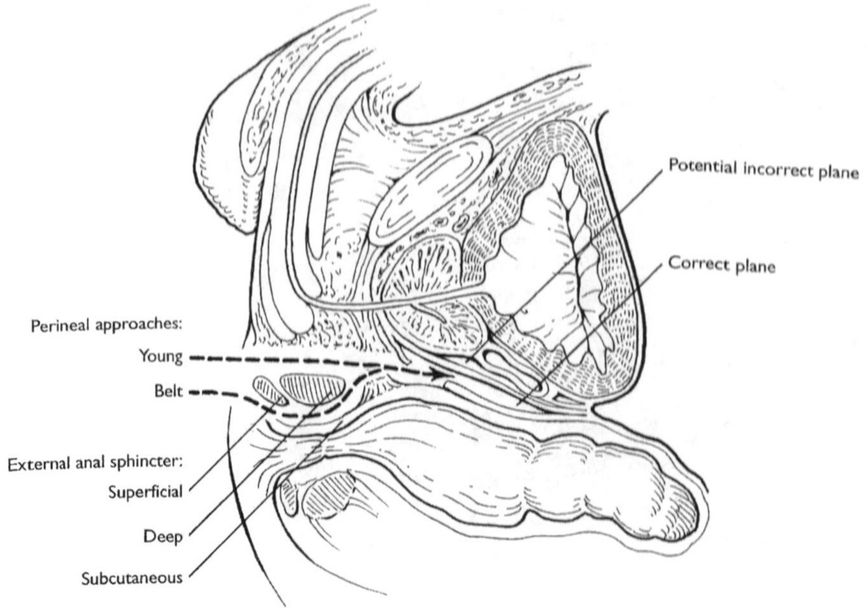

FIGURE 3 The Young and Belt perineal approaches to the prostate. (From Haas CA and Resnick MI [56], used with permission)

III. RESURGENCE OF RADICAL PERINEAL PROSTATECTOMY

Radical perineal prostatectomy has enjoyed a recent increased interest due to exceedingly low mortality, very acceptable morbidity, the ability to spare both cavernous erectile nerves, selective exclusion of pelvic lymphadenectomy in patients with low-risk of lymphatic involvement, and equivalent long-term cancer control compared to retropubic prostatectomy [10–11]. Radical perineal prostatectomy also results in lower operative time, mean blood loss, recovery, narcotic use, hospital stays, and periods of convalescence compared to the retropubic approach [12–13]. While recent interest in minimally invasive laparoscopic prostatectomy has increased the procedure has not demonstrated any advantage over perineal prostatectomy in terms of morbidity, bleeding, transfusion rate, hospital stay, cost, or efficacy [14]. Acquired knowledge for predicting disease stage by PSA level, clinical stage, and Gleason pathological score [15] has produced the ability to predict cancer involvement of the pelvic lymph nodes. This has made it possible to selectively exclude staging lymphadenectomy [16–17]. The development of laparoscopic techniques of pelvic lymph-node sampling in the early 1990s has also obviated the necessity of open lymphadenectomy [18–19].

TABLE 1 Relative Advantages of Perineal and Retropubic Prostatectomy

Perineal	Retropubic
Less pain	Easier for large glands
Shorter hospital stay	Easier to spare nerves
Lower cost	Pelvic lymph node dissection via the same incision
Less blood loss	Lower rectal injury rate
Shorter OR time	Wider anterior margins
Better apical exposure	
Better posterior and lateral exposure	
Easier anastomosis	
Easier in obese patients	
Avoidance of an abdominal incision	

(Modified from Harris MJ, Thompson IM (57), used with permission)

Modifications to radical perineal prostatectomy that incorporate many of the observations of the retropubic approach have enabled bilateral cavernous nerve sparring and equivalent potency outcomes comparable to the retropubic approach [20–21]. In addition, despite the fact that most urologists are unfamiliar with this approach, radical perineal prostatectomy can be learned as easily as the more common retropubic prostatectomy [22]. The perineal approach also avoids an abdominal incision and provides better visualization of the vesicourethral anastomosis [23–24]. With mobilization of the prostate within the lateral pelvic fascia and less anterior dissection, avoidance of Santorini's plexus and the dorsal vein complex leads to a relatively avascular surgical field with decreased surgical blood loss when compared to retropubic prostatectomy [25]. Postoperative bleeding in the prostatic fossa is usually managed conservatively, with quick tamponade of offending vessels due to the limited perineal cavity. Nonabdominal incisions, often no more than 10 cm, lead to rapid recovery and minimal morbidity. Relative advantages of radical perineal versus retropubic prostatectomy are summarized in (table 1).

IV. PATIENT SELECTION

In this authors' experience, there are few relative, and almost no absolute, contraindications to this procedure in patients with a high probability of localized prostate cancer. Intolerance of the exaggerated lithotomy position secondary to severe respiratory dysfunction or severe lower extremity disability disallows perineal prostatectomy. Among these disabilities are ankylosis, unstable artificial hip replacements, and severe coxarthrosis [26]. Large prostates (>100 grams), especially in a narrow pelvis with short distances between the ischial tuberosities, and severe hemorrhoids or anal fissures are relative difficulties associated with radical perineal prostatectomy, so surgery should be performed by an experienced surgeon. Patients with a high likelihood of having positive surgical margins based on serum PSA and biopsy information (tumor grade and volume) are not offered radical curative surgery, whereas patients with an expected noncancer survival of greater than 15 years without evidence of metastatic disease are considered candidates. Those with a biopsy Gleason score of 8 or less, a PSA level below 20 ng/mL, and are without palpable bilateral disease are offered radical perineal prostatectomy. Laparoscopic pelvic lymphadenectomy is excluded if the PSA is less than 10 ng/mL and the Gleason score is less than 7 in the presence of unilateral disease. Laparoscopic lymphadenectomy typically is performed immediately before prostatectomy under the same anesthesia [25,27–29]. The patient is repositioned while processing the frozen section specimens of lymph nodes. The procedure is terminated if metastatic disease is identified in the lymph nodes.

V. PREOPERATIVE CARE

Blood for transfusion is not routinely cross-matched preoperatively because blood loss is usually limited; however, a type and screen is obtained on all patients preoperatively. Because of the risk for rectal injury during the procedure, a full bowel preparation is administered that provides primary closure of any inadvertent injury and the completion of the surgery. The patient is instructed to consume a regular diet until the day before surgery. The afternoon before the procedure, the patient is requested to consume 4L of polyethylene glycol (GoLYTELY® Braintree Laboratories Inc. Braintree, MA) and is administered neomycin, 1.0 g orally, at 12:00, 2:00, 4:00, 6:00, 8:00, and 10:00p.m. Knee-high antithromboembolic stockings are placed without sequential compression devices in the preoperative staging area, and the patient is administered 1.0 g of intravenous cefazolin in the operating room. Patients with penicillin allergy are administered gentamicin at a dose of 2 to 5 mg/kg body weight.

VI. ANESTHESIA

Anesthetic techniques are discussed with the patient preoperatively. Regional and general anesthesias are acceptable options. Limitations of regional anesthesia are related to the position of the patient. The positioning used by the authors is not as exaggerated as the traditional placement used to perform the perineal approach, allowing the use of regional anesthesia. Regional anesthesia may be provided as a spinal or epidural. The best results are obtained if the block is at the level of T8 to T10. Bupivacaine (Marcaine® or Sensorcaine®, Astra Zeneca LP, Wilmington, DE) is the preferred agent for the patient who elects, and is a candidate for, regional anesthesia.

VII. POSITION

Sequential compression devices are placed on the lower leg for the duration of the procedure. The patient is positioned supine so that the sacrum is well over the break of the operating table. When the leg section of the table is lowered, the buttock is off the table edge. Allen stirrups are secured allowing 2 inches on the rail for the attachment of the Thompson retractor. With the Allen stirrups at the level of the patient's legs in the supine position, the feet are placed in well padded stirrups to protect all pressure points. The stirrups are then elevated simultaneously. The patient is placed in a modified exaggerated dorsal lithotomy position, and the final position of the legs is reached when the upper thigh is approximately at a 75° angle with the spine (figure 4). This position slightly elevates the perineum and places it at a right angle to the floor. The perineum, anus, and scrotum are shaved, and the area of the anterior abdomen below the umbilicus, scrotum, penis, perineum, anus, and both thighs to the level of the midthigh are prepared with povidone-iodine (Betadine®, Purdue Frederick, Stamford, CT.) in the standard fashion. A sterile towel is sewn from the 9 o'clock to 3 o'clock position around the anus at the mucocutaneous pigmentation line with a 2–0 silk suture. Perineal and leg drapes are placed next. The upright of the Thompson® retractor is fixed to the edge of the bed on the patient's left, keeping most of the upright sterile in front of the drapes. The use of a headlight is helpful because it is often difficult to direct the operating room lights into the small perineal incision.

VIII. TECHNIQUE

A. Incision and Initial Exposure of the Prostate

A curved Lowsley tractor is placed into the bladder and its wings are opened (figure 5). A curvilinear incision is made approximately 2 to 3 cm ventral to the mucocutaneous pigmentation line of the anus, starting from a position just medial to the ischial tuberosity to a position medial to the contralateral ischial tuberosity (figure 6). This modification reduces postoperative pain because it protects the incision from direct pressure while the patient sits. The subcutaneous tissues, fat, and Colles' fascia are incised sharply along the same curvilinear direction as the skin incision. Electrocautery, followed by blunt dissection, is employed to open and develop each ischiorectal fossa lateral to the central tendon. An index finger is directed from one fossa toward the other, ventral to the rectum. This exposes the central tendon, which is divided over the index finger with electrocautery (figure 7). The horizontal fibers of the superficial external anal sphincter are dissected then retracted ventrally by an appendiceal retractor. This allows for a

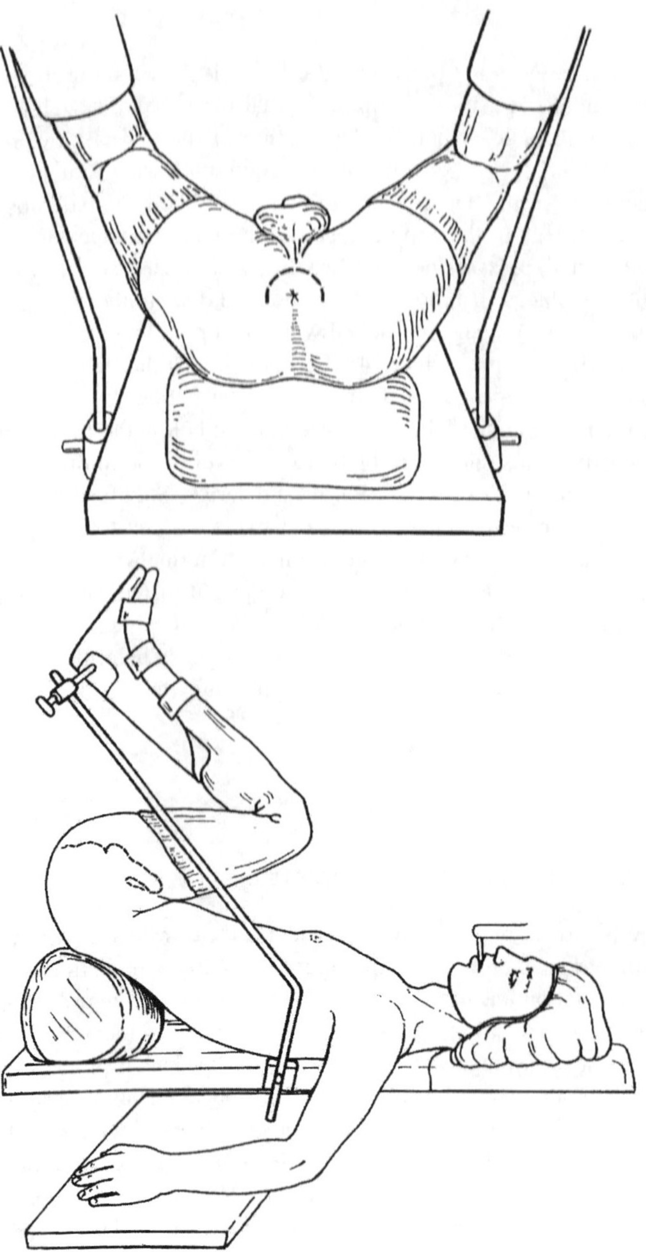

FIGURE 4 The exaggerated lithotomy position. (From Haas CA and Resnick MI [56], used with permission)

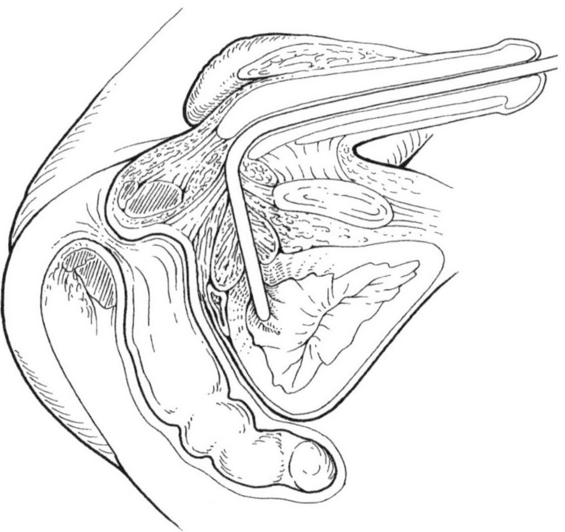

FIGURE 5   Sagittal view of the perineum showing correct placement of the curved Lowsley tractor. (From Haas CA and Resnick MI [56], used with permission)

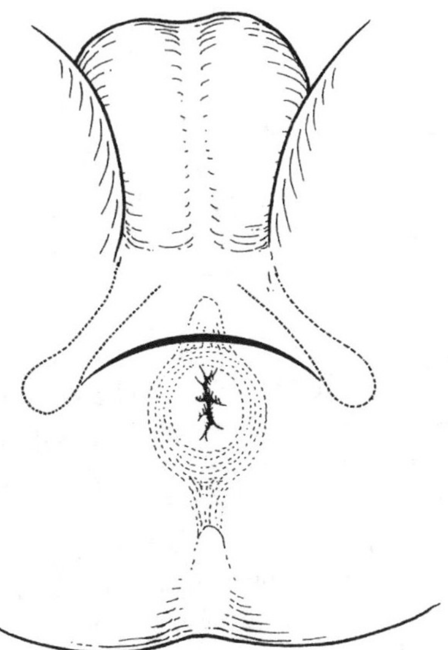

FIGURE 6   The curvilinear skin incision is made approximately 1 to 2 cm above the anal verge, medial to both ischial tuberosities. (From Haas CA and Resnick MI [56], used with permission)

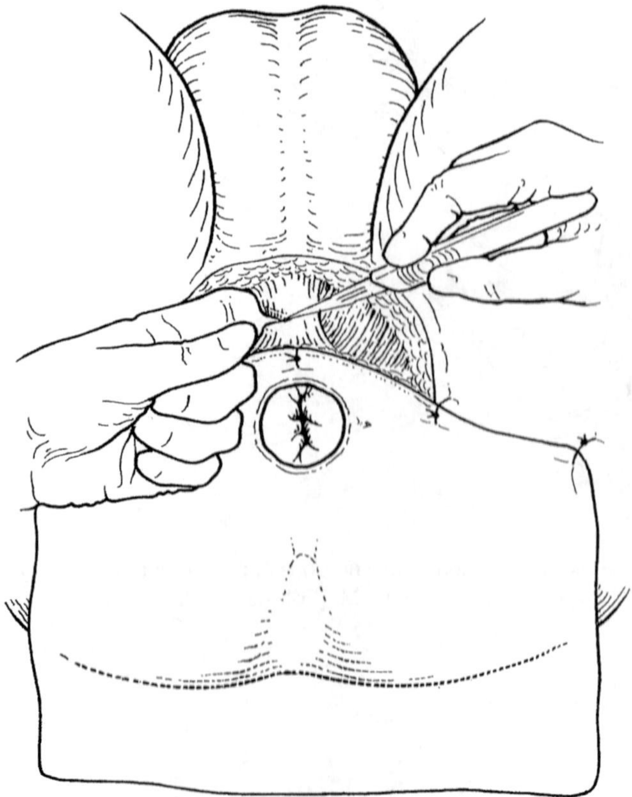

FIGURE 7 The index finger exposes the central perineal tendon, which is sharply incised. (From Haas CA and Resnick MI [56], used with permission)

Belt subsphincteric dissection along the anterior rectal surface toward the prostate (figure 8). The longitudinal fibers of the rectum are identified, and then a wet sponge is used to place gentle dorsal traction on the rectum. This plane is developed and followed proximally along the ventral wall of the rectum with blunt dissection until the rectourethralis muscle is identified (figure 9). The lateral edges of this muscle can be identified by placing vertically oriented scissors in a cephalad direction on either side of the rectourethralis muscle and spreading the surrounding connective tissue. Traction is not applied on the Lowsley tractor to avoid tenting of the rectum as the rectourethralis muscle is divided sharply, with scissors, close to the apex of the prostate. This maneuver must be performed carefully to prevent rectal injury. Once the rectourethralis muscle is divided, the rectum falls dorsally. Denonvilliers' fascia is identified by its shiny white appearance, and an assistant

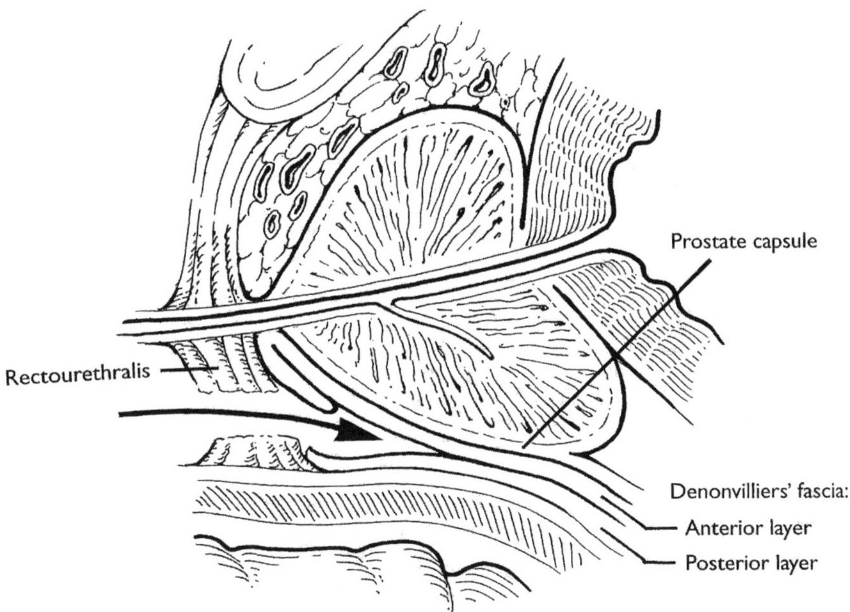

FIGURE 8 Sagittal view of the perineum showing the proper plane of posterior dissection. (From Haas CA and Resnick MI [56], used with permission)

places gentle pressure on the Lowsley tractor toward the anterior abdominal wall. This maneuver delivers the prostate into the incision. Blunt dissection is used to separate the rectum from the prostate. The proper posterior plane is between Denonvilliers' fascia attached to the dorsal surface of the prostate and the ventral rectal fascia (also known as the "posterior leaf" of Denonvilliers' fascia) (figure 8). Cephalad dissection in this plane is continued to the base of the prostate, exposing the posterior vesicoprostatic junction (figure 10).

B. Continued Prostate Dissection and Preservation of the Cavernous Neurovascular Bundles

Resumed traction on the Lowsley tractor toward the anterior abdominal wall allows displacement of the prostate into the incision. If preservation of the neurovascular bundles is intended, a scalpel should be used to incise the ventral rectal fascia (posterior leaf of Denonvilliers' fascia) in the midline, vertically from the base to the apex of the prostate (figure 11a). Careful lateral dissection with gentle lateral traction preserves the cavernous nerves located at the posterolateral edge of the prostate between the layers of ventral rectal and Denonvilliers' fascia, improving postoperative potency [20] (figure 11b).

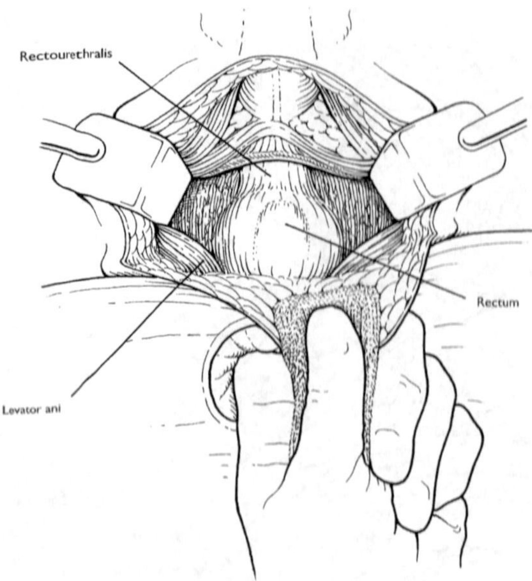

FIGURE 9 Dissection along the longitudinal fibers of the rectal wall exposes the rectourethralis muscle. (From Haas CA and Resnick MI [56], used with permission)

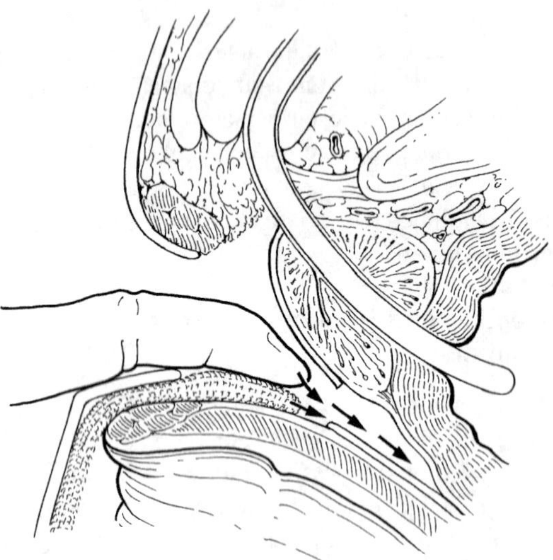

FIGURE 10 Sagittal view demonstrating the correct plane of posterior dissection. (From Haas CA and Resnick MI [56], used with permission)

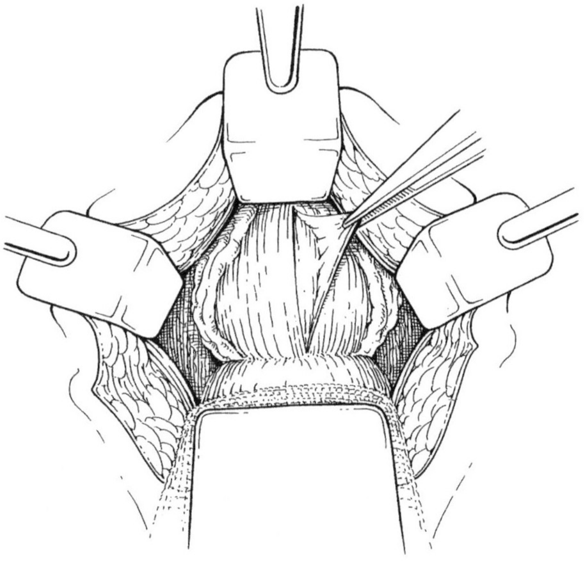

Figure 11 a A vertical incision in Denonvilliers' fascia enables preservation of the neurovascular bundles. (From Haas CA and Resnick MI [56], used with permission)

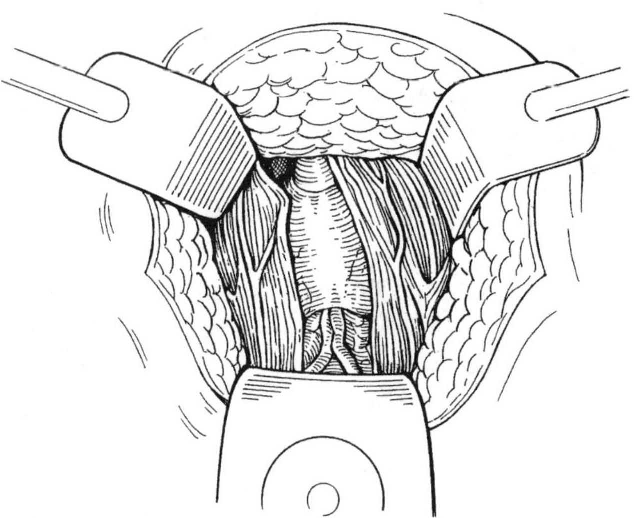

Figure 11 b Left-sided cavernosal nerves are preserved while periprostatic tissues lateral to the levators are included in the right-sided wide excision. (From Harris MJ and Thompson IM [57], used with permission)

Attention is then focused on the prostatic apex and urethra. The Lowsley tractor can be palpated within the urethra, and a right-angle clamp is placed with the open points facing cephalad on either sides of the urethra to dissect the neurovascular bundles off the urethra as they course distally. A scalpel is used to incise the posterior aspect of the urethra over the Lowsley tractor (figure 12), and the curved Lowsley tractor is replaced with the straight Lowsley tractor, which is placed through the prostatic urethra into the bladder. With moderate traction on the straight Lowsley tractor and the right-angle clamp beneath the remaining intact urethra, the remaining anterior portion of the membranous urethra is sharply transected from the apex of the prostate. The Thompson retractor is attached to the previously placed upright, and four blades are placed in the 6, 9, 12, and 3 o'clock positions. This action provides excellent exposure for the remainder of the procedure (figure 13).

Blunt and sharp dissection over the anterior prostate is performed in the direction from the apex of the prostate toward the bladder neck (figure 14). Traction on the Lowsley tractor brings the prostate toward the incision, aiding

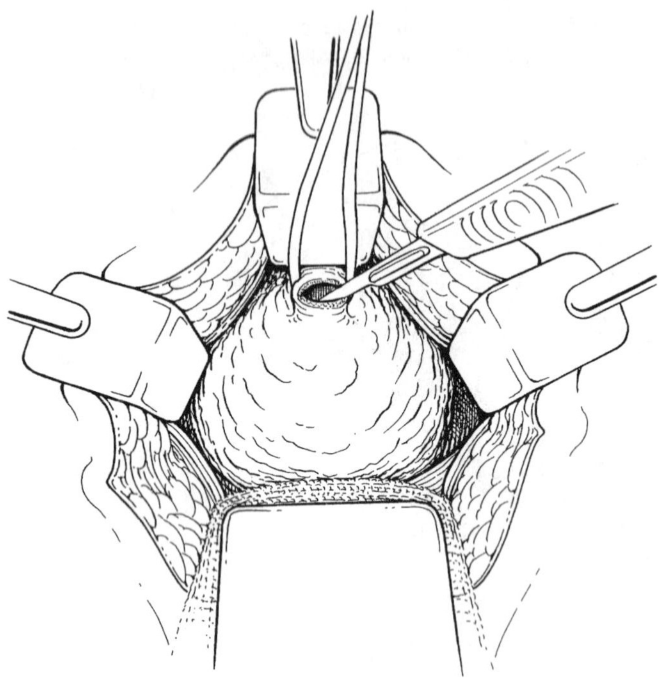

FIGURE 12   Incised posterior urethra just distal to the prostatic apex. (From Haas CA and Resnick MI [56], used with permission)

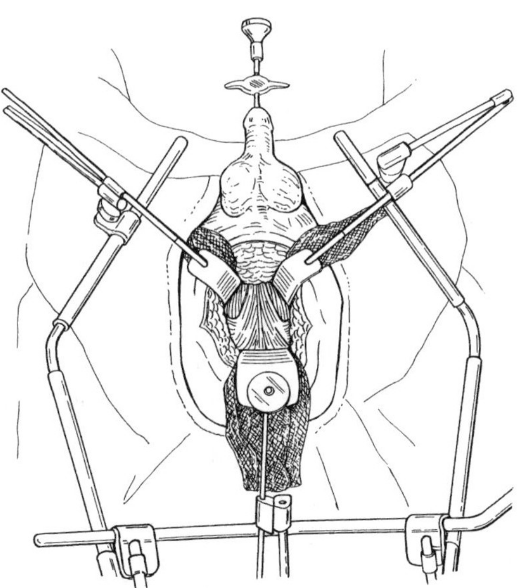

FIGURE 13   Utilization of Thompson® retractor. (From Harris MJ and Thompson IM [57], used with permission)

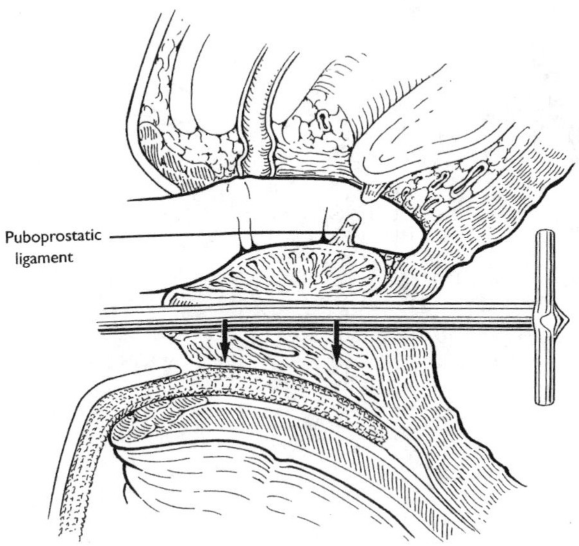

FIGURE 14   Sagittal view demonstrating the correct plane of anterior dissection. (From Haas CA and Resnick MI [56], used with permission)

in this portion of the dissection. Care is taken not to carry the dissection too far ventrally, as the dorsal vein complex would be encountered. In rare instances, the dorsal vein complex is violated; the resulting bleeding can be secured with 3–0 absorbable sutures directed toward the pubic symphysis in a figure-eight fashion. The puboprostatic ligaments, seen during this part of the dissection, should be sharply divided. Palpation of the wings of the Lowsley tractor aids in defining the junction of the bladder neck and the prostate base. Once identified, this junction is developed further with blunt and sharp dissections, preserving the bladder neck. The dissection is continued and the bladder entered anteriorly (figure 15). The Lowsley tractor is removed from the urethra, and a long right-angle clamp is passed retrograde through the prostatic urethra and through the bladder neck. A 14F red-rubber catheter is grasped with the open right-angle clamp and pulled through the prostatic urethra, the ends grasped with a Kelly clamp. Traction on the catheter delivers the prostate toward the incision, and

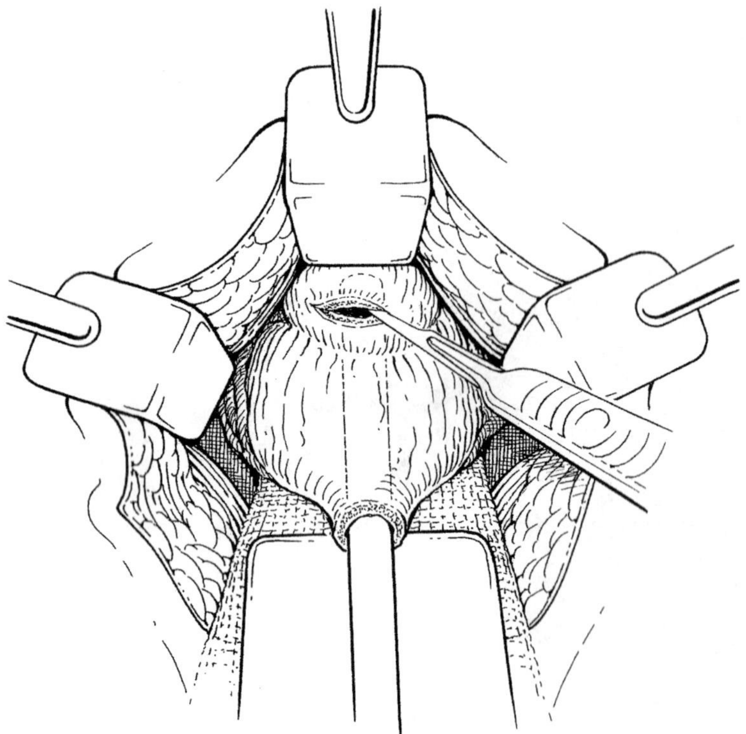

FIGURE 15   The incision of the anterior bladder with a straight Lowsley tractor in place. (From Haas CA and Resnick MI [56], used with permission)

dissection of the anterior bladder neck is continued circumferentially around the prostatic base (figure 16). Identifying the ureteral orifices are not routinely necessary, unless the dissection inadvertently involves the trigone posteriorly. The use of parental indigo carmine or ureteral stents can aid in identifying the orifices, if necessary. The lateral attachments and neurovascular pedicles are identified as they course toward the base of the gland and are dissected, divided between right-angle clamps, and secured with 3–0 chromic catgut ties. If a nerve-sparing procedure is performed, the pedicles should be divided close to the prostate without compromising the surgical margin. Electrocautery is avoided during this phase of the procedure. The dissection is continued posteriorly at the bladder neck to separate it completely from the prostate, and the red-rubber catheter repositioned

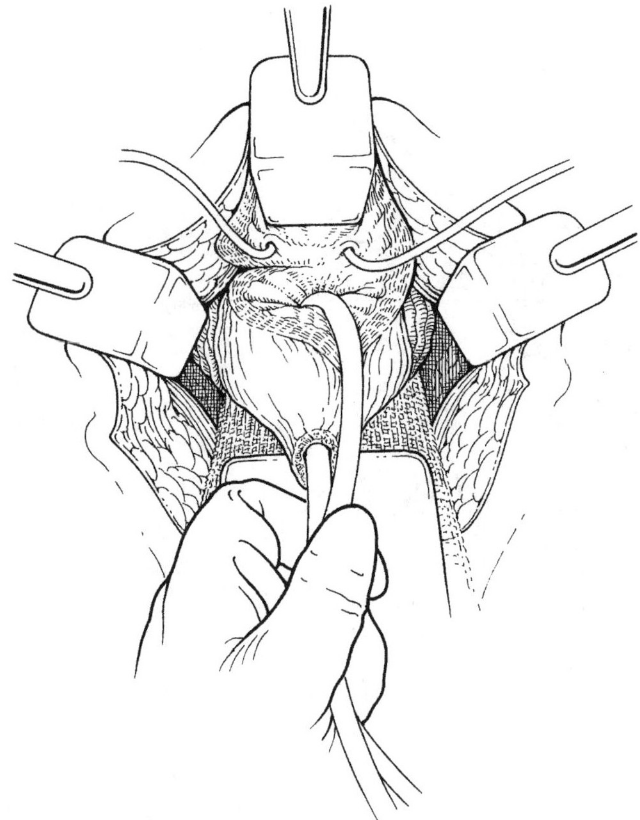

FIGURE 16   The bladder neck is incised with care to avoid the ureteral orifices. (From Haas CA and Resnick MI [56], used with permission)

so that traction on the entire prostate is achieved. This traction is accomplished by passing a right-angle clamp along the posterior surface of the prostate in the midline, from caudad to cephalad, and directing the tips around the prostatic base toward the anterior surface of the prostate between the vasa. Then, the 14F red-rubber catheter is grasped with the right angle and wrapped around the prostate. This allows for continued traction on the prostate toward the incision, exposing the remaining attachments.

C. Dissection of the Vas Deferens and Seminal Vesicles

Attention is directed toward the ampullae of the vas deferens and seminal vesicles (figure 17). These areas are identified easily with traction on the prostate, and

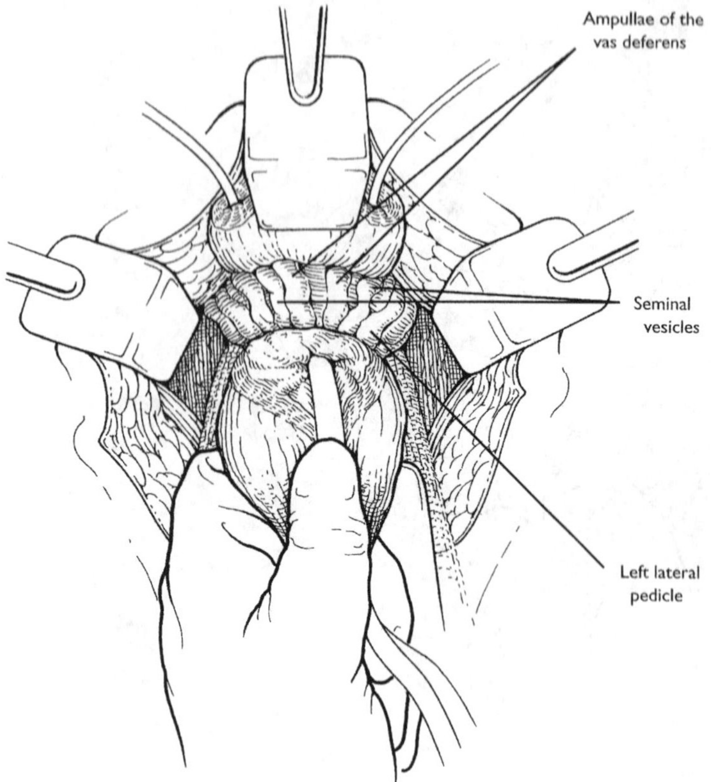

FIGURE 17   Dissection of the posterolateral prostate reveals the lateral vascular pedicles, seminal vesicles, and ampullae of the vas deferens. (From Haas CA and Resnick MI [56], used with permission)

each vas is grasped with a right-angle clamp, bluntly dissected proximally, and then divided with electrocautery. Similarly, each seminal vesicle is grasped with a right-angle clamp and blunt dissection is used to remove them, dividing and ligating the seminal vesicle artery with 3–0 chromic suture. At this point the surgical specimen, including the prostate and seminal vesicles, is removed completely. The incision and empty prostate bed is inspected for hemostasis.

D. Vesicourethral Anastomosis

At times, though infrequently, it is necessary to reconstruct the bladder neck before performing the anastomosis. This procedure is accomplished with simple interrupted 3–0 polyglycolic acid sutures placed posteriorly in a "tennis-racquet" fashion (figure 18). Attention should be given to the ureteral orifices to prevent

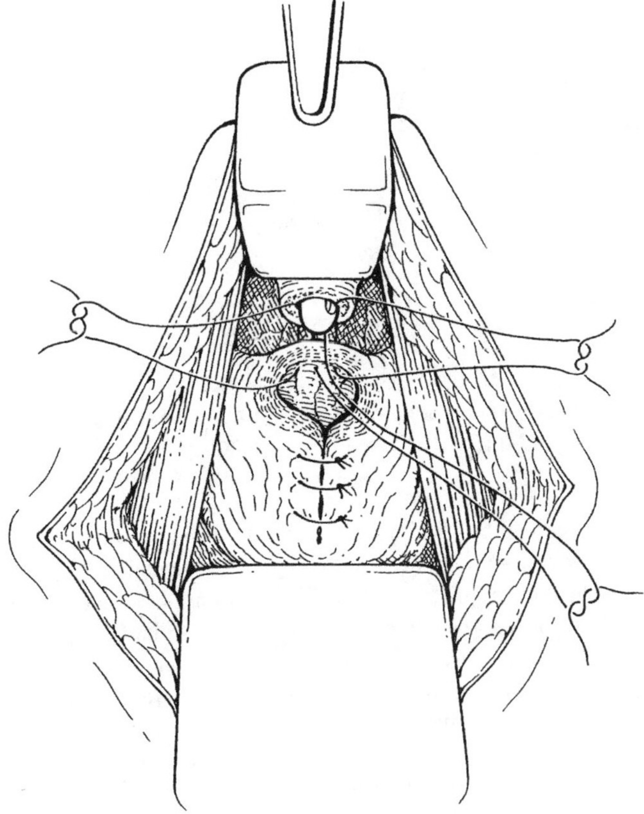

FIGURE 18   Bladder neck reconstruction and anterior vesicourethral anastomosis. (From Haas CA and Resnick MI [56], used with permission)

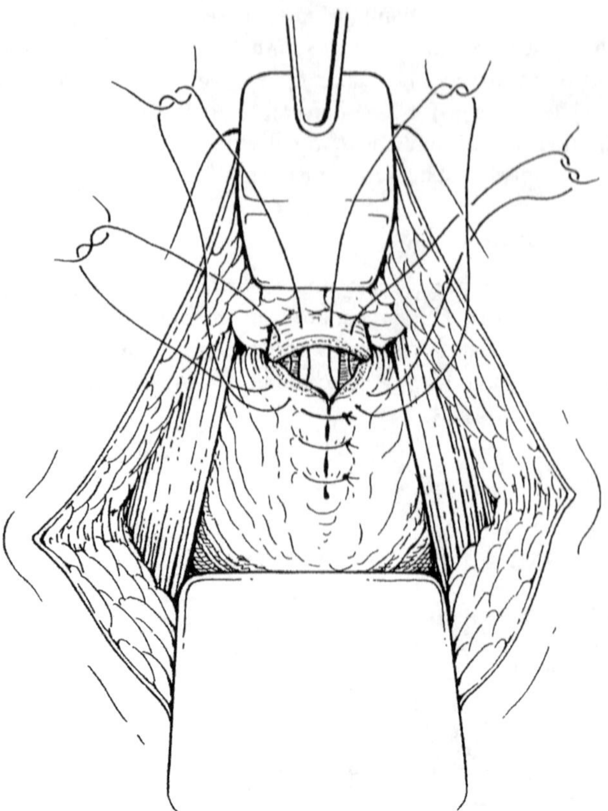

FIGURE 19 Closure of the posterior portion of the vesicourethral anastomosis. (From Haas CA and Resnick MI [56], used with permission)

damage. The retractor placed at the 12 o'clock position is now removed to facilitate identification of the membranous urethra. The red-rubber catheter used to retract the prostate is placed retrograde through the penile urethra, and the end of the catheter at the level of the glans is grasped with a Kelly clamp to prevent it from being pulled through the urethral meatus. This catheter serves several purposes: it helps the surgeon to identify the membranous urethra accurately, it prevents injury to the permanent catheter balloon due to an inadvertently placed anastomotic needle, and it enables retraction of the urethra so that the anastomotic sutures can be placed accurately. The vesicourethral anastomosis is initiated on the anterior side, placing a 3–0 polyglycolic acid suture at the 12 o'clock position. All sutures are placed with the knots tied on the outside of the anastomosis. Continuing in an interrupted fashion, the anterior anastomosis is completed with

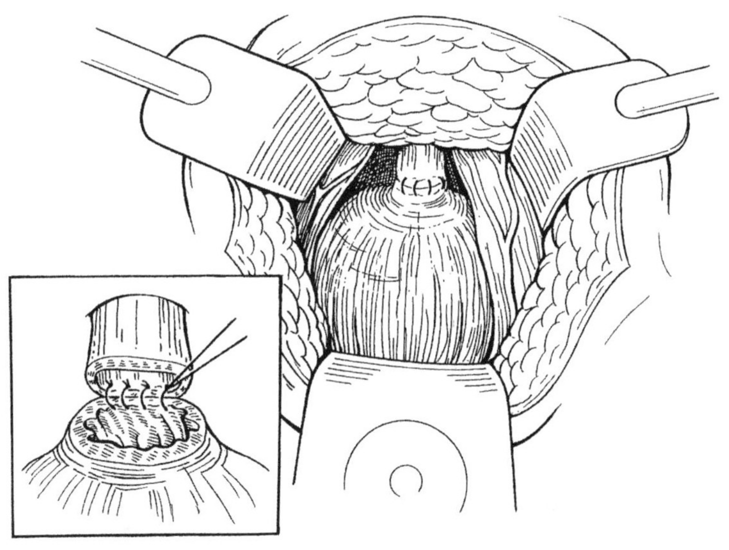

Figure 20 Completion of vesicourethral anastomosis. *Inset:* anterior vesicourethral anastomosis being completed. (From Harris MJ and Thompson IM [57], used with permission)

sutures placed at the 2 and 10 o'clock positions on the bladder neck and urethra. Gentle traction on the red-rubber catheter in a direction opposite of the intended suture allows for excellent exposure and accurate needle placement. The red-rubber catheter is then replaced with a 22F Silastic catheter, which is passed into the bladder. The 5-mL balloon is inflated with 15 mL of sterile water, and sutures are placed at the 4, 6, and 8 o'clock positions to complete the posterior portion of the anastomosis (figure 19 and 20).

E. Closure

After inspection for hemostasis and rectal injury, a Penrose drain is placed near the anastomosis and brought through the incision. Closure is performed by reapproximating the levator ani muscles with simple interrupted 2–0 chromic sutures, taking care to avoid the neurovascular bundles. The central tendon is reapproximated with 2–0 absorbable sutures, as is Colles' fascia, and the skin is closed with interrupted simple or vertical mattress sutures of 4–0 chromic (figure 21). For the surgeon who is familiar with this procedure, operative times are usually less than 1 hour.

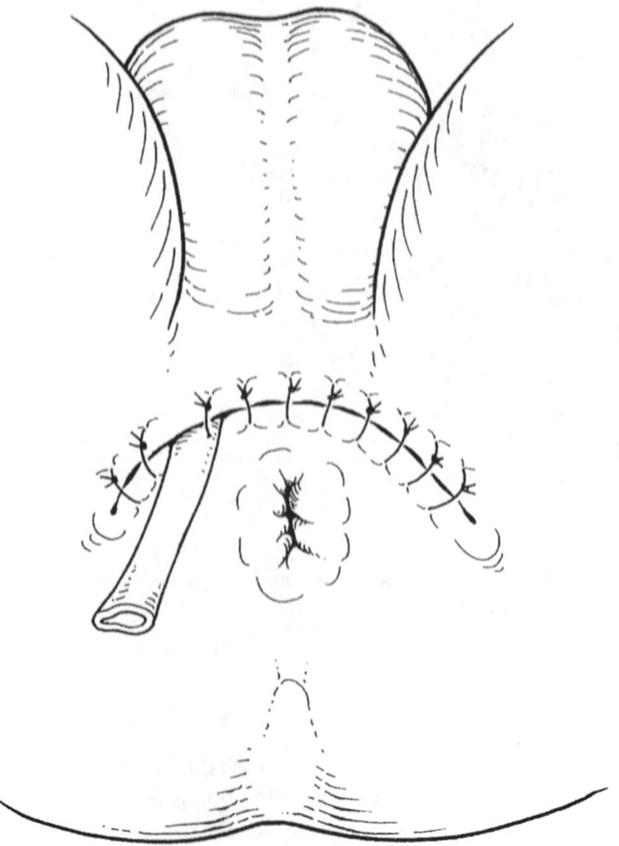

FIGURE 21   Skin closure with Penrose drain placement. (From Haas CA and Resnick MI [56], used with permission)

IX. POSTOPERATIVE CARE

The postoperative care of patients undergoing radical perineal prostatectomy is identical regardless of whether the patient has had a laparoscopic lymphadenectomy or not. After recovering from anesthesia, the patient is started on a clear liquid diet the same day and advanced to a regular diet within 24 hours. Oral narcotics are often sufficient for analgesia; intravenous narcotics are rarely required. The authors no longer provide epidural postoperative analgesia for prostatectomy patients because it is excessive. Ambulation is encouraged the evening of surgery and incentive spirometry is used to help prevent atelectasis. Lower extremity sequential compression devices are not used routinely postoperatively due to early ambulation. All patients are started on docusate postoperatively, and this regimen is maintained until the patient discontinues the use of oral narcotics. Prophylactic antibiotics are administered while the patient retains the Foley catheter. Avoiding rectal instrumentation, stimulation, or medication insertion is mandatory, and, when absolutely necessary, only gentle irrigation of the catheter is performed. The Penrose drain is routinely removed on postoperative day 1. Approximately one-third of the patients are discharged on postoperative day 1, and most are discharged on postoperative day 2. The catheter remains in place for 3 weeks.

X. OUTCOMES OF RADICAL PERINEAL PROSTATECTOMY AND COMPARISON TO RADICAL RETROPUBIC PROSTATECTOMY

A review of contemporary studies on the radical perineal prostatectomy was performed and is summarized in Tables 2 and 3. Most investigations are retrospective and not randomized, however, together they are able to draw some adequate conclusions. The radical perineal prostatectomy, in most studies, is equivalent to radical retropubic prostatectomy in terms of oncological control demonstrated by biochemical PSA failure, positive margin status, and cancer-free survival. Additionally, the perineal approach offers comparable rates of urinary continence and potency. Most investigators agree that there is less blood loss and transfusion rates when performing a radical perineal versus a retropubic prostatectomy.

A. Operative Mortality

Mortality in the 90-day postoperative period for patients less than 65 years of age is approximately 0.2% [30]. Frazier et al. did not report any postoperative mortality in a series of 122 radical perineal prostatectomies [31]. Similarly, Weldon and colleagues [21] reported no deaths in 220 men undergoing radical perineal prostatectomy. Haab et al. did not report any postoperative mortality in their series of 35 radical perineal prostatectomies [32].

B. Rectal injury

In a retrospective study comparing perineal and retropubic radical prostatectomy, Haab and coworkers [32] noted rectal injury in 1 of 35 patients in the perineal group and in 1 of 36 in the retropubic group. The rate of rectal wall injuries has been reported as high as 11% in patients undergoing radical perineal prostatectomy, however, these injuries are treated effectively with primary closure and usually with little consequence [33–34]. Infrequently, rectal injuries that are recognized and repaired intraoperatively or injuries that are unrecognized at the time of surgery may result in rectocutaneous fistulas. Significant leakage can occur

TABLE 2 Oncologic Control: A Comparison Between Radical Perineal Prostatectomy (RPP) and Radical Retropubic Prostatectomy (RRP)—A Review of the Recent Literature

Authors	EBL (mL)			Incontinence (%)			Impotence (%)			Urethral strictures (%)			Rectal injury (%)		
	RPP	RRP	p	RPP	RRP	p	RPP	RRP	p	RPP	RRP	p	RRP	RPP	p
Lance et al. (2001) (89)	802	1575	< 0.001	35.2 (@ 47.1 m)	40.1 (@ 41.1 m)	0.34	91.8 (@ 47.1 m)†	91.1 (@ 41.4 m)†	0.83	3.5*	9.3*	0.13	4.9	0	0.01
Ruiz-Deya et al (2001) (42)	n/a	n/a	n/a	7 (@ 1 y)	n/a	n/a	59 (@ 18 m)*	n/a	n/a	3	n/a	n/a	2	n/a	n/a
Sullivan et al. (2000) (43)	416	1138	<0.001	47 (@ 1 y)	56 (@ 1 y)	n/s	n/a	n/a	n/a	10	19	n/a	2.5	0	n/c
Kaller et al. (1999)	n/a	n/a	n/a	n/a	n/a	n/a	n/a	n/a	n/a	1*	n/a	n/a	3.5	n/a	n/a
Weldon et al. (1997) (21)	600	n/a	n/a	5 (@ 10 m)	n/a	n/a	30 (@ 2 y)††	n/a	n/a	1	n/a	n/a	1	n/a	n/a
Haab et al. (1994) (82)	n/a	n/a	n/a	18 (@ 6 m)	18 (@ 6 m)	n/c	97 (@ 3 m)‡	89 (@ 3 m)‡	n/c	0	5	n/c	3	3	n/c
Harris et al. (1996) (57)	n/a	n/a	n/a	2.5 (@18 m)	n/a	n/a	50□	n/a	n/a	5/3□	n/a	n/a	n/a	n/a	n/a
Frazier et al. (1992) (31)	565	2000	<0.001	4	4	n/c	22.7 (@ 1 y)‡‡	n/a	n/a	7	8	n/c	n/a	n/a	n/a

m = months
y = years
n/a = not available
n/c = not calculated
n/s = not significant
ADT = antiandrogen deprivation therapy
all PSA values in ng/mL
* overall margins not significant, however RPP had significantly higher positive anterior and bladder neck margins while RRP had significantly higher posterior positive margins
† PSA >0.2, p=0.44 for entire Kaplan-Meier log rank test
‡ PSA failure (>0.5)
†† 32.4 months in patients with preoperative PSA, 48 months in the era before preoperative PSA
** in pT2 tumors, RPP had a significantly higher rate of positive margins (43% versus 29%)
$ mean age of the combined RRP and RPP groups
‡‡ complete seminal vesicle excision, a confounding variable when multivariate analysis was applied, as no difference in PSA failure was found (p0.02)

TABLE 3 Selected Morbidities Following Radical Perineal Versus Retropubic Prostatectomy: A Review of the Recent Literature

Authors	Study Design and significant factors	No. patients			Mean Age (yrs)		Mean Followup (mo)			PSA Failure			Margin Positive (%)	
		RPP	RRP	RRP	RRP	p	RRP	RRP	RRP	RRP	P	RRP	RRP	p
Lance et al. (2001) (39)	retrospective, nonrandomized case matched multiinstitutional (Uniformed Services Urology Research Group)	190	190	62.2	63.7	0.02	47.1	42.9	12.90% (@ 47.1 m)	17.60% (@ 42.9 m)	0.25	43.1	39.5*	0.67
Sullivan et al. (2000) (43)	retrospective, nonrandomized single institution 71/77% (RRP/RPP) got ADT preoperative significantly lower preoperative PSA in the RPP group (6.48 vs. 11.65)	79	59	64.6	81.7	n/a	17–60	17–60	17% (@ 60 m)†	30% (@ 60 m)†	0.44†	9	7	n/s
Iselln et al. (1999) (10)	retrospective, single institutional	1242	0	65.2	n/a	n/a	32.4–48††	n/a	8/35/65% (@ 5 yrs) for organ confined, specimen confined and margin-positive disease‡	n/a	n/a	22.9	n/a	n/a
Boccoo-Gibod et al. (1998) (44)	retrospective, non randomized single institution	48	46	65	64	25	25	n/a	67% (@ 25 m)	67% (1 @ 25 m)	n/s	56**	61**	n/s

(continued)

TABLE 3 Continued

Authors	Study Design and significant factors	No. patients			Mean Age (yrs)		Mean Followup (mo)			PSA Failure			Margin Positive (%)		
		RPP	RRP	RRP	RRP	p	RRP	RRP	RRP	RRP	P	RRP	RRP	RRP	p
Theodorescu et al. (1998) (47)	retrospective, non randomized single institution non nerve sparring RPP short followup no information on margin status or final pathologic stage	31	56	63$	63$	n/a	10.9	10.9	45.20% (@ 10.9 m) ‡‡	17.90% (@ 10.9 m) ‡‡	<0.0023	n/a	n/a	n/a	n/a
Harris et al. (1996) (57)	retrospective, single institution	84	n/a	n/a	n/a	n/a	12	n/a	2% of pT2 (@ 12 m) 4% (@ 12m) of stage B C1 or C2	n/a	n/a	13	n/a	n/a	
Haab et al. (1994) (32)	retrospective, non randomized single institution	35	36	64.7	65.6	n/a	3	3	n/a	n/a	n/a	37	48	>0.1	
Frazier et al. (1992) (31)	retrospective nonrandomized single institution	122	51	65.3	65.8	0.74	n/a	n/a	n/a	n/a	n/a	29	31	0.803	

m = months
y = years
n/a = not available
n/c = not calculated
n/s = not significant
† no comment on nerve-sparring status
¥ nerve-sparring, no comment on unilateral versus bilateral
* bladder neck contractures
†† bilateral nerve-sparring
‡ nerve-sparring was not done during RPP; no comment on nervesparring during RRP
□ 50% of unilateral nerve sparring procedures; 5% bladder neck contracture/3% distal pendulous urethral stricture
‡‡ unilateral or bilateral nerve-sparring RPP
ADT = androgen deprivation therapy

with these fistulas. Effective management includes a short period of bowel rest followed by a low-residue diet. If spontaneous closure does not result, simple excision of the small remaining fistula can be performed several months later [34–36]. A recent report has suggested that patients undergoing radical prostatectomy experience fecal incontinence more frequently than has been recognized [37]. Although this observation has not been the authors' experience, Bishoff and coworkers [37] have reported that 10% of patients undergoing a retropubic procedure and 15% undergoing a perineal operation experience fecal incontinence at least monthly.

C. Operative Blood Loss

Blood loss during radical perineal prostatectomy is significantly less than blood loss incurred during radical retropubic prostatectomy. Dissection during perineal prostatectomy is often below the plane of the endopelvic fascia, thereby avoiding the multiple venous complexes that inhabit that level. Notably, the dorsal venous complex and Santorini's plexus are often anterior to the plane of dissection, thus are reflected cephalad and not transected as during radical retropubic prostatectomy. Many studies have supported the lower blood loss during perineal prostatectomy. Frazier and coworkers [31] studied 173 patients in a nonrandomized fashion and reported that the operative blood loss in patients undergoing radical perineal prostatectomy was significantly less than the blood loss in patients undergoing radical retropubic prostatectomy (565 mL versus 2000 mL, respectively, p <0.001). Similarly, in a randomized study of patients undergoing radical prostatectomy following radiotherapy failure, Zippe and Rackley [38] reported that patients in the radical perineal group had an average blood loss of 550 mL versus 1475 mL in the radical retropubic group. Lance et al. [39] also noted significantly less average surgical blood loss (802 cc versus 1575 cc respectively) and transfusion amount in the perineal approach compared to retropubic approach.

D. Other Morbidity Factors After Radical Perineal Prostatectomy

Weldon et al. reported that 18% of their prostatectomies experienced adverse events, although few were serious: anastomotic strictures were reported in 1%, proctotomy in 1%, transient peripheral neuropathy in 2%, and prolonged urinary extravasation in 2%. Transient lower extremity neurapraxia increases with the length of the operation, and, therefore, with time in the extended lithotomy position, as noted by Price et al [40]. They noted a 21% incidence of neurapraxia after a mean of 188 minutes of operative time. However, Keller reported a 0% incidence of neurapraxia in 284 prostatectomies with a mean operative time of 99 minutes [41]. Keller hypothesized that exaggerated lithotomy positioning over 180 minutes may lead to an increase occurrence of postoperative neurapraxia.

Frazier and coworkers [31] reported the complication rates for patients undergoing radical prostatectomy by the perineal or retropubic approach, and noted that the rate of hospital complications was similar for the two groups (4% versus 5%, respectively), as was the rate of long-term complications (12% versus 14%, respectively). Anastomotic strictures for the perineal approach were reported in 7%, and urethral-rectal fistulas in 1%. Haab reported an 11% complication rate at 3 months; rectal injury occurred in 3%, urinary fistula in 3%, wound infections in 6%, and anastomotic strictures in 0% [32]. Ruiz-Deya and colleagues [42] reported on 250 consecutive radical perineal prostatectomies. Of the last 100 patients, 91 were discharged under 23 hours, with 13 patients leaving the same day of surgery. This study demonstrates the rapid recovery potential of patients following radical perineal prostatectomy and the minimal morbidity associated with this procedure.

E. Cancer Outcomes

Radical prostatectomy is currently being performed on disease that appears at earlier stages than prostate cancer of the past. Recent articles reviewing cancer control are thus examining a population of patients who present with their cancers at significantly earlier stages than older studies. Subsequent results of contemporary studies are therefore shifted to conclusions favoring higher overall survival after surgery, as stage of the disease significantly affects cancer prognosis. Radical perineal prostatectomy has been shown to offer effective oncological control for locally confined disease. Iselin and colleagues [10] retrospectively reviewed 1242 patients over a 22-year period and demonstrated an 82% 15-year cancer-specific survival in organ- or specimen-confined cases after perineal prostatectomy. Overall positive margin rate was 23% (reduced to 14% in the PSA era). This study used cancer-specific survival rather than the more common PSA biochemical failure as a major endpoint. Lance and coworkers [39] designed a case-matched retrospective review, comparing radical perineal prostatectomies with retropubic prostatectomies, where each group comprised 190 patients. Lance and coworkers found no significant differences between the two groups in terms of biochemical recurrence (12.9% perineal versus 07.6% retropubic), organ-confined disease (55.3% perineal versus 57% retropubic), and overall positive margins (39.5% perineal versus 43.1% retropubic) over a mean follow-up of approximately 40 months. Separating the positive margins by location, higher posterior positive margins were found in the retropubic group compared to the perineal group (25% versus 12%, respectively), while the perineal group risked more margin involvement at the bladder neck and anterior prostate compared to the retropubic group (22% versus 10%, and 10% versus 3%, respectively). In a retrospective review of 122 radical perineal and 51 radical retropubic prostatectomies, Frazier and colleagues [31] found no difference in the rate of positive margins (29% retropubic versus 31% perineal, respectively, p = 0.803). These researchers then evaluated the incidence of positive margins in various locations and found no difference between the two groups with respect to bladder, urethral, or seminal vesicle involvement, nor did they find a difference between the two groups with respect to capsular perforations. Confirming the above studies, Sullivan and colleagues [43] also did not find a difference in the margin rates between the retropubic versus the perineal approach (11.9% versus 11.4%, respectively).

Boccon-Gibod et al [44]. performed a retrospective analysis of 48 perineal and 46 retropubic prostatectomies of patients with T1c and T2a disease. The rate of positive margins was not significantly different (56% in the perineal group and 61% in the retropubic group). When examining pT2 disease, however, the rate of surgically induced positive margins (via capsular incision) was significantly greater in the perineal group when compared with the retropubic group (43% versus 29% respectively, p <0.05). However, biochemical survival (PSA <0.1 ng/mL) was equivalent in the retropubic and perineal groups (67% at a mean followup of 25 months). The authors suggested that the limited exposure of the surgical field during perineal prostatectomy led to an increase in iatrogenic capsular incisions, exposing the malignancy to the margins. Interestingly, the overall frequency of positive surgical margins and biochemical failure between the two surgical approaches were not different despite the increased capsular incision rate of the perineal approach. The higher rate of positive margins in subcapsular pT2 disease suggests transcapsular surgical incision is a fault, suggested by some [45], when utilizing the original technique of perineal prostatectomy described by Young. Contradicting Bocon-Gibod et al. is a pathological study of whole mount prostate specimens from Korman and colleagues [46]. They compared 45 retropubic and 27 perineal prostatectomy specimens using 0.4 cm cross-sections of the entire prostate. The positive margin rate (22% perineal versus 16% retropubic, p = 0.53), capsular incision rate (4% each group), and minimal distances of the tumor to the posterolateral margins (1.72/1.91 mm perineal versus 2.13/1.72 mm retropubic, p = 0.62/0.24 for right and left sides respectively) were not significantly different. They also noted no significant differences in location of the positive margins between the perineal and retropubic groups.

Theodorescu and colleagues [47] found a significant difference favoring retropubic prostatectomy in terms of biochemical failure in their retrospective, nonrandomized study. In the short mean follow-up of 10.9 months, 45.2% of the perineal group versus 17.9% of the retropubic group had persistent PSA elevations >0.2 ng/mL. They also pointed out that incomplete seminal vesicle excision in the perineal group was a significant factor leading to PSA failure in multivariate analysis. When the seminal vesicles were properly excised, there was no significant difference between the retropubic and perineal approaches in terms of biochemical PSA failure. Of note, they did not factor margin positivity status [48] or final pathological stage (i.e., seminal vesicle involvement) in the multivariate model comparing the two surgical approaches.

Weldon and coworkers [49] reported the results of 200 consecutive radical perineal prostatectomies. In these patients with clinical T1 and T2 disease, the overall rate of positive margins was 44%. The rate of positive margins was 7%, 16% and 25% for the apex, posterolateral, and anterior prostate, respectively. These values were compared with the rates in a series of patients undergoing radical retropubic prostatectomy [50–52]. The perineal group had fewer positive apical margins (7% versus 10% to 48%) and posterolateral margins (16% versus 26% to 44%); however, a higher incidence of positive anterior margins was found in the perineal group (25% versus 2% to 10%). It was theorized that 45% of the positive anterior margins could have been avoided by sharply dividing the puboprostatic ligaments ventral to the capsule, thereby avoiding avulsion of the anterior prostatic capsule and exposing the underlying malignancy [49]. The authors have since employed this approach with their patients.

F. Urinary Continence

Continence rates are traditionally believed to be superior for radical perineal prostatectomy when compared to radical retropubic prostatectomy, but this difference has not been proved in a controlled study. The authors believe that, in all likelihood, the two procedures are comparable in this regard. Patients are instructed that final continence status may not be reached until 1 year, and evaluation is not performed in patients who remain incontinent until that time. The rate of incontinence following radical perineal prostatectomy is reported to range from 4% to 8% [21,29,53–55]. Weldon [21] and coworkers reported that continence returned in 23% of patients by 1 month, 56% by 3 months, 90% by 6 months, and 95% by 10 months. All of the patients who were incontinent were older than 69 years. Age greater than 69 years was the only variable significantly related to continence. The authors defined incontinence as needing to use a pad every day. The continent patients did not use pads on a routine daily basis. Frazier et al. found no difference between the continence rates of radical perineal prostatectomy versus retropubic prostatectomy (4% each) [31]. Similarly, Haab and coworkers [32] reported that continence returned in 71% of patients at 3 months and in 88% at 6 months after radical perineal prostatectomy. In comparison, 88% of patients who underwent radical retropubic prostatectomy were continent at 6 months. Lance et al. [39] failed to appreciate any significant difference in incontinence rates between the retropubic versus perineal approach (40.1% versus 35.2% respectively at 41.1 and 47.1 months). Ruiz-Deya and colleagues [42] reported a 12.3% incontinence rate after perineal prostatectomy at 6 months, with 5.3% requiring the use of more than one pad per day, and with 7% only requiring the use of pads during strenuous activity. The total incontinence rate came down to

7% after 12 months from surgery. Zippe and Rackley [38] reported a 4% incontinence rate for patients undergoing prostatectomy following radiation failure in the perineal and retropubic groups. Bishoff and colleagues found that patients undergoing the perineal approach had a higher rate of immediate continence, and fewer of these patients failed to return to full continence when compared with patients undergoing the retropubic approach [37]. Sullivan et al. found similar pad use between perineal and retropubic groups, however, 72% of the perineal groups leaked less than once per week whereas 56% of the retropubic group leaked more than once per week [43]. Gray et al. [54] utilized validated questionnaires (AUA symptom score and the Urinary Function Questionnaire for men after radical prostatectomy) to study a population of 209 men who underwent either radical retropubic or perineal prostatectomy. They noted a 57% complete continence (no urine leakage) rate for both groups at a median of 2.7 years from surgery. When continence was defined as no urinary leakage or minimal urinary leakage, 75% of men satisfied these criteria. At 2 years, there was a higher likelihood of patients undergoing perineal prostatectomy to be completely continent, however, this difference disappears when continence was defined as no urinary leakage or minimal urinary leakage. Otherwise, there was no difference in urinary continence between the retropubic and perineal approaches.

G. Potency

Patients are warned of decreased potency, which may take up to 24 months to return postoperatively, but pharmacologic and nonpharmacologic aids are started as soon as the patient desires. Weldon and coworkers [21] reported potency results in a prospective study of 220 patients undergoing radical perineal prostatectomy. They performed nerve sparring operations on 50 select patients who had full preoperative erections and low risks of positive posterolateral margins. In this group, 70% remained potent, defined as having erections able to repeatedly achieve vaginal penetration for a prolonged period of time. Return of potency occurred in 50% of patients at 1 year and in 70% at 2 years. There was no statistical difference between patients who underwent unilateral nerve-sparring versus bilateral nerve-sparring procedures (68% versus 73%, respectively). Frazier and coworkers [48] reported on patients who underwent nerve-sparing radical perineal prostatectomy; of 22 unilateral or bilateral nerve sparring prostatectomies, 17 (77.3%) were potent more than 1 year postoperatively. They defined potency as the ability to achieve adequate vaginal penetration. In the study by Lance et al. [39], there was no significant difference between postoperative impotency rates for radical retropubic prostatectomy and radical perineal prostatectomy (91.1% versus 91.8%, after 41.4 versus 47.1 month followup, respectively). No comment, however, is made on whether nerve sparring was utilized in either approach. Ruiz-Deya et al [42]. retrospectively analyzed 250 consecutive perineal prostatectomies, and attempted nerve sparring in a younger subset of 54 patients with adequate erections preoperatively. Forty-one percent of these patients were potent 18 months following surgery. Ruiz-Deya and colleagues defined potency as vaginal penetration without the use of erectile aids. They also suggest that in large prostates being removed through the perineal route, unilateral nerve sparring may be advantageous over bilateral nerve sparring in order to avoid the stretching of both neurovascular bundles during removal of the prostate.

XI. SUMMARY

The resurgence of the radical perineal prostatectomy for the treatment of localized prostate cancer has been facilitated by the current emphasis on reducing medical costs, the identification of more cases of localized disease, the selected use of lymphadenectomy, and the use of laparoscopic techniques to perform node sampling. This technique provides a cost-effective, low-morbid, and efficacious surgical method of treating patients with localized prostate cancer.

REFERENCES

1. Stephenson RA. Prostate cancer trends in the era of prostate-specific antigen: an update of incidence, mortality, and clinical factors from the SEER database. Urol Clin North Am 2002; 29(1):173–181.
2. Weyrauch HM. Perineal Prostatectomy. In Weyrauch HM, Ed. Surgery of the Prostate. Philadelphia: W.B. Saunders, 1959:172–228.
3. Herman JR. Urology a view through the retrospectoscope. Hagerstown: Harper & Row, 1973:115.
4. Young HH. The early diagnosis and radical cure of carcinoma of the prostate: being a study of 40 cases and presentation of a radical operation which was carried out in four cases. Bull Johns Hopkins Hosp 1905; 16:315.
5. Belt E. Radical perineal prostatectomy in early carcinoma of the prostate. J Urol 1942; 78:287.
6. Belt E, Ebert CE, Surber AC. A new anatomic approach in perineal prostatectomy. J Urol 1939; 41:482.
7. Walsh PC, Donker PJ. Impotence following radical prostatectomy: insight into etiology and prevention. J Urol 1982; 128:492–494.
8. Reiner WJ, Walsh PC. An anatomical approach to the surgical management of the dorsal vein and Santorini's plexus during radical retropubic surgery. J Urol 1979; 147:1574.
9. Walsh PC, Lepor H, Eggleston JC. Radical prostatectomy with preservation of sexual function: anatomical and pathological considerations. Prostate 1983; 4:473.
10. Iselin CE, Robertson JE, Paulson DF. Radical perineal prostatectomy: oncological outcome during a 20-year period. J Urol 1999; 161:163–168.
11. Parra RO. Analysis of an experience with 500 radical prostatectomies in localized prostate cancer. J Urol 2000; 163:284–285.

12. Scoleri MJ, Resnick MI. The technique of radical perineal prostatectomy. Urol Clin North Am. 28 2001(3):521–533.

13. Gibbons RP. Radical perineal prostatectomy. In: Walsh PC, Retik AB, Vaughan ED, Wein AJ, Eds. Campbell's Urology. 8th ed. St. Louis: W.B. Saunders, 2002:3131.

14. Guillonneau B, Vallancien G. Laparoscopic radical prostatectomy: the Montsouris experience. J Urol 2000; 163:418–422.

15. Partin AW, Kattan MW, Subong EN, Walsh PC, Wojno KJ, Oesterling JE, Scardino PT, Pearson JD. Combination of prostate-specific antigen, clinical stage, and Gleason score to predict pathological stage of localized prostate cancer. J Am Med Assoc 1997; 277:1445–1451.

16. Bishoff JT, Reyes A, Thompson IM, Harris MJ, St Clair SR, Gomella L, Butzin CA. Pelvic lymphadenectomy can be omitted in selected patients with carcinoma of the prostate: development of a system of patient selection. Urology 1995; 45: 270–274.

17. Parra RO, Isorna S, Perez MG, Cummings JM, Boullier JA. Radical perineal prostatectomy without pelvic lymphadenectomy: selection criteria and early results. J Urol 1996; 155:612.

18. Schuessler WW, Vancaillie TG, Reich H, Griffith DP. Transperitoneal endosurgical lymphadenectomy in patients with localized prostate cancer. J Urol 1991; 145: 988–991.

19. Kerbl K, Clayman RV, Petros JA, Chandhoke PS, Gill IS. Staging pelvic lymphadenectomy for prostate cancer: a comparison of laparoscopic and open techniques. J Urol 1993; 150:396–399.

20. Weldon VE, Tavel FR. Potency-sparing radical perineal prostatectomy: Anatomy, surgical technique and initial results. J Urol 1988; 140:559–562.

21. Weldon VE, Tavel FR, Neuwirth H. Continence, potency and morbidity after radical perineal prostatectomy. J Urol 1997; 158:1470–1475.

22. Mokulis J, Thompson I. Radical prostatectomy: is the perineal approach more difficult to learn?. J Urol 1997; 157:230.

23. Jewett HJ. The case for radical perineal prostatectomy. J Urol 1970; 103:195–199.

24. Dees JE. Radical perineal prostatectomy for carcinoma. J Urol 1970; 104:160–162.

25. Levy DA, Resnick MI. Laparoscopic pelvic lymphadenectomy and radical perineal prostatectomy: a viable alternative to radical retropubic prostatectomy. J Urol 1994; 151:905–908.

26. Gillitzer R, Thäroff JW. Relative advantages and disadvantages of radical perineal prostatectomy versus radical retropubic prostatectomy. Crit Rev Oncol Hematol 2002; 43:167–190.

27. Lerner SE, Fleischmann J, Taub HC, Chamberlin JW, Kahan NZ, Melman A. Combined laparoscopic pelvic lymph node dissection and modified Belt radical perineal prostatectomy for localized prostate adenocarcinoma. Urology 1994; 43:493.

28. Parra RO, Boullier JA, Rauscher JA, Cummings JM. The value of laparoscopic lymphadenectomy in conjunction with radical perineal or retropubic prostatectomy. J Urol 1994; 151:1599.

29. Thomas R, Steele R, Smith R, Brannan W. One-stage laparoscopic pelvic lymphadenectomy and radical perineal prostatectomy. J Urol 1994; 152:1174.

30. Optenberg SA, Wojcik BE, Thompson IM. Morbidity and mortality following radical prostatectomy: a national analysis of Civilian Health Medical Program of the Uniformed Services Beneficiaries. J Urol 1995; 153:1870–1872.

31. Frazier HA, Robertson JE, Paulson DF. Radical prostatectomy: the pros and cons of the perineal versus the retropubic approach. J Urol 1992; 147:888.

32. Haab F, Boccon-Gibod L, Delmas V, Toublanc M. Perineal versus retropubic radical prostatectomy for T1, T2 prostate cancer. Br J Urol 1994; 74:626.

33. Boeckmann W, Jakse G. Management of rectal injury during perineal prostatectomy. Urol Int 1995; 55:147.

34. Lassen PM, Kearse WS. Rectal injuries during radical perineal prostatectomy. Urology 1995; 45:266.

35. Lassen PM, Mokulis JA, Kearse WS, Caballero RL, Quinones D. Conservative management of rectocutaneous fistula following radical perineal prostatectomy. Urology 1996; 47:592.

36. Resnick MI. Editorial Comments. Urology 1996; 47:594.

37. Bishoff JT, Motley G, Optenberg SA, Stein CR, Moon KA, Browning SM, Sabanegh E, Foley JP, Thompson IM. Incidence of fecal and urinary incontinence following radical perineal and retropubic prostatectomy in a national population. J Urol 1998; 160:454–457.

38. Zippe CD, Rackley RR. Non-nerve sparing radical prostatectomy in the elderly patient: perineal versus retropubic approach [abstract 359]. J Urol 1996; 155:400A.

39. Lance RS, Freidrichs PA, Kane C, Powell CR, Pulos E, Moul JW, McLeod DG, Cornum RL, Brantley Thrash. A comparison of radical retropubic with perineal prostatectomy for localized prostate cancer within the Uniformed Services Urology Research Group. BJU 2000; 87:61–65.

40. Price DT, Vieweg J, Roland F, Goetzech, Spalding T, Iselin C, Paulson DF. Transient lower extremity neurapraxia associated with radical perineal prostatectomy. A complication of the exaggerated lithotomy position. J Urol 1998; 160:1376–1378.

41. Keller H. Comment: Re: Transient lower extremity neurapraxia associated with radical perineal prostatectomy. A complication of the exaggerated lithotomy position. J Urol 1999; 162:171.

42. Ruiz-Deya G, Davis R, Srivastav SK, Wise A, Thomas R. Outpatient radical prostatectomy: impact of standard perineal approach on patient outcome. J Urol 2001; 166:581–586.

43. Sullivan LD, Weir MJ, Kinahan JF, Taylor DL. A comparison of the relative merits of radical perineal and radical retropubic prostatectomy. BJU 2000; 85:95–100.

44. Boccon-Gibod L, Ravery V, Vordos D, Toublanc M, Delmas V, Bocon-Gibod L. Radical prostatectomy for prostate cancer: the perineal approach increases the risk of surgically induced positive margins and capsular incisions. J Urol 1998; 160:1383–1385.

45. Weldon VE. Comment in. J Urol 1999; 161(4):1287.

46. Korman HJ, Leu PB, Huang RR, Goldstein NS. A centralized comparison of radical perineal and retropubic prostatectomy specimens: is there a difference according to the surgical approach?. J Urol 2002; 168:991–994.

47. Theodorescu D, Lippert MC, Broder SR, Boyd JC. Early prostate-specific antigen failure following radical perineal versus retropubic prostatectomy: the importance of seminal vesicle excision. Urology 1998; 51:277–282.

48. Walsh PC. Comment in. J Urol 1998; 160(1):269–270.
49. Weldon VE, Travel FR, Neuwirth H, Cohen R. Patterns of positive specimen margins and detectable prostate-specific antigen after radical perineal prostatectomy. J Urol 1995; 153:1565.
50. Epstein JI, Pizov G, Walsh PC. Correlation of pathologic findings with progression after radical retropubic prostatectomy. Cancer 1993; 71:3582.
51. Rosen MA, Goldstone L, Lapin S, Wheeler T, Scardino PT. Frequency and location of extracapsular extension and positive surgical margins in radical prostatectomy specimens. J Urol 1992; 148:331.
52. Stamey TA, Villers AA, McNeal JE, Link PC, Freiha FS. Positive surgical margins at radical prostatectomy: importance of the apical dissection. J Urol 1990; 143:1166.
53. Gibbons RP, Correa RJ, Brannen GE, Mason JT. Total prostatectomy for localized prostate cancer. J Urol 1984; 131:73.
54. Gray M, Petroni GR, Theodorescu D. Urinary function after radical prostatectomy: a comparison of the retropubic and perineal approaches. Urology 1999; 53:881–890.
55. Reiter RE, deKernion JB. Epidemiology, etiology, and prevention of prostate cancer. In: Walsh PC, Retik AB, Vaughan ED, Wein AJ, Eds. Campbell's Urology. 8th ed.. St. Louis: W.B. Saunders, 2002:3003–3005.
56. Haas CA, Resnick MI. Radical perineal prostatectomy: late division of seminal vesicles. In: Resnick MI, Thompson IM, Eds. Surgery of the Prostate. New York: Churchill Livingstone, 1998:131–148.
57. Harris MJ, Thompson IM. Radical perineal prostatectomy: early dissection of seminal vesicles. In: Resnick MI, Thompson IM, Eds. Surgery of the Prostate. New York: Churchill Livingstone, 1998:149–165.

EDITORIAL COMMENTARY

Michael J. Harris

Northern Institute of Urology, Traverse City, Michigan, USA

In the foregoing chapter, Drs. Feng and Resnick provide an excellent review of the history of the perineal approach to radical prostatectomy in the United States. Similarly, they discussed the stage migration that has resulted since the widespread use of the prostate-specific antigen (PSA) in the early detection of prostate cancer. Pelvic lymphadenectomy is infrequently indicated in the management of patients presenting with newly diagnosed, clinically localized prostate cancer. Likewise, the increasing number of men presenting with minimal volume cancers are better candidates for cavernosal nerve preservation. Drs. Feng and Resnick thoroughly reviewed the technique of radical perineal prostatectomy incorporating late dissection of the vas and seminal vesicals, similar to the 1905 description by Young [1].

     This commentary will focus on an anatomic technique of radical perineal prostatectomy that utilizes Young's suprasphincteric approach to the pelvic floor,

Belt's early dissection of the seminal vesicals and Weldon's method of cavernosal nerve preservation [2,3]. Data presented has been prospectively accumulated since 1993. The data are analyzed every 1 to 2 years and alterations of the technique are incorporated based upon the analysis of these data to improve clinical outcomes. The operative technique presented in this editorial has evolved significantly since our first description in 1995 [4].

Mechanical bowel prep is accomplished on the day prior to surgery with a Fleets Phosphosoda prep, CB Fleet Company, Lynchbag VA. On the morning of surgery, a 1% Neomycin enema is administered. Second-generation cephalosporin antibiotic is infused preoperatively. Thromboembolic deterrent hose and pneumatic compression stockings are applied prior to induction of either a general or spinal anesthetic. The patient is positioned in the lithotomy position utilizing Yellow Fin or Allen Alan Medical Systems, Acton MA stirrups to support the legs. The risk of lower extremity neuropraxia is increased if candy cane stirrups, which do not adequately support the weight of the leg, are utilized. A six-inch jellyroll is used to elevate the sacrum. The perineum should be adequately exposed without excessive tension on the hamstring muscles and does not need to be parallel with the floor. (Figure 4 in this chapter)

A curved incision is placed with the apex in the midperineum and the ends one centimeter medial to the ischial tuberosities and at least one centimeter anterior to the anus. If the incision is more posterior, there is greater risk for anal canal dysfunction [5,6]. The central tendon is divided and the ischiorectal space developed. By entering this space well anterior of the anal canal, using Young's suprasphincteric approach, the midline raphe of the bulbospongiosus muscle is encountered. Midline attachments to the raphe are divided with cautery and the raphe is exposed posteriorly to the fibrous confluence of the perineum where the levator ani and rectourethralis converge. By elevating the fibrous confluence with forceps, and with a finger in the O'Conor-Sullivan (American V Mueller, Chicago, IL) rectal sheath for identification of the rectum, the fibrous confluence is divided with cautery exposing the fine, pink, vertical fibers of the rectourethralis muscle. Using scissors partly open, the rectum is carefully swept posteriorly away from the prostatic apex while thinning the rectourethralis fibers. Remaining fibers are divided to expose the pearly white layer of Denonvilliers' fascia overlying the apex of the prostate. The rectum is swept posteriorly off of Denonvilliers' fascia deep to the tips of the seminal vesicals. The plane of entry into the pelvis lateral to the prostate is along the medial surface of the levator ani muscles. All of the periprostatic tissues to the levator ani muscles are removed with the prostate in a wide excision case. In cases of nerve preservation, the periprostatic tissues include the cavernosal nerves that will be spared. A Thompson (Thompson Surgical Inc, Traverse City MI) retractor or other similar low-profilie retractor system is used to provide excellent exposure. (See Figure 13 in this chapter.)

Denonvilliers' fascia is incised transversely from seminal vesical to seminal vesical 1 cm from the base of the prostate with electrocautery. A vein retractor is used to elevate the prostate revealing the vas and seminal vesicals. The vas is grasped and dissected for 3–5cm and divided. The seminal vesical is grasped on the medial side and pulled medially revealing the lateral aspect. Scissors are placed just lateral to the seminal vesical and spread. This maneuver usually completes the seminal vesical dissection and the vessel at its tip is clipped or sealed with Ligasure (Valley lab, Boulder, CO) and divided (Fig. 1).

In wide excision cases, endopelvic fascia is scored overlying the bladder neck and the Ligasure is used to seal the pedicles such that all periprostatic tissue is taken with the prostate. In nerve sparing cases, Denonvilliers' fascia is incised with a knife from the midline at the apex to a point overlying the base of the prostate near the seminal vesical. Denonvilliers' fascia with associated cavernosal nerves and periprostatic tissues are sharply and carefully dissected off of the prostate laterally from apex to base (Fig. 2). The proximal pedicle is isolated medial to the nerve bundles and sealed with Ligasure and divided (Fig. 3). The bladder base is pushed off of the prostate with a peanut dissector. A natural plane of dissection opens that preserves the bladder neck.

Once the nerves are separated from the prostate and the posterior dissection is complete, the plane of nerve preservation is extended to the apex of the prostate.

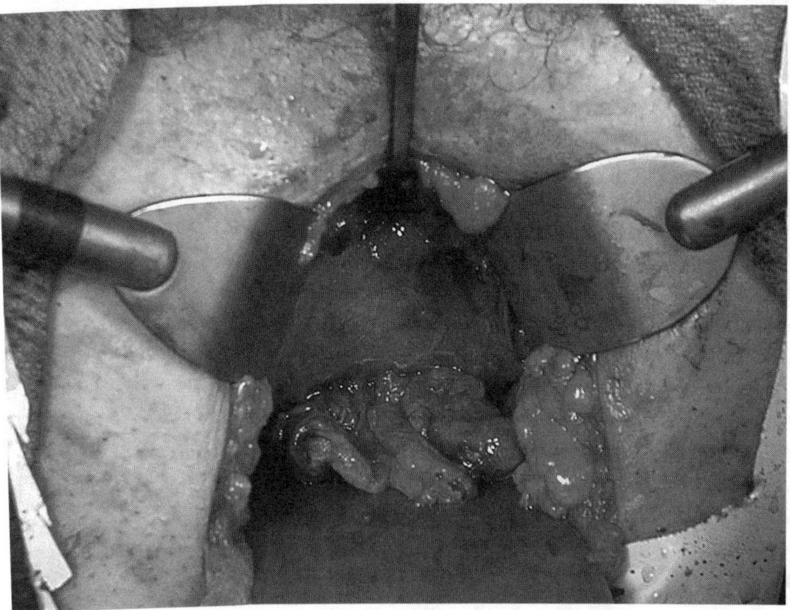

FIGURE 1   The right seminal vesical is pulled medially while the vessel at its tip is clipped. The posterior bladder neck is revealed just below the vein retractor.

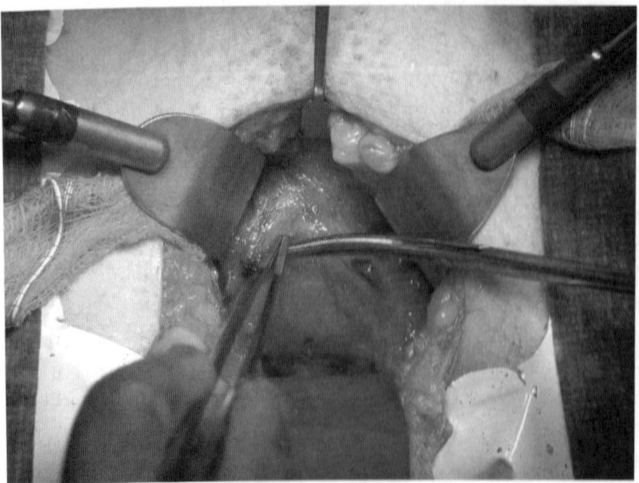

FIGURE 2   Cavernosal nerve preservation starts with a delicate incision in Denonvilliers' fascia followed by careful, sharp dissection of the plane between the prostate and the fascia. The nerves are invested in Denonvilliers' fascia. This plane of dissection is extended around the prostate to the puboprostatic ligaments, anteriorly and the bladder neck proximally.

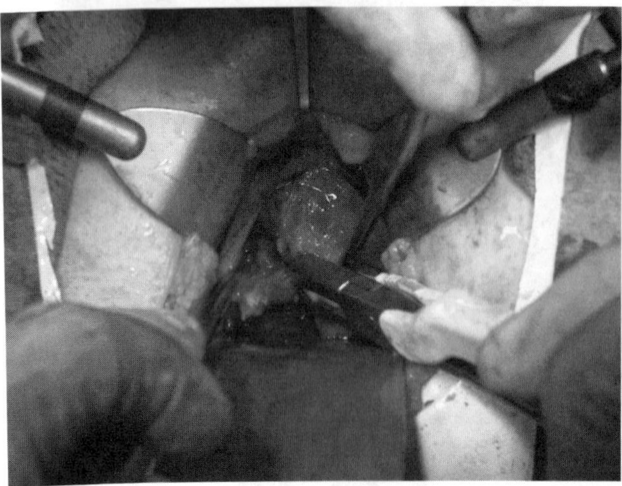

FIGURE 3   Ligasure is applied to the proximal pedicle while the right-sided cavernosal nerve bundles are carefully retracted laterally away from the Ligasure device.

The urethra is gently separated from surrounding tissues by a long-tyne right-angled clamp that is passed around the membranous urethra and carefully opened. The peanut dissector is "rolled" along the urethra into the apex of the prostate to separate the urethra up to the veru montanum. The urethra is divided leaving a 1.5-cm length at the pelvic floor (Fig. 4).

To reduce the risk of anterior positive margins, the puboprostatic ligaments are divided several millimeters away from the anterior aspect of the prostate with electrocautery [7]. The bladder neck is pushed off of the anterior aspect of the prostate with a peanut dissector. The bladder neck is circumferentially separated from the prostate and a 1cm length of urethra is dissected out of the prostate with associated urethral smooth muscle. The urethra is then divided (Fig. 5).

An end-to-end anastomosis is accomplished with two separate running 3-0 absorbable, synthetic monofilament sutures starting near the midline anteriorly and running to the midline posteriorly, where they are tied without tightening the circumference of the anastomotic portion of the urethra. An 18 French catheter is placed (Fig. 6). If the bladder neck needs "tennis-racquet" reconstruction, the described running anastomosis is accomplished and then the cystoplasty is reinforced with a second layer of absorbable sutures.

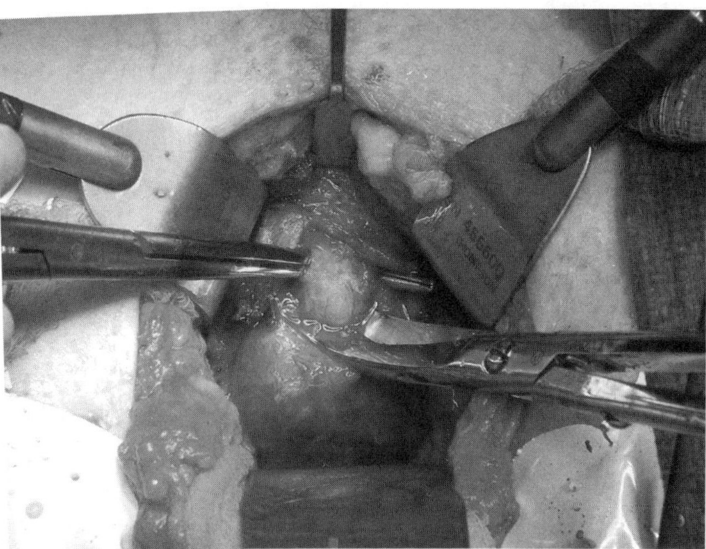

FIGURE 4   In this case of bilateral cavernosal nerve preservation, the urethra is dissected out of the apex of the prostate. It is important to avoid excessive traction to the urethra during this dissection. The nerve bundles are seen behind the exposed portions of the right-angle clamp. The apex of the prostate is below the Jorgenson scissors.

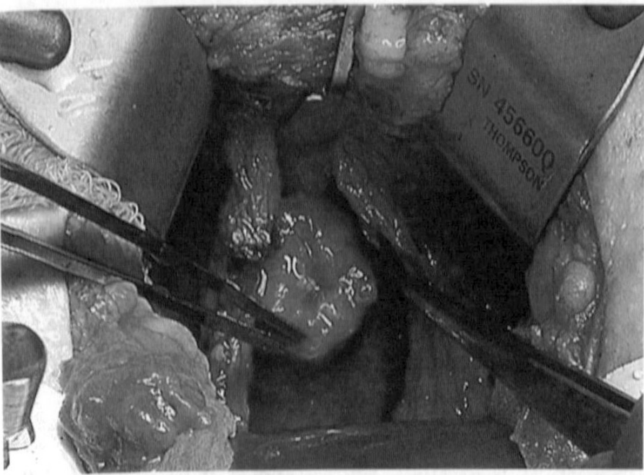

FIGURE 5   The urethra is dissected out of the prostate base for a 1-cm length. Preservation of the bladder neck and proximal urethra allows for end-to-end urethrourethrostomy. In this picture, the intact bladder neck and proximal urethra are seen between bilateral Cavernosal Nerve bundles.

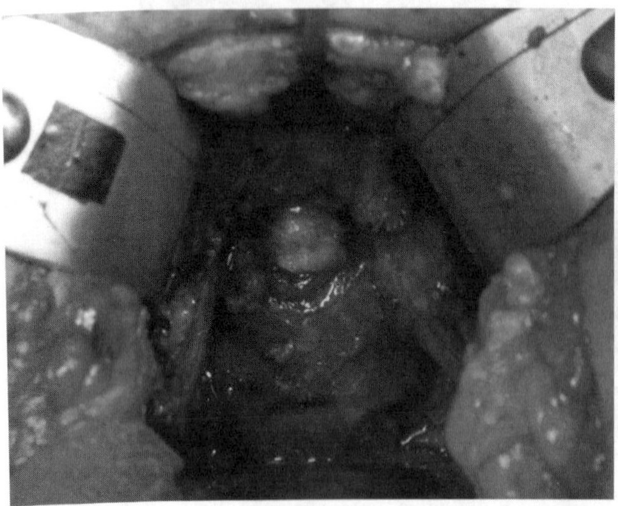

FIGURE 6   Bilateral cavernosal nerve preservation is complete. The nerve bundles are lateral to the anastomosis. The membranous urethra is attached to proximal prostatic urethra with two separate running 3-0 absorbable monofilament sutures. In this photo, the anastomosis is nearly complete and the sutures are seen on the membranous urethra side of the urethrourethrostomy.

The wound is closed in layers with a penrose drain exiting the corner of the incision. The skin is closed with a running subcuticular suture. On the day of surgery, the patient resumes diet and ambulation. On the morning after surgery, the penrose drain is removed, his postoperative teaching is completed, and he is discharged home. A cystogram is performed on the 4th day after surgery and, if no extravasation is noted, the catheter is removed. Activities are liberalized at that time.

PATIENT CHARACTERISTICS

Data on 558 men with cT1-2 prostate cancer who underwent radical perineal prostatectomy by one surgeon is accumulated prospectively. Modifications of technique based upon data analysis have lead to progressive improvement in outcomes over the past 9 years. The average patient age is 65.4 years (range 41–86). The average prebiopsy PSA is 6.6 (range 0.3–29.9) and biopsy Gleason Score is 6.3. The average prostate weight and cancer weight are 49.0 gm and 8.8 gm, respectively, and are based upon specimen weight and percent involvement with cancer. Seven patients underwent pelvic lymphadenectomy and all were negative for metastatic disease on frozen section analysis.

CANCER CONTROL

Two hundred nineteen men of the 558 who underwent radical perineal prostatectomy have PSA data beyond 4 years of actual follow-up. Ninety-five percent and eighty percent of men with organ-confined and specimen-confined (clean margins with extracapsular disease) tumors are free of biochemical evidence of recurrent disease, respectively. Seventy-four percent versus forty-three percent of men with focal vs. nonfocal margins positive in the absence of seminal vesical invasion remain free of biochemical evidence of recurrence at 4 years of actual follow-up. Only 20% of men with seminal vesical invasive disease have an undetectable PSA at 4 years of actual follow-up. Four men underwent prostatectomy despite occult metastatic disease that was apparent on permanent section of lymph nodes after initially negative frozen section analysis. PSA detectability by stage over 6 years of actual follow-up is shown in Figure 7.

While 36% of cases have extracapsular disease and an average 8.8 gms of cancer, positive margins are seen 16.3% of cases without seminal vesicle invasion and 18% overall. Margins are focally (less than 1 mm^2) positive in 8.9%, isolated and nonfocal in 4.3% and multifocal in 3.1% of cases. Positive margins are noted at the apex, anterior, bladder neck, and bladder base along the seminal vesicals in 5.1%, 2.6%, 3.1%, and 2.8%, respectively (Fig. 8).

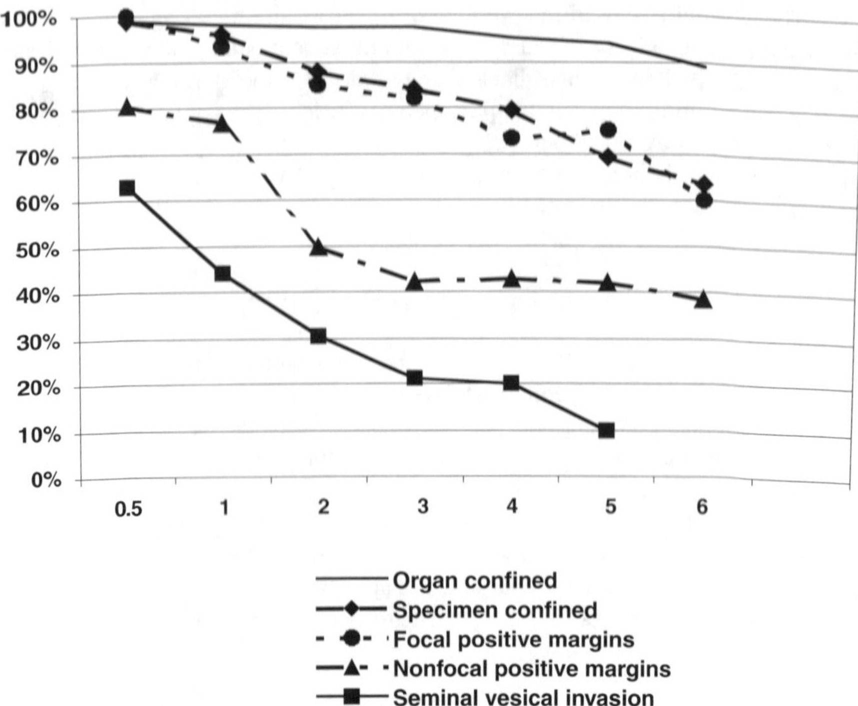

FIGURE 7   This graph demonstrates the percent of men with undetectable PSA by number of years after radical perineal prostatectomy. The solid line represents organ confined, clean margin cases; solid diamonds represent specimen confined; solid circles represent focal (< 1 mm^2) positive margins; solid triangles represent nonfocal (> 1 mm^2 or multiple) positive margins; solid squares represent seminal vesical invasion.

URINARY CONTINENCE

From February 1995 to January 2002, bladder neck and proximal urethral preservation was intended in all patients. An interrupted suture urethrourethrostomy with 8–10 sutures was then accomplished. If the proximal urethra was inadequate, than an interrupted suture urethrovesicostomy is performed without eversion. As a default, last resort, bladder neck reconstruction with a two-layer ''tennis-racquet'' cystoplasty precedes urethrovesicostomy. Over that time period, the catheter was removed initially 17 days, and later 8 days after surgery. By the first month, second month, fourth month, sixth month, and first year, 38%, 53%, 74%, 85%, and 96%, respectively, of patients are free of pad use. Two-and-one-half percent of patients use one pad daily for minimal stress incontinence and 1.5% use more

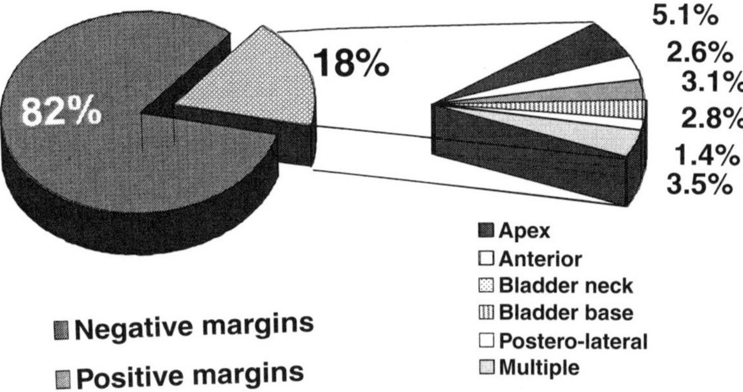

FIGURE 8 Sites of positive margins including cases with seminal vesical invasion. Overall, 18% of patients have positive margins. The apex and bladder neck are the most common sites of positive margins in 5.1% and 3.1% of all patients.

than one pad daily after the first year. "Socially dry" continence preceded "totally dry" continence by 6–8 weeks during the first six months after surgery. Eight men were treated with 1–5 collagen implants while 6 (1.2%) received artificial sphincters (Fig. 9).

Since January 2002, when bladder neck and proximal urethra are spared, a running urethrourethrostomy is performed as described in the above operative description. In all 38 men, the cystograms were normal at 4 days and their catheters removed at that time. Two men developed urinary retention and were recatheterized for 2 and 8 days. Three men developed delayed urethrocutaneous drainage that resolved spontaneously with replacement of the catheter (Fig. 10).

RETURN OF ERECTILE FUNCTION

Criteria for consideration of cavernosal nerve preservation are based upon the staging by sextant biopsies (medial and lateral cores in each sextant). Initially, only fully potent men with unilateral, nonapical tumors are offered nerve preservation of the contralateral nerve bundle. Since July 2001, bilateral nerve preservation has been performed in selected patients as noted previously. A spontaneous "partial erection" is defined as penile tumescence with erotic stimulation inadequately rigid for vaginal penetration. An "adequate erection" is defined as an erection adequate to complete vaginal intercourse with or without the use of sildenafil. With the introduction of sildenafil, men with erections that are only adequate when sildenafil is used are offered nerve preservation. Additionally, some men can complete intercourse without silde-

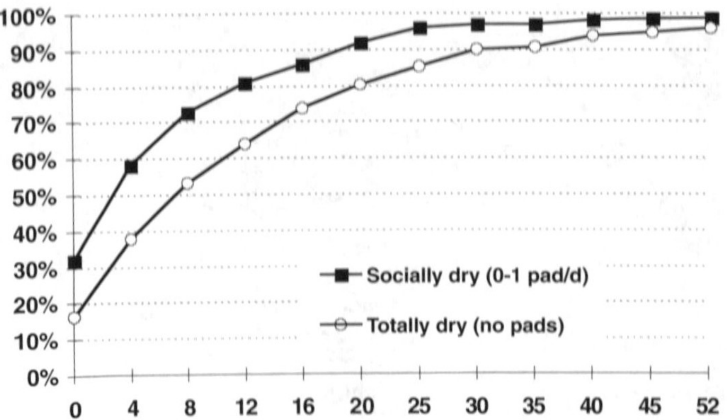

FIGURE 9   Socially dry (0–1 pad daily, solid squares) and Totally dry (no pad use, open circles) in weeks after catheter removal. This graph represents the results of 439 men from February 1995 to December 2001. The initial intent is to spare the bladder neck and proximal urethra and a generous stump of membranous urethra for an ***interrupted-suture*** urethrourethrostomy. If the proximal urethra is not sufficient, then the urethrovesicostomy is to an intact bladder neck without eversion. The "default" technique is a "tight" tennis-racquet closure before urethrovesicostomy followed by a second layer of suture to reinforce the tennis-racquet portion. The catheter is removed 8–17 days after surgery.

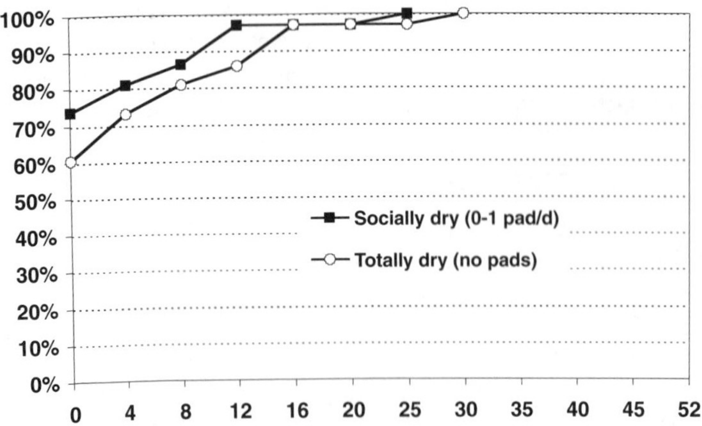

FIGURE 10   This graph represents 38 men who underwent preservation of bladder neck and proximal urethra and membranous urethra for ***running*** urethrourethrostomy. The percent of men who are "socially dry" or "totally dry" time in weeks after catheter removal. The catheter is removed on postoperative day 4.

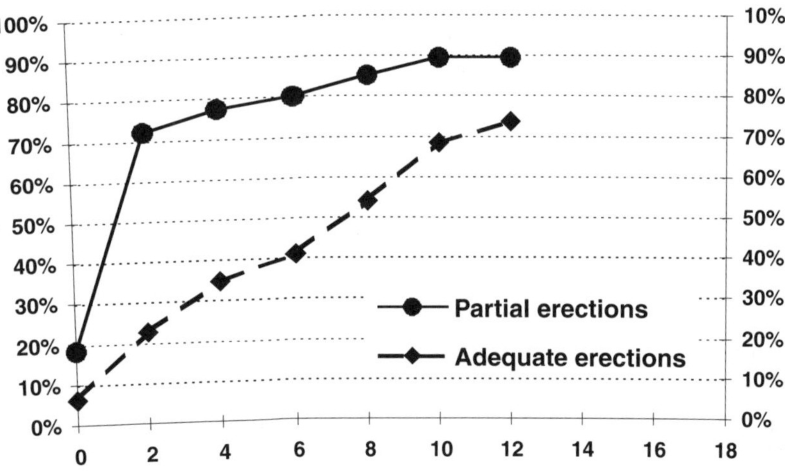

Figure 11 Partial and adequate spontaneous erectile function by months after radical perineal prostatectomy with bilateral cavernosal nerve preservation.

nafil, however, prefer the improved rigidity with its use. While the use of sildenafil is greater after surgery than before, the preoperatively "sildenafil-dependent" men are not segregated from the men that did not use sildenafil before surgery in this database. Figure 11 demonstrated the time to partial and adequate spontaneous erections in bilaterally nerve-spared men. Figure 12

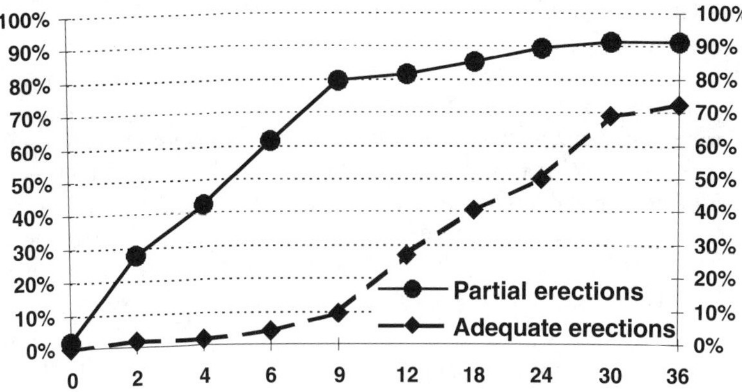

Figure 12 Partial and adequate spontaneous erectile function by months after radical perineal prostatectomy with unilateral cavernosal nerve preservation.

TABLE 1. Oncologic Characteristics of Prebiopsy PSA, Pathologic Gleason Score, Patient Age, Prostate and Tumor Size and Rate of MarginP. Note that Despite Selecting Patients for Nerve-Sparing with Smaller Cancers, the Positive Margin Rate Increases.

Nerves spared	None	Unilateral	Bilateral	Total
N	469	54	35	558
Age	66.3	61.5	58.8	65.4
PSA (ng/mL)	6.8	5.7	4.6	6.6
Path Gleason score	6.5	6.1	6.2	6.4
Prostate size (gms)	49.8	47.4	41.1	49.0
Cancer size (gms)	9.5	6.7	2.8	8.8
positive margins (%)	18.6	11.1	37.1	19.0

demonstrates the time to partial and adequate spontaneous erections in unilaterally nerve-spared men.

Sofer reported that nerve-sparing techniques did not increase the risk for positive surgical margins [8]. Conversely, an increased risk of positive surgical margins is seen in bilaterally nerve-spared men despite smaller average tumor size as compared to unilateral nerve preservation or bilateral wide excision cases (Table 1).

In an effort to select appropriate ''nerve-sparing'' candidates, additional 3-dimensional information is obtained in this author's practice. During prostate ultrasound and biopsy, specimens are isolated by sextant to six separate containers. The medial and lateral cores are inked with green and blue ink at the capsular ends, respectively. This biopsy protocol provides anatomic localization of tumor sites that may be proximate to the cavernosal nerves that course along the postero-lateral aspect of the prostate. Despite this process of understanding tumor location as best possible, and selecting candidates carefully for nerve-sparing with clean margin cancer excision as a first priority, the risk of positive margins is still higher in the bilaterally nerve-spared men. While some of these positive margins are secondary to surgical trauma caused by applying a ring clamp to the apex of the prostate during bladder neck dissection, one must be aware of the possibility of the increased risk of positive margins when removing the prostate without any periprostatic tissues.

COMPLICATIONS

Distal urethral strictures and anastomotic strictures have occurred in 2% each. Office cystoscopic evaluation and dilation resolved most strictures with 3 patients undergoing internal urethrotomy under anesthesia. One patient developed a recurrent urethrocutaneous fistula, which required excision and Gracilis muscle interposition flap. He is continent and cancer-free 9 years later. One man has experienced anal incompetence, while 2–4% note mild fecal urgency or valsalva related flatus. One man experienced a transcient ischemic event and another a mild stroke on the day of discharge, requiring an extra day of neurologic tests and initiation of rehabilitation. No cardiac or pulmonary complications occurred. There were no perioperative deaths. No patients developed lower extremity neuropraxia. Two percent of patients had rectal injuries that were all identified, repaired with a two-layer closure and recovered without adverse sequelae. No specific alteration in post-operative management is undertaken in men with repaired proctotomies, as all men are prepped for this possible complication.

COST ISSUES

Most cases are completed between 75 and 120 minutes with less than 10% taking longer or shorter time. The length of hospital stay declined in recent years as a nursing care pathway was instituted and improvements in preoperative teaching resulted in a steady decline in the length of stay. The average length of hospital stay of the most recent 300 patients is 1.1 days. In the past 300 patients, 95% are discharged on the morning after surgery and 5% on the second postoperative day. Average hospital charges were $4,889 in 1999 and 2000. Blood banking of autologous blood type and screening for potential transfusion are not performed. Post-operative lab testing of any type is rare.

CONCLUSION

Radical perineal prostatectomy as nicely outlined in the foregoing chapter by Drs. Feng and Resnick, or by the above description, can provide a minimally invasive method of achieving treatment goals competitive with retropubic and laparoscopic approaches. Every surgeon should monitor his/her own results and improve their operating technique based upon the evaluation of their outcomes. While radical prostatectomy is a difficult operation with competing objectives (wide excision for cancer control versus minimal excision for preservation of urinary and erectile function), careful attention to detail and reassessment of technique will help our patients maintain good quality of life after cancer surgery.

REFERENCES

1. Young HH. The early diagnosis and radical cure of carcinoma of the prostate. Being a study of 40 cases and presentation of a radical operation which was carried out in four cases. Bull Johns Hopkins University 1905; 16:315–321.

2. Belt E. Radical perineal prostatectomy in early carcinoma of the prostate. J Urol 1942; 48:287–297.

3. Weldon VE, Tavel FR. Potency-sparing radical perineal prostatectomy: Anatomy, surgical technique and initial results. J Urol 1988; 142:559–562.

4. Harris MJ, Thompson IM. The anatomical radical perineal prostatectomy: an individualized approach to the treatment of men with clinically localized prostate cancer. Monographs in Urology. Medical Directions Publishing Co. Inc. Monteverde FL. Stamey Thomas A, Ed. Vol. 16, 1995.

5. Bishoff JT, Motley G, Optenberg SA, Stein CR, Moon KA, Browning SM. Incidence of fecal and urinary incontinence following radical perineal and retropubic prostatectomy in a national population. J Urol 1988; 160:454–458.

6. Dahm P, Silverstein AD, Weizer AZ, Young MD, Vieweg J, Albala DM, Paulson DF. A longitudinal assessment of bowel related symptoms and Fecal incontinence following medical prostatectomy. J Urol 2003; 169:2220–2224.

7. Weldon VE, Tavel FR, Neuwirth H, Cohen R. Patterns of positive specimen margins and detectable prostate specific antigen after radical perineal prostatectomy. J Urol 1995; 153:1565–1569.

8. Sofer M, Hamilton-Nelson KL, Schlesselman JJ, Soloway MS. Risk of positive margins and biochemical recurrence in relation to nerve-sparing radical prostatectomy. J Clin Onc 2002; 20:1853–1858.

EDITORIAL COMMENTARY

Robert P. Gibbons

Section of Urology and Renal Transplantation, Virginia Mason Clinic, Seattle, WA, USA

Feng and Resnick have provided a detailed and well-illustrated description of the technique of radical perineal prostatectomy. They have also prepared a comprehensive and well-referenced discussion on its morbidity and outcomes compared with radical retropubic prostatectomy.

GENERAL

Surgery is curable only if all the tumor is removed. Surgery is necessary only if the cancer will inflict morbidity or shorten the patient's expected survival. I believe the appropriate patient for radical prostatectomy is one whose disease is confined to the prostate, has an expected survival longer than the natural history of the cancer (15 years), has no significant surgical risk factors, and, after a discussion of these issues and treatment options, wishes to undergo surgery. I would add to the discussion by the authors that the perineal route is particularly advantageous in patients who have undergone prior low abdominal or pelvic surgery, especially if a mesh has been used.

A simple office test to see if the occasional patient with hip ankylosis or marked obesity can be placed in the exaggerated lithotomy position is to have him lie supine on the examining table and bring his knees to his chest. The inability to do this is a contraindication to the procedure.

Patients given the GoLYTELYP bowel prep, as described by the authors, often complain more of the bowel prep than of the surgery, and take a longer time to regain their normal bowel pattern and stool consistency than if they just give themselves a Fleet enema at 9:00PM the evening before surgery. The rectum seems equally well prepared either way.

PROCEDURE

Neurapraxia of the lower and upper extremities is minimized if during positioning the knees are kept as extended as the stirrups allow, the buttocks are supported to achieve the desired lithotomy position rather than forcing the legs alone to maintain the position, and the upper arms are not extended more that 45° away from the body.

"Tricks" to better illuminate the depths of the perineal incision include a lighted sucker or a fiber-optic light cable that can be held with a clamp or by hand, or attached to the self-retained retractor.

The authors describe and illustrate (authors' figures 8, 10) how to develop a plane between Denonvilliers' fascia by keeping the anterior layer attached to the prostate and the posterior layer attached to the rectum. This later facilitates mobilization of the neurovascular bundles. My preference, however, is to keep both layers attached to the prostate to reduce the risk of a positive margin at this location [1], (figure 1).

A technical advantage of radical perineal prostatectomy is the clear exposure and access to the apex of the prostate to optimize the complete removal of this critical margin and allow precise transection of the urethra. The presence of the Lowsley retractor allows the apex of the prostate and adjacent urethra to be readily palpated. I suggest that, at this point, minimal dissection be performed and the urethra not be encircled to avoid injury to the region of the primary continence mechanism, the striated urethral sphincter [2,3].

A curved Heaney needle holder significantly aids in the placement of most sutures placed inside the perineal field of surgery. Those sutures placed in the vesicourethral anastomosis include a 1-mm segment of mucosa to reduce the formation of an anastomotic stricture. The total number of sutures placed across the anastomosis can be reduced by the use of a "figure-of-eight" suture placed in the manner of Jewett on the posterior bladder closure (Figure 2) [4]. This affords a watertight closure that allows the catheter to be removed on postoperation day 10.

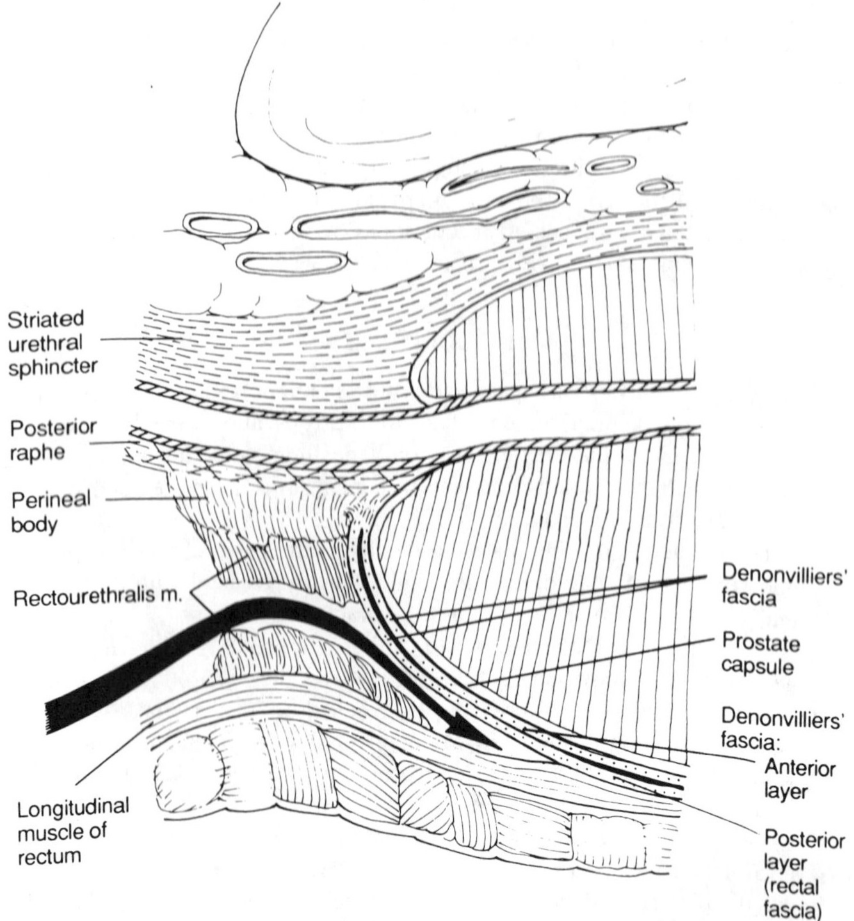

FIGURE 1 Relationship of the rectum, recto-urethralis muscle, striated urethral sphincter, Denonvilliers' fascia, and apex of the prostate. An extended, wide-field radical dissection leaves both of Denonvilliers' layers attached to the rectum (authors' reference 13). (Reproduced with permission from Elsevier)

The authors note, "Operative times are usually less than 1 hour." In my hands and with the most experienced help, it is 90 minutes—longer when teaching a resident or fellow.

Rectal injury, although infrequent, does occur more often during radical perineal than radical retropubic prostatectomy. This generally is not a problem in the patient prepared with a bowel prep and in whom the opening is noticed

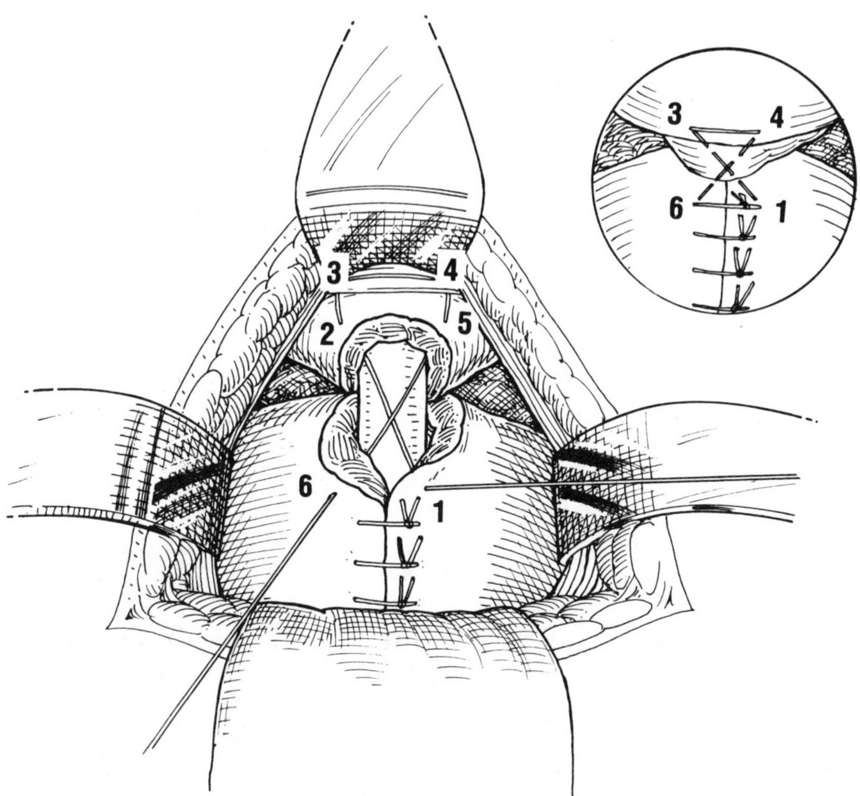

FIGURE 2 Jewett's "figure-of-eight" closure of the posterior vesico-urethral anastomosis provides a watertight closure with a minimum number of sutures across the anastomosis [4]. (Reproduced with permission from the American Urological Association Update Series, vol. 13, lesson 5. American Urological Association Office of Education, Houston. 1994)

and closed at the time of injury. To repair, the edges are freshened, and the mucosa is closed with a running suture of 4-0 monofilament absorbable sutures, turning the mucosa inward toward the lumen. A second layer of interrupted 4-0 monofilament nonabsorbable sutures is placed in Lembert's manner to invert the first layer. These sutures are placed approximately 4 mm apart. The proctotomy and operative site are copiously irrigated with 1 L of normal saline containing an antibiotic such as 1 g cefazolin sodium (Ancef). Anal dilation is *not* performed because the colorectal literature indicates that anal dilation itself can result in fecal incontinence in up to 20% of patients [5,6]. Some surgeons use digital guidance during radical perineal prostatectomy, which, if not done gently and without excessive sphincter stretch, could possibly explain the higher risk of monthly fecal incontinence episodes in radical perineal prostatectomy patients (16%) vs. in radical retropubic patients (8%) (authors' reference 37). If a rectal injury has occurred, the patient receives nothing by mouth for 3 days after surgery and is then given a soft diet for 2 days. The drain is left in for 5 days. Parenteral gentamicin and cefotetan are continued until the drains are removed. The patient is given a stool softener but no mineral oil or other cathartic.

CANCER OUTCOMES

In 1996, we reported, in abstract form, about our single institution's (10 urologists) experience, over a 33-year time period, documenting the efficacy of total prostatectomy in selected patients with clinically localized prostate cancer [7]. This report was based on 463 consecutive patients treated with radical perineal (368) or radical retropubic (95) prostatectomy and *followed a minimum of 5 years.* Median follow-up was 9.6 years with a mean of 10.8 years. Most of the patients had been diagnosed clinically prior to the availability of PSA, but PSA follow-up was available for 320 out of 321 patients alive at the time of the report. Results are seen in Table 1. The positive margin rate was 16%, with an additional 12% with positive seminal vesicles. Sixty-three percent had organ-confined disease. Recurrence-free survival was 68% at 10 years, 56% at 15 years, and 47% at 20 years following surgery. There was no significant difference by type of operation. Thirty-one patients (6.7%) died of prostate cancer (1.6–27 years/median 8.6) following surgery. Contemporary studies of radical perineal prostatectomy performed on patients with earlier (PSA-detected) stage of prostate cancer should result in even better results.

Urinary Incontinence

In our 1984 report (author's reference 53), 92% of the patients reported to their urologist that they had normal urinary control by 6 months following radical perineal prostatectomy. An independent staff member who was not involved in their care performed another survey in 1991–1992 assessing urinary control 1 year following radical perineal prostatectomy. Three percent reported total urinary incontinence and another 9% reported the occasional use of a protective pad.

Potency

Weldon's group (authors' reference 21) has developed strict criteria for recommending nerve-sparing radical perineal prostatectomy. Using these criteria,

TABLE 1. Long-term efficacy of radical prostatectomy in the management of clinically localized prostate cancer. 463 consecutive patients (368 radical perineal, 95 radical retropublic) followed a minimum of 5 years (median follow-up 9.6 years/mean 10.8 years). No significant difference by type of operation (7).

Median age—63.0 years (45–76)
Operative mortality—0.4%

Pathologic Findings:
Organ Confined (pT1–T2)—63%
Capsule Invasion = 9%
Positive Margin = 16%
Positive Seminal Vesicle = 12%

Recurrence Rate (observed at mean follow-up of 10.8 years):
Local = 11% (0.75–17.8 years/median 4.8)
Distant ± Local = 13% (0.25–19.5 years/median 6.4)
PSA Only = 20% (64/321) of patients followed > 5 years
Overal = 35%

Survival:

	10 Years	15 Years	20 Years
Overall	78%	60%	41%
Recurrence-free	68%	56%	47%
Disease-specific	95%	89%	83%

potency returned by 24 months in 70% of patients who were fully potent before surgery. My own experience with nerve-sparing radical perineal prostatectomy is limited. Several of my initial patients were found to have a positive margin somewhere along the course of the reflected posterior layer of Denonvilliers' fascia, which, I felt, was iatrogenic. I also found it frustrating that the side of the gland felt by palpation or biopsy to be less involved with tumor and therefore "OK" to perform a unilateral nerve-sparing modification proved to have a positive margin. Others shared these findings [8,9]. Combining these observations with the knowledge that patients with positive surgical margins have PSA failure rates significantly higher than patients with specimen-confined disease restrained me from becoming enthusiastic with nerve-sparing radical perineal prostatectomy. Indeed, positive margin rates 24% higher in patients undergoing nerve-sparing versus non-nerve-sparing radical perineal prostatectomy have been reported. [10]. Even with strict patient selection, patients must understand and accept some increased risk of a positive margin with this modification. In my practice, not many men who elected to undergo surgery wished to take this small but potential risk—indeed, their primary desire was to increase the odds of "getting rid" of *all* the cancer. Even when extended bilateral non-nerve-sparing prostatectomy is performed, 7% of patients surveyed have erections satisfactory for intercourse (authors' reference 53). Nearly all (98%) of the surveyed patients noted that the sensation of orgasm was intact postoperatively, allowing excellent rehabilitation with a penile prosthesis.

SUMMARY

The many advantages of radical perineal prostatectomy have been known for many years (authors' Table 1) [11]. Laparoscopic radical prostatectomy has again renewed interest in a minimally invasive surgical approach to the increasing number of patients with PSA-detected, low-stage, low-grade prostate cancer. However, laparoscopic radical prostatectomy has proved to be technically demanding, with a steep learning curve [12–14]. It has not demonstrated any advantages over the more easily learned and less expensively performed radical perineal prostatectomy where the long-term cancer control rates are well known (authors' references 10,14,22). Radical prostatectomy effectively halts the natural progression of prostate cancer in the vast majority of properly selected men who undergo this operation via either the perineal or retropubic approach. Side effects are similar, but the perineal approach is associated with less pain, less blood loss, and shorter hospitalization.

REFERENCES

1. Villers A, McNeal JE, Freiha FS, Gibod L, Stamey TA. Invasion of Denonvilliers' fascia in radical prostatectomy specimens. J Urol 1993; 149:793–798.
2. Myers RP, Goellner JR, Cahill DR. Prostate shape, external striated urethral sphincter in radical prostatectomy: the apical dissection. J Urol 1987; 138:543–550.
3. Myers RP. Male urethral sphincteric anatomy and radical prostatectomy. Urol Clin North Am 1991; 18:211–227.
4. Hodges CV. Vesicourethral anastomosis after radical prostatectomy: Experience with the Jewett modification. J Urol 1977; 118:209–210.
5. Speakman CTM, Burnett SJD, Kamn MA, Bartram CI. Sphincter damage following anal dilatation revealed by anal endosonography. Br J Surg 1991; 78:1429–1430.
6. Corman ML. Colon and Rectal Surgery. Philadelphia: Lippincott-Raven, 1998: 285–343.
7. Bundrick WS, Gibbons RP, Weissman RM, Correa RJ. The long-term efficacy of radical prostatectomy in the management of localized prostate cancer [abstr 990]. J Urol 1996; 155(suppl):558A.
8. Rosen MA, Goldstone L, Lapin S, Wheeler T, Scardino PT. Frequency and location of extracapsular extension and positive surgical margins in radical prostatectomy specimens. J Urol 1992; 148:331–337.
9. Litwiller SE, Djavan B, Klopukh BV, Richier JC, Roehrborn CG. Radical retropubic prostatectomy for localized carcinoma of the prostate in a large metropolitan

hospital: Changing trends over a 10-year period (1984–1994). Urology 1995; 45: 813–822.

10. Trapasso JG, Weiss JP, Blaivas JG, Stember DS, Ravitz GA. Nerve-sparing radical perineal prostatectomy: Effect on margin status [abstr 1283]. J Urol 2000; 163(suppl):289.

11. Belt E, Ebert CE, Surber AC. A new anatomic approach in perineal prostatectomy. J Urol 1939; 41:482–497.

12. Gill IS, Zippe C, Savage S, Sung GT. Laparoscopic radical prostatectomy: the video [abstr V53]. J Urol 2000; 163(suppl):356.

13. Guillonneau B, Cathelineau X, Barret E, Rozet F, Vallancien G. Morbidity of laparoscopic radical prostatectomy: Evaluation after 210 procedures [abst 619]. J Urol 2000; 163(suppl):140.

14. Rassweiler J, Seemann O, El Quaran M, Sentker L, Stock C. Laparoscopic Radical Prostatectomy—early experience with the first 40 cases [abstr 622]. J Urol 2000; 163(suppl):141.

EDITORIAL COMMENTARY

Philipp Dahm and David F. Paulson

Division of Urology, Department of Surgery, Duke University Medical Center, Durham, North Carolina, USA

Resnick and Feng have provided an elegant description of their technique for radical perineal prostatectomy (RPP). Review of this manuscript and comparison with the original article of Hugh Hampton Young will quickly demonstrate how much and how little this surgery has changed in the intervening years. Although the basic surgical principles remain the same, many important technical details have been added. These details have resulted in the significantly decreased morbidity and favorable functional outcomes of modern RPP. The outlined suggestions as to the conduct of this operation deserve to be read and incorporated by all surgeons intending to perform this procedure, who each will, without doubt, find additional technical modifications to bring to the table. Over the years, we have modified our surgical approach many times at our institution, as will all surgeons as they seek to improve on outcome. In the following pages, we will outline a few technical modifications that one may wish to consider.

In our experience, the patient is optimally positioned in full-exaggerated lithotomy position. This position places the prostate approximately 18 inches above the cardiac silhouette. Such positioning reduces the venous pressure and venous backflow, contributing to a reduction in overall blood loss. This position also permits the surgeon to take full advantage of the greatest distance from the inferior arch of the pubis and the greatest breadth of the inverted V of the pubic rami. While lower extremity neuropraxia is a recognized complication of this position [1], it is rarely observed in patients with an operating time of less than two hours.

The incision is carried in a large inverted U behind the anus on either side. This permits the anus and rectum to be dropped far posterior and allows maximum exposure of the prostate. Once the incision is made and the ischial rectal fossa has been developed, the central tendon is digitally mobilized and divided at the point of its insertion on the perineal body. The central tendon is later reattached to the perineal body at the time of closure, thereby restoring the perineal anatomy to its preoperative status.

After division of the central tendon, the rectum will drop posterior. The prostate is approached over the external anal sphincter, the rectourethralis identified in the midline and placed on traction by the use of a gloved finger in the rectum. In our current practice, the rectourethralis is no longer completely divided, but the most external fibers nipped with a curved scissors, and the avascular space within the two lateral leaves of the rectourethralis separated in the midline. This leaves the rectourethralis available for closure over the anterior rectal fascia at the time of closure, a factor that may contribute to fecal continence in the early postoperative period. As emphasized by the authors, active manipulation of the Lowsley tractor during this phase of the procedure significantly aids the surgeon in orientating himself with the perineal anatomy.

As the lateral fibers of the rectourethralis are separated, the surface of the prostate will come into view. The next most important portion of this procedure is exposure of the prostate and its apex in the midline. One or both neurovascular bundles can be effectively spared, or not, as the clinical situation dictates. However, posterior exposure of the prostate apex allows the surgeon to encircle the urethra with a right angle clamp and liberate the urethra from the ventral prostatic notch, thereby preserving the maximum portion of urethral length. Achieving maximal urethral length is likely an important factor that impacts upon the degree of postoperative continence that may be achieved [2].

Following removal of the prostate, a wide margin of bladder neck is removed. After years of bladder neck preservation and years of wide resection of the bladder neck, we believe that there is no difference in the postoperative continence rates [3]. The bladder neck is reconstructed in a racket handle fashion from 6 o'clock with absorbable sutures, snug around a regular 18 French catheter. In our opinion, a small amount of postoperative stricture may be more preferable to a lax anastamosis. The urethra is brought to the reconstructed bladder neck with 4–0 absorbable sutures and is buttressed with anterior and posterior Vest sutures that are tied below the skin after the modification of Dees [4]. It may be possible to omit these Vest sutures, however, they provide a degree of comfort for the surgeon should the catheter become dislodged in the early postoperative period.

Outcome data demonstrates that cancer control is equivalent to other institutional series whether based on histopathologic grade or local extent of disease [5–7]. The notion that RPP may be associated with an increased incidence of iatrogenic margins when compared to RRP [8] has recently been refuted in a centralized, blinded comparison of whole-mount RPP and RPP specimens [9]. The capsular incision rate was 4% in both groups. Furthermore, no difference between RPP and RRP specimen was observed with regard to the distance between pT2 or pT3 tumors and the posterolateral margin.

Functional outcomes in terms of continence are at least equivalent to those of RRP [10,11]. A recent longitudinal assessment of patients at our institution using a validated self-assessment instrument found the median time to recover urinary continence to be 3.0 to 3.3 months, depending upon the type of definition of continence that was applied. Despite the low incidence of rectal injury in RPP in the hands of an experienced surgeon, patient preparation should include a full mechanical and antibiotic bowel prep. This practice permits primary repair of all but the most extensive rectal injuries associated with gross fecal spillage. Intraoperative recognition of the injury, though, is paramount, and, for this reason, we routinely perform a digital rectal exam prior to reconstructing the perineal body. Closure is then performed in at least two layers of viable tissue using absorbable, monofilament suture material.

A study by Bishoff et al. reported a fecal incontinence rate of up to 15% in patients following RPP [12], an observation that prompted us to perform a prospective study to evaluate the incidence of bowel related symptoms and complaints, and fecal incontinence in particular. We found an unexpectedly high prevalence of involuntary stool leakage of some degree in 11.5% of patients prior to any form of treatment. Postoperatively, compared to their individual baseline, 7.7% and 3.9% of patients reported worsened symptoms of fecal incontinence after 6 and 12 months, respectively. Patients who denied preoperative fecal incontinence had a postoperative incidence of involuntary stool leakage of only 2.9% by 12 months following RPP, a figure significantly lower than previously reported. Based on these findings, we conclude that fecal incontinence and bowel-related symptoms may indeed be more prevalent in the early postoperative period following RPP compared to baseline, yet resolve for the majority of patients.

Contemporary RPP is a truly minimally invasive approach when it comes to postoperative analgesia requirements, recovery of bowel function, length of hospital stay, and time to recover full activity [10]. As such, it should continue to be taught to residents and offered to patients seeking curative treatment for organ-confined disease. The decreasing need for performing bilateral lymph node dissections in patients of the PSA-era is likely to further promote the renaissance of this approach. The authors should be commended for their excellent description of modern RRP, as well as their state of the art review of the contemporary literature.

REFERENCES

1. Price DT, Vieweg J, Roland F, Coetzee L, Spalding T, Iselin C, Paulson DF. Transient lower extremity neurapraxia associated with radical perineal prostatectomy: a complication of the exaggerated lithotomy position. J of Urol 1998; 160: 1376–1378.
2. Coakley FV, Eberhardt S, Kattan MW, Wei DC, Scardino PT, Hricak H. Urinary continence after radical retropubic prostatectomy: relationship with membranous urethral length on preoperative endorectal magnetic resonance imaging. J Urol 2002; 168:1032–1035.
3. Srougi M, Nesrallah LJ, Kauffmann JR, Nesrallah A, Leite KR. Urinary continence and pathological outcome after bladder neck preservation during radical retropubic prostatectomy: a randomized prospective trial. J Urol 2001; 165:815–818.
4. Thrasher JB, Paulson DF. Reappraisal of radical perineal prostatectomy. European Urology 1992; 22:1–8.
5. Lance RS, Freidrichs PA, Kane C, Powell CR, Pulos E, Moul JW, McLeod DG, Cornum RL, Brantley Thrasher J. A comparison of radical retropublic with perineal prostatectomy for localized prostate cancer within the Uniformed Services Urology Research Group. BJU Int 2001; 87:61–65.
6. Sullivan LD, Weir MJ, Kinahan JF, Taylor DL. A comparison of the relative merits of radical perineal and radical retropubic prostatectomy. BJU Int 2000; 85:95–100.
7. Frazier HA, Robertson JE, Paulson DF. Radical prostatectomy: the pros and cons of the perineal versus retropubic approach. J of Urol 1992; 147:888–890.
8. Boccon-Gibod L, Ravery V, Vordos D, Toublanc M, Delmas V. Radical prostatectomy for prostate cancer: the perineal approach increases the risk of surgically induced positive margins and capsular incisions. J of Urol 1998; 160:1383–1385.
9. Korman HJ, Leu PB, Huang RR, Goldstein NS. A centralized comparison of radical perineal and retropubic prostatectomy specimens: is there a difference according to the surgical approach?. J Urol 2002; 168:991–994.
10. Weldon VE. Technique of modern radical perineal prostatectomy. Urology 2002; 60:689–694.
11. Harris MJ, Thompson IM. The anatomic radical perineal prostatectomy: a contemporary and anatomic approach. Urology 1996; 48:762–768.
12. Bishoff JT, Motley G, Optenberg SA, Stein CR, Moon KA, Browning SM, Sabanegh E, Foley JP, Thompson IM. Incidence of fecal and urinary incontinence following radical perineal and retropubic prostatectomy in a national population. J of Urol 1998; 160:454–458.

EDITORIAL OVERVIEW

Kenneth B. Cummings

Feng and Resnick provide strong arguments favoring radical perineal prostatectomy (RPP) in a PSA era where patient selection and the need for pelvic lymphadectomy may be avoided. Their elegant anatomic illustration of the technique provides the basis for understanding and applying this surgical procedure. Continence data for RPP is equal or superior to that of radical retropubic prostatectomy (RRP) [1], while potency data for RPP compared to RRP in the better series exhibits a significant advantage for RRP in that the best RPP series reflects a 70% preservation of potency [2].

Further, the comprehensive review of outcomes for RPP demonstrate the procedure to be competitive to RRP with respect to cancer control when reported in established series [3].

Gibbons advocates the importance of an adequate cancer operation as a first priority. As such, he prefers leaving the Denonvellier's fascia in its entirety on the prostate and seminal vesicles, to reduce the risk of positive surgical margins. He remains unenthusiastic with respect to nerve-sparing RPP, citing positive margin rates 24% higher in patients undergoing nerve sparing vs. nonsparing RPP [4].

Harris has been a student of the RPP and has modified his approach from his 1995 description. From 1995 to January 2002, bladder neck and proximal urethral preservation was intended in all patients. He performed a urethrourethrostomy with 8 to 10 sutures. He ultimately removed the urethral catheter in eight days and reports pad-free continence rates of 96% at one year.

His anatomic technique for RPP employs Young's suprasphincteric approach to the pelvic floor [5], Belt's early dissection of the seminal vesicles [6] and Weldon's method of cavernosal nerve preservation [7].

Dehm and Paulson describe their modification to the Feng-Resnick technique.

The apical dissection is in the midline, with one or both nervovascular bundles preserved. They describe encirclement of the urethral from the perineal approach with a right-angle clamp permitting liberation of the urethra from the "prostate notch," achieving maximal urethral length and thereby improving continence. Potency rates are not reported.

REFERENCES

1. Harris MJ, Thompson IM. Radical perineal prostatectomy, early dissection of seminal vesicles. In: Resnick MI , Thompson IM, Eds. Surgery of the Prostate. New York: Churchill Livingstone, 1998:131–165.

2. Weldon VE, Tavel FR, Neuwirth H. Continence, potency and morbidity after radical perineal prostatectomy. J Urol 1997; 158:1470–1475.
3. Islin CE, Robertson JE, Paulson DF. Radical perineal prostatectomy: Oncological outcome during a 20-year period. J Urol 1999; 161:163–168.
4. Trapasso JG, Weiss JP, Blaivas JG, Stember DS, Ravitz GA. Nerve-sparing radical perineal prostatectomy: effect on margin status (abstr 1283). J Urol 2000; 163(suppl):289.
5. Young HH. The early diagnosis and radical cure of carcinoma of the prostate: being a study of 40 cases and presentation of a radical operation, which was carried out in four cases. Bull Johns Hopkins Hosp 1905; 16:315.
6. Belt E. Radical perineal prostatectomy in early carcinoma of the prostate. J Urol 1942; 78:287.
7. Weldon VE, Tavel FR. Potency-sparing radical perineal prostatectomy: anatomy, surgical technique and initial results. J Urol 1988; 140:559–562.

3

Laparoscopic Radical Prostatectomy

Sidney C. Abreu, Andrew P. Steinberg, and Inderbir S. Gill
Cleveland Clinic Foundation, Cleveland, Ohio, USA

1. INTRODUCTION

Since Millin reported the first retropubic approach for prostate surgery in 1947 [1], the urological community has concentrated their efforts on learning and refining this technique. Although radical retropubic prostatectomy remains an intricate operation, several anatomical discoveries in the past twenty years have changed the face of this surgery. As such, it has evolved from an unpopular operation with significant morbidity into an anatomically precise dissection [2].

Recently, laparoscopy has been incorporated into the urological armamentarium as an alternative technique for the treatment of localized prostate cancer. Laparoscopic radical prostatectomy (LRP) aims to simulate the open retropubic approach [3]. Due to its enhanced visualization and magnification, laparoscopy has the potential to have a favorable impact on the morbidity and functional sequelae related to this operation.

In the initial report of LRP by Schuessler et al. in 1991 [4], the authors concluded that the laparoscopic procedure ''offers no advantage over open surgery'' mainly because of the extreme length of operative time (mean 9.4 hours) [5]. However, in the past 3 years, improvement in laparoscopic skills, confidence, and technology has turned LRP into an efficient day-to-day practice at selected centers. In this endeavor, enormous credit goes to the French team of Guillonneau and Vallencien from Montsouris [6], who ultimately pioneered, and validated, the technique of LRP.

At our institution, we have been developing the technique of LRP to duplicate the principles of the open radical retropubic technique practiced in the United States today [7]. Our experience with LRP approaches 250 cases, and includes experience in both transperitoneal and extraperitoneal approach. In this chapter, we describe our step-by-step laparoscopic radical prostatectomy technique, highlighting some modifications incorporated by our team and discussing how each step is related to the anatomical and functional outcome of this challenging procedure.

2. PATIENT SELECTION

Proper patient selection is paramount in achieving adequate surgical and oncological outcomes. As such, patients need to fulfill two sets of criteria.

Criteria for Undergoing Radical Prostatectomy

The laparoscopic approach follows the well-established oncological principles for the open radical prostatectomy. Therefore, like in most centers that routinely performed conventional open prostatectomy, this approach is reserved for patients with clinically localized prostate (T1, T2) cancer. The surgical treatment of advanced stages (T3, T4) remains controversial.

Criteria for Undergoing Laparoscopy

Prior hormone treatment or localized radiation therapy will increase the potential for operative morbidity. However, in our experience, they are no longer a formal contraindication for the laparoscopic approach. A large prostate gland will also raise the level of technical difficulty. Nonetheless, we have performed this procedure successfully in patients with a prostate glands weighting up to 220 grams. Previous abdominal surgery, such as appendectomy, is not an absolute contraindication for the laparoscopic technique either; however, difficulty may be encountered while gaining intraperitoneal access. Extra care should be taken during initial trocar insertion. Obesity is not, in itself, a contraindication to the laparoscopic approach, although it significantly increases the level of technical difficulty. Our heaviest patient has weighted 350 pounds.

3. PREOPERATIVE PREPARATION AND PATIENT POSITION

Two bottles of magnesium citrate are self-administered by the patient at home on the afternoon before surgery. The patient reports to the hospital on the morning of the procedure. Broad-spectrum intravenous antibiotics and subcutaneous heparin are given. Bilateral sequential compression devices are placed routinely. The patient is placed in a modified lithotomy position (thighs abducted) with the arms adducted to facilitate simultaneous abdominal and perineal access. The abdomen, penis, scrotum, upper thighs, and perineal region are prepared with iodine-based disinfectant and draped. A Foley catheter is inserted in the sterile field and the bladder drained. The table is set in a Trendelenburg position, with the degree of head-down inclination varying depending on the proposed approach [8].

4. PORT PLACEMENT

The Montsouris transperitoneal approach for LRP was described by Guillonneau and Vallencien [8]; the reader is refered to their article for an in-depth description.

At the Cleveland Clinic, five ports are arranged in a ''fan'' configuration in the pelvic area (Figure 1). In this port configuration, the surgeon uses the 12 mm port and the 5 mm port inserted respectively along the right and left lateral border of the rectus muscle, approximately 2 fingerbreadths below the umbilicus.

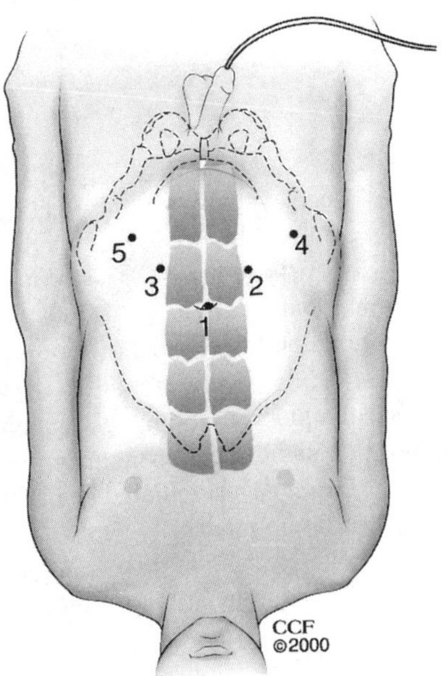

FIGURE 1   For either the transperitoneal or the extraperitoneal approach, 5 ports are employed in a "fan" array.

5 mm ports are placed 2 fingerbreadths medial to each anterior superior iliac spine and are used by the assistant for retraction and suction purposes.

5. LAPAROSCOPIC ROUTE SELECTION

As the laparoscopic technique for radical prostatectomy evolved, three different approaches to the prostate gland were described. Initially, Guilloneau and Vallencien described a *transperitoneal posterior approach*, in which the dissection initially commences at the rectovesical cul-de-sac [8]. A transverse peritoneotomy is created at the second peritoneal fold in the rectovesical cul-de-sac, and the seminal vesicles and vas deferens are mobilized circumferentially using bipolar electrocautery. At the Cleveland Clinic, we initially explored this posterior transperitoneal approach for LRP. However, in an attempt to bring the laparoscopic technique more in line with the open procedures, we shifted our technique to a pure *extraperitoneal approach* [11,12]. However, in our hands, the extraperitoneal approach allows a smaller working space and was found to be technically demanding and skill intensive [13]. Our current approach of choice for LRP is the *anterior transperitoneal approach* [14]. In this technique, no dissection is performed at the rectovesical cul-de-sac. Access to the Retzius' space is gained after the bladder is mobilized anteriorly. Although this modified route transgresses the peritoneal cavity, it allows a more familiar view of the landmarks with minimal bowel manipulation [10,14].

6. SURGICAL TECHNIQUE

For the transperitoneal approach, the bladder is distended with 200 ml of saline through the indwelling Foley incision located medial to the ipsilateral medial umbilical ligament (Figure 2). The horizontal part of the U-incision is located high on the undersurface of the anterior abdominal wall. This helps to prevent inadvertent bladder injury and to preclude the parietal peritoneum from hanging in front of, and thereby compromising, the surgical view. Circumferential dissection of the bladder is performed in a virtually avascular plane, involving dissection of delicate fibrofatty septae. Once the symphysis pubis has been visualized, the bladder is actively emptied using the bulb syringe. Dissection is initiated laterally on either side, completely exposing the endopelvic fascia bilaterally.

For the extraperitoneal approach, a trocar-mounted balloon dissection device (US Surgical, Norwalk, CT) is used for rapid and atraumatic creation of a working space in the extraperitoneum (Figure 3).

An incision is made on the anterior rectus fascia just below the umbilicus, and the trocar-mounted balloon is inserted and advanced down toward the pelvis under the rectus aponeurosis until the pubic bone is reached. At this point, the tip of the trocar is gently pushed underneath the pubic bone, entering the transver-

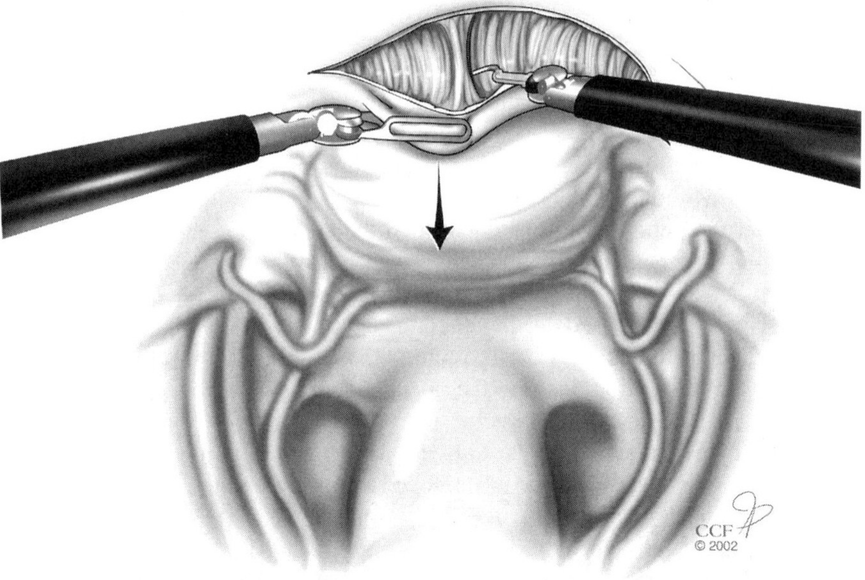

FIGURE 2 Exposure of Retzius' space during the transperitoneal anterior approach. Any kind of dissection is no longer performed at the rectovesical space.

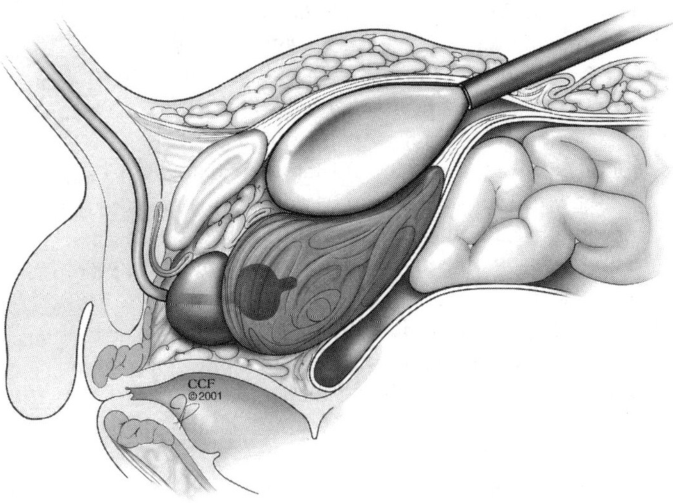

FIGURE 3 Air is instilled into the balloon to develop the prevesical working space.

salis fascia to reach the prevesical space. Typically, only 200–300 ml of air are instilled into the balloon for inflation. The laparoscope is inserted to ensure the adequate positioning of the balloon.

Following dilation, the balloon is deflated and removed. A 10-mm Bluntip trocar (Origin Medsystems, Menlo Park, CA) is inserted as the primary port to assure an airtight seal, which, in our experience, is more difficult to achieve with a standard Hasson cannula [15].

After the puboprostatic ligaments and the endopelvic fascia on either side are exposed and the superficial dorsal vein is controlled, the prostate is retracted tautly to the left side, placing the right endopelvic fascia on the stretch. The endopelvic fascia is incised distally up to the lateral-most puboprostatic ligament. Visualization of the apex of the prostate is the endpoint of this dissection. We minimize any dissection distal to the prostate apex, such as to not compromise this nerve-rich, sphincter-active zone.

The Foley catheter is replaced by an 18 Fr metallic urethral sound. A 2–0 vicryl stitch with a CT-1 needle is employed to ligate the dorsal vein. This stitch is placed in a back-hand manner from the right to the left side, distal to the apex of the prostate, between the dorsal vein complex and the urethra. In order to avoid inadvertent transgression of the urethra by the suture, the assistant pushes down the metallic sound, displacing the urethra posteriorly. A back-bleeding stitch is placed across the anterior surface of the prostate base, and the tails of this stitch are cut somewhat long.

The long tails of the previously placed back-bleeding stitch are grasped and tautly retract anteriorly, thus elevating and "fixing" the base of the prostate. The bladder is tautly retracted cephalad, thereby placing the anterior bladder neck on traction. The precise anatomic location of the junction between the prostate and the bladder neck is not well defined under laparoscopic visualization. The absence of landmarks for the bladder neck identification is overcome by a combination of maneuvers: close laparoscopic visualization usually identifies the area where the prevesical fat ends, signifying the prostatovesical junction. Gentle blunt dissection with the elbow of the J-hook eletrocautery tip also aids to define this junctional area. Repeated in-and-out movements of the metallic urethral dilator, with its curved tip pointing anteriorly, provides another clue where the prostate ends and where the bladder begins.

At the presumed prostatovesical junction, a horizontal incision is created using J-hook eletrocautery. The initial dissection aims to develop the plane laterally on each side of the bladder neck. The anterior bladder neck is divided in the midline, and the tip of the urethral dilator is delivered through the cystotomy into the space of Retzius.

Upon transecting the anterior bladder neck, the remaining posterior bladder neck is clearly seen. Using a J-hook electrocautery, the posterior bladder neck is scored away from the ureteral orifices. The posterior bladder neck is then grasped in the midline with a laparoscopic Allis and gently retracted cephalad. The plane between the posterior bladder neck and the prostate is developed with a J-hook electrocautery. Care should be taken to avoid inadvertent creation of a "button hole" on the posterior bladder wall.

We do not make a major effort to spare the bladder neck, which may result in a positive surgical margin at this location. However, a carefully dissected bladder neck can avoid the extra step of bladder neck reconstruction.

The incision on the posterior bladder neck is deepened for approximately 2–4 mm until the anterior layer of the Denonvilier's fascia is encountered. The surgeon must create a wide enough transverse incision to avoid "digging into a hole." The anterior layer of the Denonvilier's fascia is incised and the vasa deferentia are identified, grasped with a laparoscopic Allis clamp, and retracted cephalad (Figure 4). Dissection is carried along its lateral border to identify the ipsilateral seminal vesicle, which is mobilized circumferentially. The vesicular vessels are carefully secured using a combination of harmonic scalpel and hemolock clips. This is carried distally to its junction with the prostate.

The mobilized vas deferens and seminal vesicles are tautly retracted anteriorly, which places the posterior layer of Denonviliers' fascia under traction. A

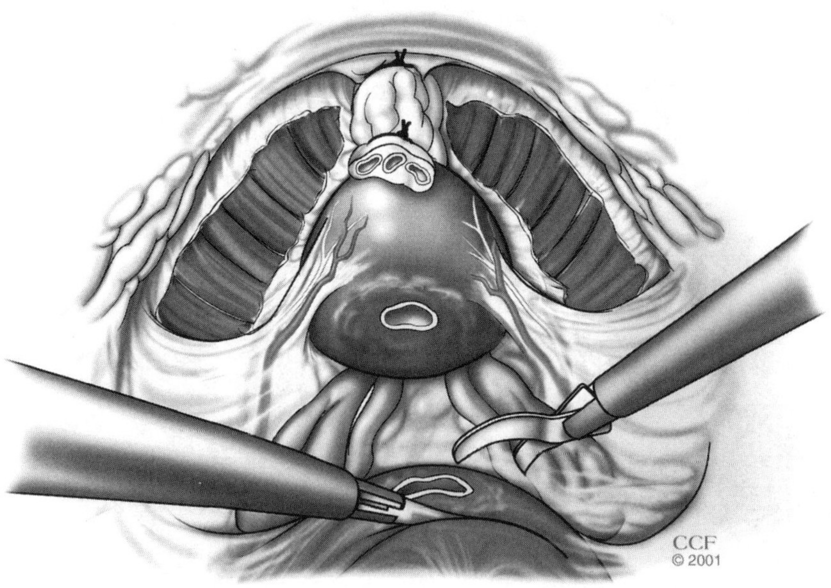

FIGURE 4　The posterior bladder neck is incised. The posterior layer of Denonvilliers' fascia is entered and the vas deferens are identified.

small horizontal incision is created and enlarged with blunt dissection. Making this incision approximately 2 to 3 mm posterior to the junction of the seminal vesicles with the prostate allows proper entry into the prerectal plane posterior to the prostate.

In a nonnerve-sparing procedure, while placing the adjacent lateral pedicle on traction, an articulating Endo-GIA stapler (vascular cartridge, 2.5 mm) is fired across each pedicle. A second Endo-GIA cartridge is employed to completely detach the lateral border of the prostate and the neurovascular bundle from the perirectal fat (Figure 5). A similar maneuver is performed on the contralateral side, leaving the prostate attached near its apex only.

The optimal technique of the nerve-sparing approach is still evolving. In this regard, we have incorporated a few technical maneuvers to improve potency outcome: (1) upon opening the endopelvic fascia, while releasing the levator muscles from the apex and lateral aspect of the prostate, no electrical energy is used near the neurovascular bundle (NVB); (2) following dorsal vein ligation, the lateral prostate fascia is bilaterally incised superficially with "cold" Endoshears in order to release the tethering of the NVB; and (3) aiming to minimize eletrocautery trauma to the NVB near the tip of the seminal vesicles, by securing

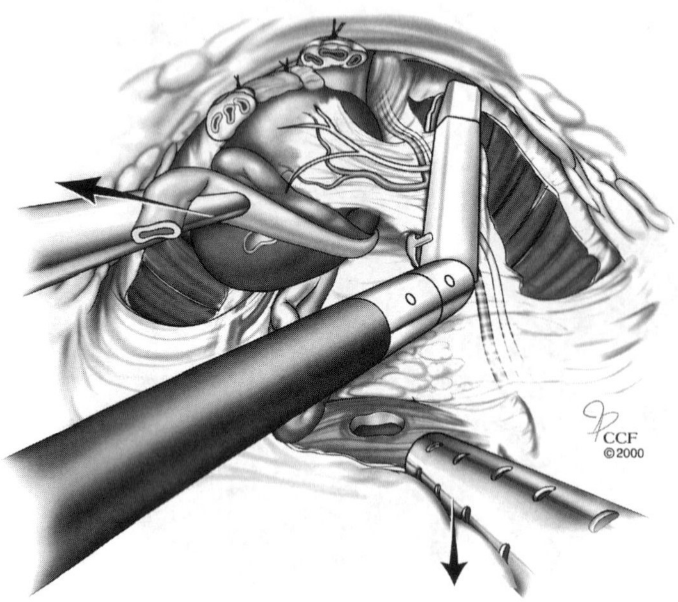

FIGURE 5 In a nonnerve-sparing procedure, an articulated Endo-GIA is used to widely transect the lateral pedicle and ipsilateral neurovascular bundle en bloc.

the vesicular artery with hemostatic locking clips (Weck Systems, Triangle Park, NC).

The nerve-sparing technique itself is performed in a combined antegrade-retrograde fashion. Initially, the lateral pedicles of the prostate are controlled with one or two 10 mm Hemolock clips (Weck Systems, Triangle Park, NC). The posterolateral edge of the prostate base is identified and the harmonic scalpel is employed to develop a plane between the gland and the NVB. The harmonic scalpel is preferred because of its limited spread of thermal energy (1–2 mm). We believe that further refinements in equipment that have no spread of any source of energy may lead to earlier recovery and higher rates of potency.

Using a laparoscopic Allis clamp, the transected base of the prostate is grasped with significant cephalad traction, placing the urethra and the dorsal vein complex on the stretch. Subsequently, the harmonic scalpel is used to divide the dorsal vein complex along the curvature of the apex of the prostate. Occasionally, the dorsal vein stitch may loosen, leading to venous bleed. However, due to the tamponade effect of the CO_2 pneumoperitoneum, the degree of hemorrhage is usually not significant, and it is controlled by placing another stitch (2–0 vicryl, CT-1 needle) around the transected dorsal vein.

After the dorsal venous complex is divided, the anterior urethral wall is identified with the aid of the metallic urethral sound. Cold Endoshears are used to transect the anterior urethral wall close to the concave notch of the prostate, which assures preservation of an excellent urethral stump. The tip of the intraurethral metallic sound is delivered through the urethral opening. The posterior urethral wall and the rectourethralis muscles are divided. During this maneuver, which completely detaches the prostate, extreme care is taken to avoid inadvertent entry into the prostatic apex and rectum. The prostate is entrapped immediately in a 10 mm Endocatch bag (US Surgical, Norwalk, CT) and placed in the abdomen until extraction at the end of the case.

The bladder neck is evaluated closely and biopsied if there is suspicion that prostatic tissue was left behind. The ureteric orifices are assessed and if there is any doubt as to their integrity, intravenous indigo carmine can be administered. A running suture (UR-6 needle, 3–0 vicryl) is employed to tighten the posterior bladder neck if necessary. Due to the superb mucosa-to-mucosa laparoscopic urethrovesical anastomosis, bladder neck eversion is not performed [9].

During open retropubic radical prostatectomy, the pubic bone impairs the visibility and access to the urethral stump, making the placement of sutures difficult. In addition, the surgeon must tie the knots in a blind field and rely on tactile sensation alone. Comparatively, during laparoscopic radical prostatectomy, all sutures are meticulously placed and tied under complete visual control [16].

In our early experience, the urethrovesical anastomosis was performed with 6 to 8 interrupted sutures. With increased laparoscopic suturing skills, we switched to a running suture technique in an attempt to decrease the anastomotic time and postoperative urinary leak [16,17]. The running suture technique frequently results in a watertight anastomosis immediately after the operation, and, thus, the urethral Foley catheter can be removed safely as early as 2 to 4 postoperative days [17].

Optimal preparation of the bladder neck and the urethral stump is paramount for the adequacy of the urethrovesical anastomosis. Two full-thickness mucosa-to-mucosa hemicircumferential running sutures are placed in a preplanned, choreographed sequence. Using 2 needle holders, an initial stitch (UR-6 with a 2–0 vicryl) is placed and tied at the 5 o'clock position, approximating the bladder neck to the urethral stump. Subsequently, this suture is run in a clockwise direction to the 11 o'clock position (Figure 6), where it is pulled toward the symphis pubis and maintained under traction by an assistant. At least 3 to 4 needle passes are necessary to create an adequate posterior plate. The metallic sound is used to guide the needle, which glides into the urethra as the sound is retracted. A 22 Fr urethral Foley catheter is advanced into the bladder. A second stitch is placed at 5 o'clock and run counterclockwise to 11 o'clock, where it is tied to the previous placed stitch.

A Jackson-Pratt drain is inserted through one of the 5-mm port sites. The specimen is extracted through an extension of the umbilical incision. Fascial

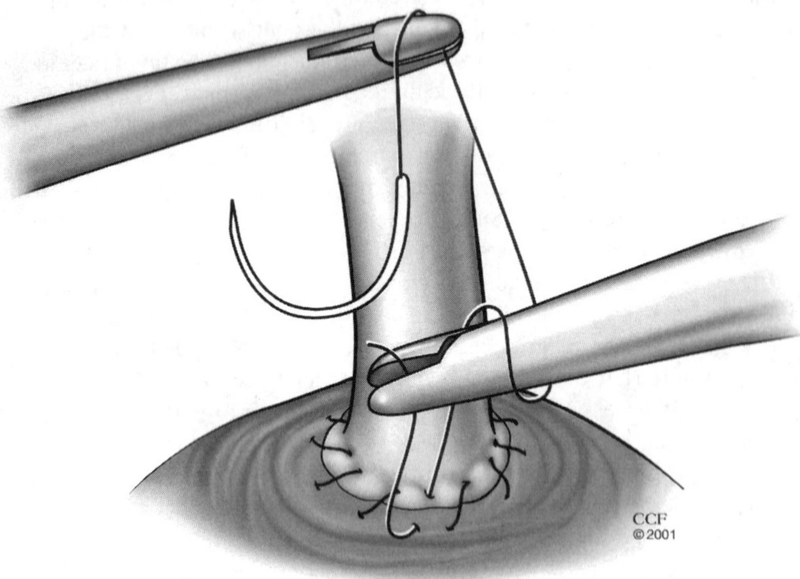

FIGURE 6   Under excellent laparoscopic visualization, a precise mucosa-to-mucosa approximation is completed during the urethrovesical anastomosis using running suture technique.

closure of the 12 mm port site is achieved with a Carter-Thomason needle device and a 0 vicryl suture.

7. INTRA-OPERATIVE DATA

High operative blood loss and transfusion is a common problem of prostate surgery. A major advantage of the LRP is the potential to reduce operative blood loss. The magnified view of the dorsal venous complex provided by the laparoscope combined with the tamponading effect of the 15 mm Hg pressure of CO_2 pneumoperitoneum are important factors which help decrease venous bleeding. The precise knowledge of the anatomy and the acquisition of experience by the surgeon are also important issues related to the reduced blood loss during LRP [18].

In a review of 1228 LRP at 6 European centers, the average blood loss was 488 mL with a transfusion rate of 3.5% [17]. The French team of Guillonneau and Vallancien also reported a mean intraoperative blood loss of 354 mL with a transfusion rate of 5.7% (20 patients) in a series of 350 LRP [18]. At the Cleveland Clinic, the average blood loss of our first 100 patients was only 322 mL [19], resulting in transfusion of 2 patients (Table 1).

8. PERIOPERATIVE COMPLICATIONS

The meticulous tissue handling and dissection during LRP have translated into low surgical and postoperative complications (Table 2) [18,19,30]. However, issues such anastomotic leak and rectal injury require more attention and are discussed in further detail below.

Anastomotic leak, which is usually defined as persistent extravasation at the anastomotic site for more than 7 days, occurs mainly because of the tear of the urethra by the suture at the anastomosis. During LRP, the magnified view may lead into an overestimation of the amount of tissue in the bite of the suture. Ideally, the depth of the suture is 4–5 mm on both bladder and urethral sides. In this manner, care must be taken to get sufficient width of tissue in the anastomosis [16].

Rectal injuries mainly occur when the rectourethralis muscle is divided after insufficient dissection between the rectum and the prostate, and less frequently when the posterior layer of Denonviliers' fascia is incised [20]. The surgeon must take caution to avoid inadvertent rectal injury during these steps. Rectal injury must be immediately recognized and repaired to avoid further consequences.

9. ONCOLOGIC RESULTS

Concerns about the high rate of positive surgical margins after LRP, even in a select group of patients with organ-confined disease, have been raised [21]. We

TABLE 1 Intraoperative Data

Author	Guillonneau(18)	Turk(30)	Hoznek(31)	Rassweiler(14)	Bollens(12)	Gill(19)
No. of patients	350	125	134	180	50	100
Approach	Transp.	Transp	Transp.	Transp.†	Extrap.‡	Transp Extrap
OR time (hr)	3.6	4.25	3.5*	4.5	4.4	4.5
Blood loss (cc)	354	185	–	1230	680	322
Transfusion rate	5.7%	2%	3%	31%	13%	2%
Open conversion	2%	0	0	4.4%	2%	1%

(*) Excludes first 20 patients
(†) With immediate access to Retzius' space
(‡) Includes 8 transperitoneal procedures

TABLE 2 Intraoperative and Postoperative Complications

	Guillonneau(20)	Turk(30)	Rassweiler(14)
No. of patients	567	125	180
Anastomotic stricture	–	2	6
Bladder injury	9	–	–
Ureteral injury	3	1	–
Ileus	6	4	5
Small bowel injury	2	1	–
Rectum injury	8	3	–
Rectourethral fistula	–	1	2
Epigastric injury	3	–	–
Iliac vein injury	–	1	–
Thrombosis*	2	3	–
Wound dehiscence	4	–	1

* Although, the combination of pelvic surgery, laparoscopic procedure, and cancer increases the risks of thrombosis, this is not clinically observed probably due to the prevention based on antithrombotic profilaxis, compression stockings, and early patient mobilization.

do agree that a rightfully strict inclusion criteria was employed by laparoscopic surgeons in their initial experiences, which may explain the larger percentage of organ-confined disease (surgical pathology) after LRP when compared with some large, open prostatectomy series. In regard to surgical margins status, we do believe that laparoscopy will likely be comparable to open surgery. To support this, our preliminary data show a drop of almost 50% on the positive surgical margin from our first 50 cases to our third 50 cases [19]. Refinements of our technique, especially the pristine dissection of the apex, were intrinsically related to this significant decrease on the rate of positive surgical margins.

Because definitive cure of prostate cancer needs a long follow-up, current available data are still quite immature. However, LRP is likely to emerge as a sound oncological alternative. Salomon and colleagues have reported a projected Kaplan-Meier biochemical (i.e., PSA) recurrence-free likelihood of 84% at three years (91% for organ-confined tumor and 81% for pT3 tumors) [22]. Guillonneau et al. have shown that in a subset of 250 patients who have undergone LRP, serum PSA remained less than 0.2 ng/mL [23]. More recently, Guillonneau and colleagues reported an oncological midterm evaluation of 1000 patients who underwent LRP. The overall actuarial biochemical progressionfree survival was 90.5% at 3 years. According to the pathological stage, the progression-free survival was 91.8% for pT2aN0, 88% for pT2bN0, 77% for pT3aN0 and 44% for pT3bN0. Patients with negative surgical margins had 94% progression-free survival, while those with positive margin status had 80% (p <0.001) [24].

10. FUNCTIONAL OUTCOME

10.1 Urinary Continence

The laparoscopic technique has the potential to improve the postoperative continence rates due to the outstanding urethrovesical anastomosis performed under
laparoscopic visualization. Guillonneau et al. reported on their first 133 patients
with at least a 1-year follow-up and found 85.5% were totally continent (no
protection needed during day or night) [18]. Five patients (3.8%) were classified
as severely incontinent. Nadu et al. have reported continence rates greater then
93% in a median follow-up of 7 months (range from 1 to 15). In this particular
study, the urethrovesical anastomosis was performed with a single circular running 3–0 polyglactin stitch. Only 15.1% of the patients had anastomotic leak on
postoperative day 2–4 cystography. No anastomotic stricture, pelvic abscess, or
urinoma were noticed in this series [17].

10.2. Potency

The anatomical course of the neurovascular bundles is well known, yet it is often
difficult to preserve one or both nerves. Laparoscopy, with its unparalleled vision
allows for excellent identification and handling of the neurovascular bundles.
The potential to improve on postoperative potency rates exists, but outcome data
with nerve-sparing techniques of LRP are sparse. Guillonneau et al. reviewed 73
of their patients who had either bilateral (46 patients) or unilateral (27 patients)
nerve-sparing LRP [25]. An impressive 74% spontaneous erection rate was reported in the bilateral nerve-sparing group, and 51% in the unilateral group, where
a follow-up ranging from 2 to 12 months was employed. Bollens et al. had a
9-month potency rate of 75% in patients who were potent preoperatively [26].
Salomon and colleagues describe a one-month positive erection rate in 40% of
patients with bilateral nerve-sparing, and in 22.2% of patients with unilateral
nerve-sparing procedures [27]. More recently, Katz et al. reported a postoperative
potency rate at 1 year in 87.5% of patients with bilateral nerve-sparing [28]. These
authors found that the overall rate of patients who had erections preoperatively and
maintained erections after surgery (53.8%) was comparable to the overall rate
for patients who underwent open surgery.

11. CONCLUSION

The lessons learned with laparoscopic renal surgery may not be valid for laparoscopic prostatectomy. From the very initial cases with laparoscopic renal surgery,
it was apparent that morbidity was markedly reduced [29]. With laparoscopic
radical prostatectomy, the avoidance of a low midline incision may not have the
same implications, and further prospective studies are necessary. Nonetheless,

diminished blood loss, excellent length of urethral stump, superb watertight urethrovesical anastomosis, and unparalleled visualization of the neurovascular bundles provided by the laparoscopic technique may allow this minimally invasive approach to overcome the already higher outcomes obtained with open radical prostatectomy.

REFERENCES

1. Millin T. Retropubic Urinary Surgery. London: Livingtone, 1947.
2. Walsh PC, Donker PJ. Impotency following radical prostatectomy: insight into etiology and prevention. J Urol 1982; 128:492–497.
3. Andriole GL. Laparoscopic radical prostatectomy. Con Urology 2001; 58:507–508.
4. Schuessler WW, Kavoussi LR, Clayman RV, Vancaille T. Laparoscopic radical prostatectomy: initial case report. J Urol 1992; 147:246A.
5. Schluesser W, Shulman P, Clayman RV. Laparoscopic radical prostatectomy: initial short-term experience. Urology 1997; 50:854.
6. Guillonneau B, Vallancien G. Laparoscopic radical prostatectomy: the Montsouris experience. J Urol 2000; 163:418–422.
7. Sung G, Meraney A, Zippe C, Gill S. Technical improvements in laparoscopic radical prostatectomy. J Urol 2001; 165(Suppl):181.
8. Guillenneau B, Vallancien G. Laparoscopic radical prostatectomy: the Mountsouris technique. J Urol 2000; 163:1643–1649.
9. Gill I, Zippe C. Laparoscopic radical prostatectomy: technique. Urol Clin North Am 2001; 28:423–436.
10. Steinberg A, Gill I. Laparoscopic radical prostatectomy. Contemporary Urol 2002; 14:34–49.
11. Raboy A, Ferzli G, Albert P. Initial experience with extraperitoneal endoscopic radical retropubic prostatectomy. Urology 1997; 50:849–853.
12. Bollens R, Bossche MV, Roumeguere T, Damoun A, Ekane S, Hoffmann P, Zlotta AR, Schulman CC. Extraperitoneal laparoscopic radical prostatectomy. Eur Urol 2001; 40:65–69.
13. Abreu S, Gill I, Kaouk J, Matin S, Meraney A, Farouk A, Steinberg A, Desai M, Zippe C, Sung G. Laparoscopic radical prostatectomy: comparison of transperitoneal versus extraperitoneal approach. J Urol 2002; 167(4, Suppl):19.
14. Rassweiler J, Sentker L, Seemann O, Hatzinger M, Rumpelt HJ. Laparoscopic radical prostatectomy with the Heilbronn technique: an analysis of the first 180 cases. J Urol 2001; 166:2101–2108.
15. Gill S. Retroperitoneal laparoscopic nephrectomy. Urol Clin North Am 1998; 25:343.
16. Hoznek A, Salomon L, Rabii R, Slama MB, Cicco A, Antiphon P, Abbou CC. Vesicourethral anastomosis during laparoscopic radical prostatectomy: the running suture method. J Endourol 2000; 14:749–753.
17. Nadu A, Salomon L, Hoznek A, Olsson LE, Saint F, Taile A, Cicco A, Chopin D, Abbou CC. Early removal of the catheter after laparoscopic radical prostatectomy. J Urol 2001; 166:1662–1664.

18. Guillonneau B, Cathelineau X, Doublet JD, Vallancien G. Laparoscopic radical prostatectomy: the lessons learned. J Endourol 2001; 15:441–445.

19. Farouk A, Gill I, Kaouk J, Matin S, Meraney A, Desai M, Abreu S, Steinberg A, Zippe C, Sung G. 150 laparoscopic radical prostatectomy (LRP): learning curve in the United the States. J Endourology 2002; 16(Suppl 1, A33):P9–2.

20. Guillenneau B, Rozet F, Cathelineau X, Frank L, Barret E, Doublet JD, Baumert H, Vallancien G. Perioperative complications of laparoscopic radical prostatectomy: the Montsouris 3-year experience. J Urol 2002; 167:51–56.

21. Walsh PC. Minimally invasive treatment of prostate cancer. J Endourol 2001; 15:447–448.

22. Salomon L, Hoznek A, Saint F, Cicco A, Antiphon P, Chopin DK, Abbou CC. Oncologic results of 100 consecutive laparoscopic radical prostatectomies. J of Urol 2001; 165(Suppl):1442A.

23. Guillonneau B, Cathelineau X, Doublet JD, et al. Short-term oncological follow-up results of laparoscopic radical prostatectomy. J Urol 2001; 165(Suppl):1346A.

24. Guillonneau B, el Fettouh H, Baumert HC. Laparoscopic radical prostatectomy: oncological evaluation after 1000 cases at Montsouris Institute. J Urol 2003; 169:1261–1266.

25. Guillonneau B, Cathelineau X, Doublet JD, et al. Prospective assessement of functional results after laparoscopic radical prostatectomy. J of Urol 2001; 165(Suppl):614A.

26. Bollens R, Bossche MV, Roumeguere T, et al. Laparoscopic radical prostatectomy: analysis of the first series of extraperitoneal approach. J of Urol 2001; 165(Suppl):1354A.

27. Salomon L, Olsson LE, Hoznek A, Antiphon P, Cicco A, Chopin DK, Abbou CC. Continence and potency after laparoscopic radical prostatectomy. J Urol 2001; 165(Suppl):390.

28. Katz R, Salomon L, Hoznek A. Patient-reported sexual function following laparoscopic radical prostatectomy. J Urol 2002; 168:2078–2082.

29. Kavoussi LR. Laparoscopic radical prostatectomy: irrational exuberance? Uroloy 2001; 58:503–505.

30. Turk I, Serdar D, Winkelmann B, Schonberger B, Loening SA. Laparoscopic radical prostatectomy. Eur Urol 2001; 40:46–53.

EDITORIAL COMMENTARY

Joseph R. Wagner

Connecticut Surgical Group/Hartford Hospital Hartford, CT, USA

Caner Z. Dinlenc

Department of Urology, Beth Israel Medical Center, New York, NY, USA

This chapter is an excellent review of Dr. Inderbir Gill's technique and experiences performing laparoscopic radical prostatectomy at the Cleveland Clinic. Just as any manuscript deservedly credits Dr. Patrick Walsh for his innovations and insights in performing retropubic radical prostatectomy, the authors rightfully cite the Montsouris group for their pioneering efforts proving laparoscopic radical prostatectomy is a safe, effective surgical option for localized prostate cancer. Currently, experienced laparoscopic groups are modifying their technique as they strive to maximize cancer control and long-term quality of life outcomes and minimize surgical morbidity. As we proctor experienced open surgeons in the laparoscopic procedure, we continue to take home "pearls" that we have successfully applied to our own laparoscopic and robotic radical prostatectomy technique. This chapter successfully shares this philosophy and makes many excellent statements on the procedure.

As evidenced by the first report on laparoscopic radical prostatectomy by Schuessler et al. in 1992 [1], laparoscopic radical prostatectomy is a technically demanding procedure. Before even an experienced laparoscopic surgeon attempts the procedure, we would recommend three steps of preparation that we believe can dramatically decrease the "learning curve."

1. Assemble a team: Laparoscopic radical prostatectomy cannot be performed by one surgeon. The assistant surgeon should understand and be able to perform the necessary laparoscopic maneuvers to perform the procedure. Ideally, this surgeon should also have a firm understanding of laparoscopy and pelvic anatomy. In the operating room, nurses familiar with the equipment and anesthesiologists well versed in the physiologic considerations of what will at first be a lengthy laparoscopic procedure are critical.
2. Observation: Take courses to enhance your skills and understanding of the procedure and visit institutions performing the procedure, noting set-up, technique, etc., to optimally prepare your team.
3. Proctor: For both the laparoscopic and robotic approach, we found that having an experienced surgeon in the room to provide verbal suggestions was invaluable during our first few cases. An increasing number of institutions are requiring that initial cases are proctored/mentored to gain credentials for complex laparoscopic procedures. Though this may seem like an obstacle, both proctors and trainees we have seen the enormous benefits in terms of reducing the initial learning curve [2].

While we, too, do not place limits on patient size, prostate size, or the presence of a large median lobe, all of these can impact the ease of the procedure. Initially, "ideal patients" should be selected. Our patient preparation and positioning is the same, and we agree both compression stockings and 5,000 units of subcutaneous heparin are recommended for DVT prophylaxis.

The first step after establishing pneumoperitoneum and port placement using the Montsouris technique is to incise the second peritoneal reflection, dissect the seminal vesicles and vasa, and finally transect the vasa. As discussed, some surgeons are abandoning this portion of the procedure and dissecting the seminal vesicles and vasa after transecting the bladder neck. Performing the bladder neck transection first is felt to decrease bowel manipulation and, in some hands, decrease the length of the procedure slightly. While we feel it is important to eventually learn this approach, as it will be necessary in certain patients in whom the second peritoneal reflection is obliterated, such as in diverticulitis, we recommend initially identifying the seminal vesicles at the beginning of the procedure. The two most difficult parts of the procedure are (1) identifying and transecting the bladder neck and (2) performing the anastomosis. Encountering an open space and the already dissected seminal vesicles after transecting the bladder neck is helpful and reassuring to the inexperienced surgeon. The extraperitoneal approach is desirable for several reasons, but should be approached cautiously by the inexperienced surgeon as the decreased room to operate can be problematic.

Although the pneumoperitoneum can temporarily tamponade venous injuries, meticulous control of the venous complex is a necessity as in open radical prostatectomy. In addition to placing a urethral sound and pushing posteriorly to place the dorsal vein stitch, we also find this maneuver very useful to stretch the urethra and aid in dissecting the apex.

The steps of robotic laparoscopic radical prostatectomy are similar with some advantages and disadvantages. Suturing is certainly easier, especially for an inexperienced laparoscopist, with the robot. Performing the procedure while sitting at a console avoids many of the musculoskeletal complaints associated with prolonged laparoscopic procedures. Disadvantages include the inability to manipulate the surgical table and patient position once the robot is in place and some loss of tactile sensation compared with the straight laparoscopic approach.

Despite increased visualization and decreased blood loss, laparoscopic prostatectomy outcome studies have not shown improved erectile function and continence compared to open studies. While the authors cite all the appropriate references, we continue to be distressed by the lack of prospective analysis using validated questionnaires. Statements such as "achieving spontaneous erections" or "continent without pads" should no longer be sufficient when excellent validated questionnaires such as the UCLA Prostate Index exist. It is incumbent upon us to obtain these data to arrive at appropriate conclusions. Although intraoperative blood loss is also a frequently cited outcome, we believe comparisons of preoperative and discharge hemoglobins would be more reliable. As for surgical margins, we have seen our rates drop approximately 9% using the laparoscopic approach compared to our open series, although this has not been the experience at all institutions.

Laparoscopic radical prostatectomy has been shown to be a feasible, safe, and reliable procedure with outcomes similar to open series thus far. While we believe we can now safely state that blood loss is less than in the open procedure, comparisons of surgical morbidity, long-term PSA outcomes, and quality of life issues must be evaluated. The laparoscopic approach has been shown to decrease the morbidity and convalescence associated with numerous open procedures, such as nephrectomy and adrenalectomy. Whether this will hold true for radical prostatectomy remains to be seen. The authors are to be congratulated for this chapter, which describes their superb technique and outcomes, as well as begins to answer some of these important questions.

REFERENCES

1. Schuessler WW, Kavoussi LR, Clayman RV, Vancaille T. Laparoscopic radical prostatectomy; initial case report. J Urol 1992; 246A.
2. Dinlenc C, Wagner J. Laparoscopic Radical prostatectomy: decreasing the learning curve, Abstract presented at the World Congress of Endourology, September 19–21, 2002, Genoa, Italy.

EDITORIAL COMMENTARY

Bertrand Guillonneau

Professor of Urology, Weill Medical College of Cornell University,
Memorial Sloan Kettering Cancer Center, New York, NY, USA

The chapter, "Laparoscopic Radical Prostatectomy," summarizes perfectly what is known and what is not known by urologic teams involved in the laparoscopic approach to "modern" radical prostatectomy.

The facts here are obvious and bolster the faith of each surgeon who has already begun the laparoscopic approach.

THE APPROACH IS MINIMALLY INVASIVE

Incisional pain for the patient is reduced to a minimum, thus allowing a more comfortable and shorter hospital stay and quicker return to normal activities than with open radical prostatectomy. In addition, even if it has not been evaluated in the various series, recovery for the patient is surprisingly rapid.

These advantages are related to the less-traumatizing surgical approach to the prostate, one that makes no significant abdominal wound. Where surgery is ablative, this advantage is common to all laparoscopic procedures, as opposed to conventional ones, from cholecystectomy to nephrectomy.

THE VIEW IS IMPROVED

There are three main reasons for this improvement. The first and most obvious one is that the camera provides an approximately 15-fold magnification of the operative field. The second reason is related to the improvement in ergonomics for the surgeon: instead of remaining deep inside, the prostate becomes directly visible on the monitor screen. The third element contributing to the improvement of view is the reduction of bleeding, confirmed objectively in all series by the observation that both the estimated blood loss and the transfusion rates are lowered. Certainly, the counter-pressure of the pneumoperitoneum helps, but because of the magnification and improved ergonomics, the surgeon can see and control the vessels more efficiently before they bleed, allowing the surgeon to operate in an almost dry operative field, which leads again to a much-improved operative view.

A more perfect vision is part of the concept of the laparoscopic approach, because, as its detractors often aver, tactile sense is decreased compared with the direct digital palpation of other methods. This handicap, however, is largely compensated for by the improved view. Improved vision is a major advantage in surgery, in general, and in prostatectomy in particular, as this procedure is not only ablative, but also reconstructive and functional.

THE QUALITY OF THE URETHROVESICAL ANASTOMOSIS IS IMPROVED

This occurs no matter what suturing technique is used, whether running or interrupted. The procedure allows a good anastomosis of the orifices, and, therefore, a quicker healing time, as the short catheterization time demonstrates.

Nevertheless, the questions, or shadow areas, are numerous. But the dedication of these teams to this procedure is still justified, as long as there is a proper evaluation of it.

APPROACH

As mentioned in this chapter, three routes can be used to perform a radical prostatectomy laparoscopically, and all are probably justified, depending on the patient, the tumor, and the experience of the surgeon.

Whenever the Douglas pouch is accessible and I want to perform a nerve-sparing procedure, I first do a direct approach to the seminal vesicles. Transperitoneally, the seminal vesicles are made superficially visible and are then easily accessible. The approach to them is quicker and safer because dissection is much more accurate. There is no traction on the vascular pedicles and they are controlled directly, so the risk of injury to the neural network in this area is limited. Furthermore, in my experience, the dissection of the seminal vesicles through the bladder neck requires more traction on the seminal vesicles and, therefore, on their pedicles, and a more lateral transsection of the prostate pedicles, which might injure the neurovascular bundles in this area.

To summarize my approach, I first dissect the seminal vesicles when I want to do a nerve-sparing procedure. Otherwise, I agree with the authors on the value of the "anterior transperitoneal approach." Because surgery should be adapted to the patient and its disease one approach doesn't generally fit every situation. With this concern, the pure extraperitoneal approach is less flexible while the transperitoneal approach allows a better adaptation case by case.

THE STRATEGY OF DISSECTION

In general, some surgeons promote a pure retrograde dissection approach, mimicking Walsh's technique. I believe that, in laparoscopy, antegrade dissection is more adaptive as the dissection is always in the axis of the surgeon's view and the instruments, allowing dissection without any traction on the periprostatic structures, particularly the neurovascular bundles. For these reasons, the antegrade approach seems, to me, more logical.

INSTRUMENTATION

Each team has developed its own instrumental tactic, from the simplest use of very few instruments—which I advocate—to use of the most complicated systems, like remote-controlled telemanipulators.

I use only bipolar forceps to control vessels. This kind of cautery is very effective on veins and arteries; has limited thermal diffusion, if vessel control is accurate; and the instruments needed are inexpensive, widely available, and reusable. At present, the real question is not what is the best energy source, or what is the best brand of clip to control the vessels without damaging the nerves! Instead, it is where should the vessels be controlled so that they are far enough away for the nerves to be safe when the instrument is applied. The debate, here, is more anatomical than instrumental.

CANCER CONTROL

Control of the cancer is the primary goal of radical prostatectomy, and the best assessment of the quality of the surgery is based on the absence of positive margins in the biopsy specimen. Surprisingly, the positive-margin rate in laparoscopic surgery seems to be roughly comparable to the retropubic procedure. Half of the margins are apical, supporting the notion that, at this location, positive margins are more likely to be due to the disease itself and to the absence of capsule in this area rather than to the surgical technique. The other sites of positive surgical margins are posterolateral, pedicular, anterior, and, more rarely, at the bladder neck. Therefore, for progress in this area, it is mandatory to limit these pitfalls as much as possible. We should admit that even the improved view is clearly not sufficient to diagnose positive margins. Because of this, I prefer to extract the specimen as soon as the prostatectomy is completed and to examine it carefully under direct vision and palpation. Anytime I have a suspicion of positive margins, frozen-section examination is performed on the specimen, and, if positive, a wider excision is made in the area of concern.

URINARY FUNCTION

Broad-spectrum antibiotic therapy is not necessary in all patients, and I have given up on systematic antibiotic prophylaxis, which I prescribe only to patients with previous history of urinary infection. The question of what is the ideal duration of catheterization has yet to be answered. It is clear that, in some patients, the catheter can be removed as soon as the second postoperative day. However, selection of these patients is difficult. Early removal of the catheter exposes patients to acute retention, with makes recatheterization necessary. Even more severe complications, like extravasation, are possible if early removal becomes the rule. In fact, a prudent attitude is to let the catheter remain at least 4 days.

The evaluation of continence after laparoscopy is as difficult as after retropubic prostatectomy because there is no single questionnaire that is widely accepted and used. In addition, the definition of continence varies among series. Nevertheless, the published data suggests that the 12-month results are in the same range as after retropubic prostatectomy—80 to 90%—but the question of the speed of recovery is still debatable, as no prospective studies have been published.

SEXUAL FUNCTION

The technique of neurovascular dissection varies widely from one surgeon to another, and, even in the most experienced of hands, the technique is still evolving. It is, therefore, not surprising that the results vary so widely in the different published series. Furthermore, evaluation of potency is one of the blurriest fields of evaluation in urology because a single definition of erection itself is not commonly accepted and different questionnaires are used for evaluation. Nonetheless, the experiences of many surgeons have confirmed that nerve-sparing surgery is technically feasible and functionally efficient. Furthermore, there are some data suggesting that the recovery time of erection is shortened, probably because magnification and the operative strategy allow a less-traumatizing dissection of the fragile structures of the neurovascular bundles.

In conclusion, laparoscopy is just one approach, and certainly not the only solution, to the problems involved in radical prostatectomy. Some problems are solved through its use; for example, pain, the quality of the urethrovesical anastomosis, and blood loss. But the problems of cancer control and functional results remain. Nevertheless, I am confident that this technique will finally solve more problems than it creates and will add to the global improvement of surgery for prostate cancer. If this occurs, there is no doubt that laparoscopy will become, in the near future, the reference approach for radical prostatectomy.

EDITORIAL OVERVIEW

Kenneth B. Cummings

Significant progress has occurred in the performance of Laparoscopic Radical Prostatectomy (LRP) since the original report by Schuessler et al. in 1992 [1], in which the authors concluded that because of the protracted operative time (mean, 9.4 hours), LRP "offers no advantage over open surgery." Gill and coauthors appropriately credit the French team of Guillonneau and Vallencien from Montsouris who brought LRP to contemporary practice [2,3].

In contrast to the original approach by the Montsouris team to the seminal vesicles, Gill prefers to transect the vesicle neck before identifying and dissecting the seminal vesicles. Their nerve sparing technique, which is still evolving, is performed in a combined antigrade–retrograde fashion. The urethral anastomosis is performed utilizing a 2-0 Vicryl suture on UR-6 needle "at least 3 to 4 needle passes with subsequent sinching are necessary in order to bring into apposition the vesical urethral junction." Margin positivity is considered by this group to be experience and operator dependent, as demonstrated by a drop of almost 50% in the positive surgical margins from their first 50 cases to their third 50 cases in their series. Urinary incontinence in their series appears competitive to open surgery. Potency rates are not competitive to the "best open RRP series."

Guillonneau focuses on the obvious advantages of LRP: (a) the approach is minimally invasive, allowing a more rapid return to normal activities than open radical prostatectomy; (b) the operator's vision is dramatically improved because of camera magnification as well as the ergonomics (the prostate, which, in open surgery, is viewed deep in the pelvis in contrast to laparoscopic surgery, in which it is displayed magnified on a screen); (c) importantly, the pneumoperitoneum dramatically reduces venous bleeding, improving over all vision, and, with magnification, permitting more precise dissection and cauterization of blood vessels; and (d) improved quality of the vesicourethral anastomosis, permitting earlier removal of the catheter.

Of note, Guillonneau, for nerve sparing, prefers to initially dissect the seminal vesicles in the pouch of Douglas when this is not obliterated by adhesions (i.e., diverticulities). Guillonneau stresses the importance of the antigrade dissection approach in laparoscopy in contrast to the pure retrograde technique of Walsh. His observation is that, in laparoscopy, the axis of dissection is in the direction of the surgeon's view.

Guillonneau contends that, with time and experience, LRP should produce equal cancer-control continence and potency and may become the referenced approach to radical prostatectomy.

Wagner and Dinlenc wisely focus on the steep learning curve for LRP and highlight approaches to shorten the duration of this learning curve and achieve technical improvement. They consistently favor the initial dissection of seminal vesicles when this is technically feasible. Nerve sparing is performed antigrade and the urethral anastomosis is performed with interrupted sutures.

REFERENCES

1. Schuessler WW, Kavoussi LR, Clayman RV, Vancaille T. Laparoscopic radical prostatectomy: initial case report. J Urol 1992; 147:246A.
2. Guillonneau B, Vallancien G. Laparoscopic radical prostatectomy: the Montsouris experience. J Urol 2000; 163:418–422.
3. Guillenneau B, Vallancien G. Laparoscopic radical prostatectomy: the Mountsouris technique. J Urol 2000; 163:1643–1649.

4

The VIP Approach to the Treatment of Localized Cancer of the Prostate: Robotic Radical Prostatectomy

Mani Menon and Ashok K. Hemal

Vattikuti Urology Institute, Henry Ford Hospital, Detroit, Michigan, USA

INTRODUCTION

Surgical management of prostate cancer has evolved over the last century. Radical perineal prostatectomy was described by Young in 1900 [1], and radical retropubic prostatectomy by Millin in 1947 [2]. In 1982, Walsh laid the foundations of contemporary anatomic radical retropubic prostatectomy, based on his earlier work delineating the anatomy of the dorsal vein complex (Reiner and Walsh) and the cavernosal nerves (Walsh, 1982) [3]. As the utilization of laparoscopy in urologic surgery expanded, Schuessler and colleagues developed the technique of laparoscopic radical prostatectomy (LRP) (1992) [4]. The procedure was lengthy and technically challenging, with the most difficult component being the urethrovesical anastomosis. It was the pioneering work of Guillonneau and Vallancien that demonstrated that LRP was safe and efficient, with excellent patient outcomes [5]. This work was rapidly followed by reports from others (Abbou et al., Rassweiler et al., Turk et al., and Gill and Zippe) that validated Guillonneau's observations [6–9]. It is now accepted that this technique, with its decreased invasiveness, translates into shorter hospital stays, decreased pain, and earlier resumption of normal activities for the patient. In expert hands, this technique is safe, quick, and efficient, providing outcomes comparable to open surgery with a fraction of the blood loss and postoperative discomfort [10–11]. However, these pioneers have also raised the following warning: LRP has a steep learning curve, and only individuals with advanced laparoscopic expertise should undertake it [9–12].

Laparoscopy may have certain inherent limitations: counterintuitive movements, rigid instruments, 2-dimensional imagery, and poor ergonomics. While these limitations can be overcome with practice, practice and more practice, they still relegate complex reconstructive procedures to the realm of a few brave surgeons. We are not among these. Therefore, we attempted to incorporate robotic assistance to the performance of laparoscopic radical prostatectomy. Based on the preliminary work of Abbou, Binder, Pasticier, and their colleagues, in 2001, our team introduced an anatomical approach to the radical prostatectomy with robotic assistance [13–15,23]. In previous reports, we showed that robotic assistance enhanced our ability to perform a laparoscopic radical prostatectomy, enabling our laparoscopically naive team to achieve results that are comparable to those of the leaders in the nonrobotic laparoscopic radical prostatectomy field, who have greater laparoscopic experience [16–18]. While our early technique faithfully mimicked the Montsouris approach of LRP, we gradually modified our technique to reflect the experience that we had gained from "open" surgery, incorporating many of the steps of conventional radical retropubic prostatectomy. We initially named our procedure Computerized Robot-Assisted Prostatectomy, until a few uncharitable observers pointed out what the acronym read. To rebut these misanthropes, we call our procedure the Vattikuti Institute Prostatectomy (VIP), and our approach, the VIP approach to the treatment of prostate cancer [19–20]. For the purposes of this chapter, VIP is radical prostatectomy performed with the da Vinci™ Surgical System and utilizing the steps that we describe. Briefly, this approach combines the techniques of a transperitoneal approach (a large working space) with those of an extraperitoneal dissection. We describe our technique in detail, highlighting certain tricks learned from (bitter?) experience.

INDICATIONS AND CONTRAINDICATIONS

Our indications for the VIP are identical to those of an open, radical prostatectomy: patients with localized prostate cancer who have biologically significant disease and a life expectancy of over 10 years. We recommend surgery to patients with nonfocal Gleason 6 and higher cancer, and a Charlson comorbidity score of less than 3. Relative contraindications for VIP include previous major abdominal surgery or a history of peritonitis; however, 32% of our cases have had previous laparotomy, and about 2% have had peritonitis. The operation is more difficult in patients who are markedly obese (BMI >40), who have undergone radiation or androgen-deprivation therapy, and who have a history of prostatitis, transurethral prostatectomy, or repeated prostatic biopsies. Large volume prostates (>80g), large median or lateral lobes, or an android pelvis may lead to a difficult dissection. Cases that have been memorably difficult include those with a history of ruptured viscera, multiple laparotomies for bowel obstruction, or prior suprapubic prostatectomy. Patients who have had herniorrhaphy with mesh are often harrowing experiences for "open" radical prostatectomy: that is not the case with robotic prostatectomy.

PREOPERATIVE PREPARATION

We prefer to wait at least 6 weeks after prostatic biopsy. Aspirin and antiplatelet agents are discontinued for at least 4 weeks prior to surgery, because even slight bleeding makes the dissection imprecise. Antibiotic prophylaxis is given prior to surgery as per hospital protocol. A combination of compression stockings and subcutaneous heparin 5000 units is utilized pre- and postoperatively during the hospital stay. A mechanical bowel preparation is not necessary; however, it's preferable to maintain a clear liquid diet and utilize a laxative one day prior to surgery.

ANESTHESIA

VIP is done under general endotracheal anesthesia using halogenated gases, i.e., isoflurane, as opposed to nitrous oxide.

PATIENT'S POSITION

The patient is supine with both arms at his side to avoid the risk of brachial plexus injury. We do not use shoulder supports as they may lead to postoperative pain. A thoracic wrap, padded with foam, is preferred. The patient is positioned in moderate lithotomy with the legs separated in flexion and abduction and a foam support under the buttocks. There is a risk of neurapraxia, usually seen only if the operation takes longer than 4 hours; therefore, adequate padding of all pressure points is mandatory (Figure 1). The table is set in extreme Trendelenburg position with the robot between the patient's legs. The table is flexed at the sacral area to improve exposure to the pelvis. A Foley catheter is placed into the bladder.

SURGICAL TECHNIQUE

The operation is performed using the da Vinci™ Surgical System (Intuitive Surgicals, Sunnyvale, CA).

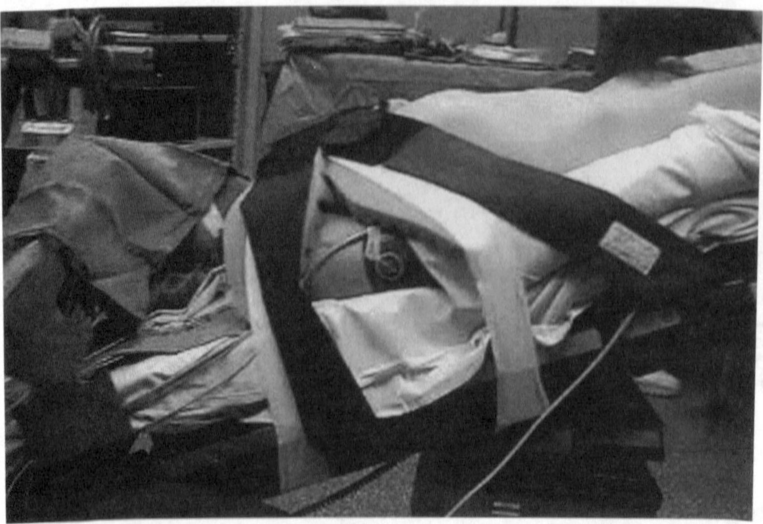

FIGURE 1   Demonstrating patient's position and support of shoulder and pressure points.

A. Pneumoperitoneum and Placement of Ports

A right-handed surgeon stands on the patient's left and vice versa. A Veress needle (Ethicon Endo-Surgery, Inc., Albuquerque, NM) is introduced from a supra or infra umbilical incision for pneumoinsufflation to a pressure of 20 mm Hg. This pressure is maintained while inserting the ports; however, the pressure is then decreased to 15 mm Hg for the remainder of the procedure. The Veress needle is replaced with a 12 mm trocar and the 3-D da Vinci laparoscope is inserted to transilluminate the abdominal wall. Four other trocars are placed under laparo-vision. Two 8 mm da Vinci trocars are placed 2.5 cm below the level of the umbilicus, pararectally on either side. A 5 mm trocar is placed on the right side between the umbilicus and the 8 mm port. A 12 mm port is then placed in the midaxillary line, about one inch above the iliac crest on the right side. A second (optional) 5 mm trocar may be placed in the left iliac fossa 3–5 cm above and medial to the anterior-superior iliac spine. This trocar allows the incorporation of a second assistant, which speeds up the operation and allows for the training of an additional surgeon. The placement of the ports is done with a 30-degree angled lens looking upward.

B. Peritoneoscopy

In previously operated cases, after placement of the first port, inspection of the abdominal cavity often reveals adhesions. These adhesions are lysed by the assistant using conventional laparoscopic instruments in order to make room for the placement of the secondary ports and also for the subsequent dissection.

C. Robotic Instruments

Robotic instruments are expensive and we use as few as possible. The minimum required are the da Vinci long-tip grasper, a hook, and two needle holders. When nerve sparing is contemplated, the articulated da Vinci bipolar coagulating forceps and scissors are used as well. Although we helped in the design of the da Vinci Pro-grasp, we now find it somewhat bulky for VIP.

D. Creation of the Extraperitoneal Working Space.

This part of the dissection is done with a 30-degree angled lens looking upward. As the patient is in the extreme Trendelenburg position, the small bowel usually falls away: however, one usually needs to take down adhesions between the sigmoid colon and the posterior peritoneum. The space of Retzius is entered through an inverted U-shaped incision on the parietal peritoneum, superior to the dome of the bladder and lateral to the medial umbilical ligaments (Figure 2). The internal inguinal ring can be seen medial to the external iliac vessels, which are covered by a lateral fold of the peritoneum. The vertical limb of the peritoneal incision is made lateral to the medial umbilical ligament and medial to the internal

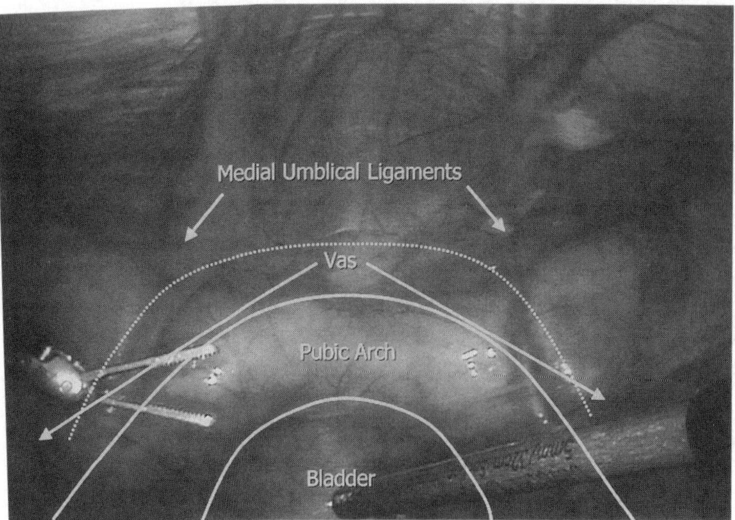

FIGURE 2   Initial peritoneoscopy revealing various anatomical landmarks: medial umbilical ligaments, vas deferens, pubic arch, and bladder.

inguinal ring. The vas deferens is seen coursing obliquely across the incision and can be retracted out of the operating field or divided prior to further dissection. The incisions are joined anteriorly, dividing the urachus and dislocating the bladder posteriorly.

A similar approach can be made completely extraperitoneally. However, we found that a purely extraperitoneal approach has two disadvantages—a limited working space and avulsion of minor capillaries when the dissection is done bluntly.

E. Pelvic Lymphadenectomy

This part of the dissection is done with the 30-degree lens angled downwards. Bilateral pelvic lymphadenectomy is performed if one or more of the following criteria are met: clinical stage T2 or higher, Gleason score equal to or greater than 7, preoperative PSA >10 ng/mL, or greater than 50% of the needle biopsy cores positive for cancer. The retroperitoneal fat is cleared off of the anterior surface of the external iliac vein. The external iliac artery is cleaned medially, and the vein is identified and carefully dissected along its inferior border. The obturator nerve is identified and serves as the posterior margin of dissection. Beginning at the pubic ramus, the lymph nodes and fatty tissues are cleaned out of the obturator fossa. Aberrant obturator vessels should be preserved if possible, as they may help maintain potency. The packet of fibro-fatty and nodal tissue, which is normally contained as one piece, is dissected toward the bifurcation of the external iliac vein.

F. Control of the Dorsal Venous Complex

This part of the dissection is done with a 0-degree lens. Once the anterior surface of the bladder is exposed, the superficial dorsal vein over the prostate is coagulated and divided (Figure 3). The fat over the prostate is swept cephalad and laterally. Endopelvic fascia is opened on either side from the semilunar gap to the prosta-tovesical junction, identified by the presence of a tongue of extravesical fat. This reveals the puboprostatic or pubovesical ligaments. Small perforating veins between the prostate and the levator ani must be cauterized. We avoid dividing the puboprostatic ligaments and dissect the urethra as little as possible. This approach has dramatically improved the time to full continence, which has averaged at 42 days for our last 200 patients. The deep dorsal vein complex is ligated with a single vertical mattress suture (0-vicryl on CT-1 needle). This suture is passed horizontally in the groove between the urethra and the dorsal vein complex, and then passed backward under the most superficial fibers of the ligament. A second suture is placed in the anterior, midprostate (Figure 4). The ends of this suture are about 2 inches long so that the assistant can grasp it and apply traction on the prostate. The neurovascular bundles and the rectourethralis are now scpa-

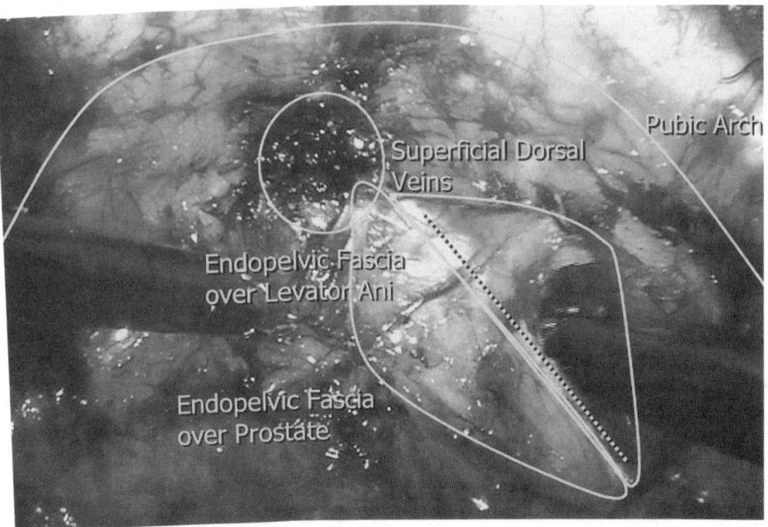

FIGURE 3 Closure view demonstrating fulgurated superficial dorsal veins, endopelvic fascia **over levator ani muscle, and spreading out over the prostate.**

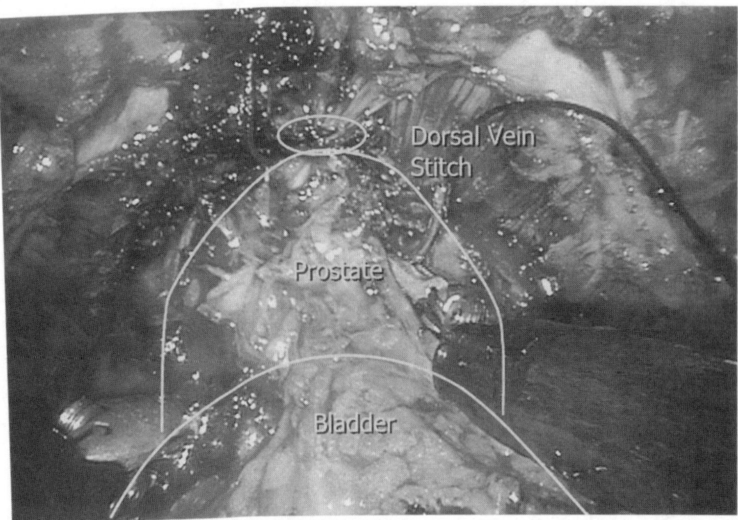

FIGURE 4 Ligated dorsal venous complex (with 0-vicryl suture on CT-1 needle), with another back-bleeding suture applied over the proximal part of the prostate.

rated from the posterior surface of the urethra using blunt dissection with the da Vinci needle holders, much in the way that the urethra is pinched off with the fingers during open prostatectomy. This is a key step because it facilitates dissection of the posterior apex and urethral transaction at a later stage.

G. Incision of the Bladder neck

This part of the dissection is done with a 30-degree angled lens directed downward. At this point, the dorsal vein and the urethra are transected during open surgery. The VIP approach deviates from this and focuses on transecting the bladder neck. Many laparoscopic surgeons consider the identification of the bladder neck as one of the most difficult parts of the operation. However, several subtle maneuvers can be used to aid this. At the midline, the bladder muscle and the prostate are in immediate contact because the bladder mucosa is continuous with the mucosa of the prostatic urethra. However, a distinct plane can be developed between the bladder and the prostate laterally, where fibroareolar and fatty tissue bridges the distance between the prostate and the bladder. Under traction, this distance can be almost 2 cm. Therefore, we start the bladder neck dissection laterally, at the junction of the lateral and anterior surfaces of the prostate (Figure 5). The left assistant pulls the prostatic suture firmly while this is done. This, aided by the downward-looking lens and the 3-D vision is usually quite adequate to identify the prostatovesical junction. We do not feel that the movement of the

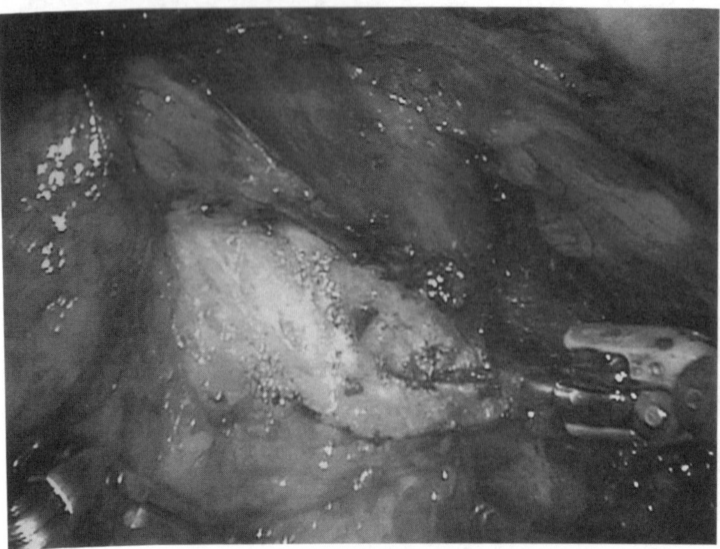

FIGURE 5 Division of bladder neck started from the lateral side.

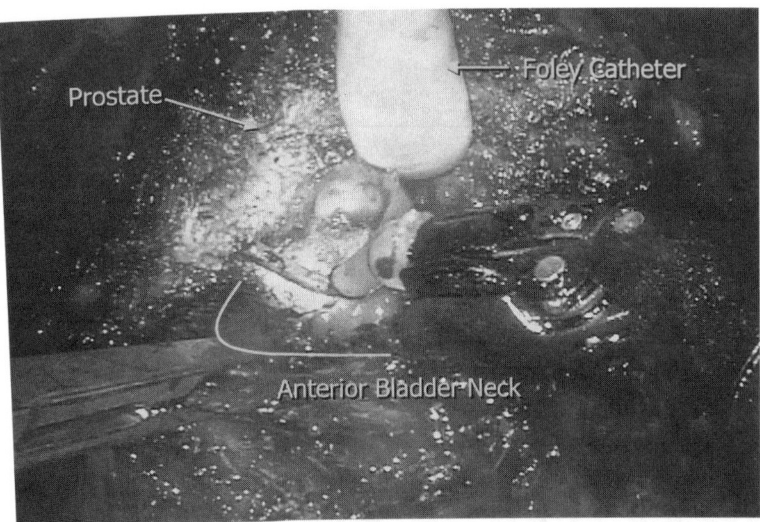

FIGURE 6 Divided anterior bladder neck and commencement of division of posterior bladder neck with the hook.

inflated balloon inside the bladder also aids in identification: rather it leads us astray, by directing the dissection to the midline. If the proper plane is entered, dissection will encounter fibrofatty tissue and very little bleeding. If, on the other hand, dissection is too close to the prostate, fibromuscular tissues that bleed annoyingly will be seen. As the dissection is deepened in the anterior midline, the shaft of the Foley catheter will be seen. The Foley balloon is deflated, and the tip of the catheter is pulled toward the ceiling by the assistant. The posterior bladder neck is now divided in the midline at the prostato vesical junction, which can be precisely identified (Figure 6). After the full thickness of the detrusor muscle has been divided, dissection is extended laterally, maintaining a clean detrusor margin for the subsequent vesicourethral anastomosis. In patients with a median lobe, its delivery outside the bladder helps in the dissection of the posterior bladder wall from the prostate.

H. Dissection of the Vas Deferens, Seminal Vesicles, Prostatic Pedicles, and Incision of Denonvillier's Fascia

This part of the dissection is done with a 30-degree lens directed downward. Division of the posterior bladder neck and incision of the anterior layer of Denonvillier's fascia lead to a window, from where ampulla of vas deferens and seminal vesicles can be dissected and pulled up. The vassal and vesicular arteries (sometimes several) can be seen clearly and should be coagulated. Both seminal vesicles

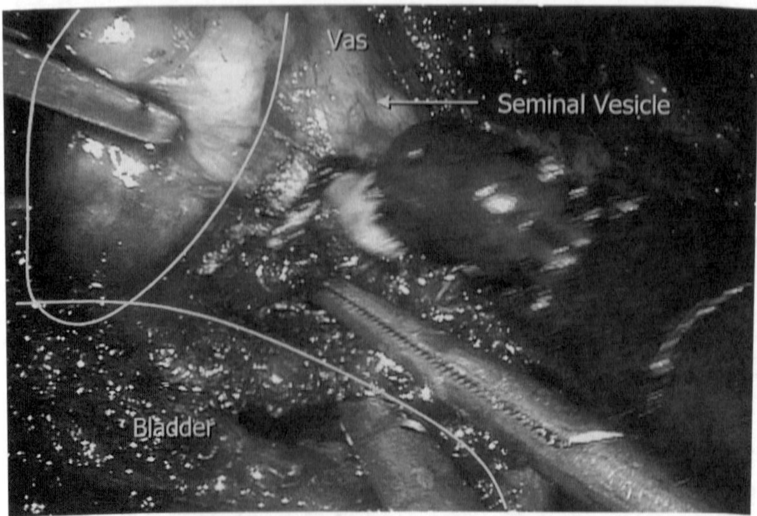

Figure 7   Divided posterior bladder neck, showing vas deferens through the window and seminal vesicle being dissected.

should be freed before commencing the dissection of the prostate (Figure 7). In some instances, the tips of the seminal vesicles are left intact to better preserve potency. In such instances, we obtain frozen sections from the transected margins of the vesicles. The prostatic pedicles are dissected on either side and divided between two hem-o-lock clips or with the help of the da Vinci bipolar cautery. The seminal vesicles are lifted up anteriorly to demonstrate the longitudinal fibers of the posterior layers of Denonvillier's fascia near the base of the prostate. The fascia is quite thick and has several layers in this location. It is incised sharply until prerectal fat is seen. We avoid the use of electrocautery for the entire posterior dissection so that the neurovascular bundles are not damaged by conducted heat. Once the proper plane is entered, we dissect in between the layers of Denonvillier's fascia to leave a protective layer of fascia over the rectum and any network of nerves that may exist in this area [28]. Although this can, in theory, lead to positive surgical margins, in over 400 patients we have not found this to be the case.

I. Nerve-Sparing

This part of surgery is done with an articulated robotic scissors and bipolar forceps. With the help of the robotic scissors, prostatic fascia is incised anteriorly and parallel to the neurovascular bundles (Figures 8 and 9). The posteriolateral surface of the prostate is cleared by dropping a layer of fascia, fat, nerves and blood

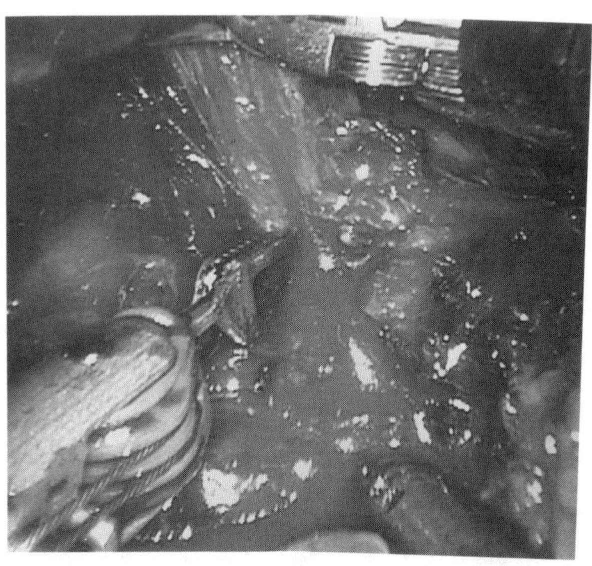

FIGURE 8 Dissection of right neurovascular bundle with bipolar forcep and articulated scissor.

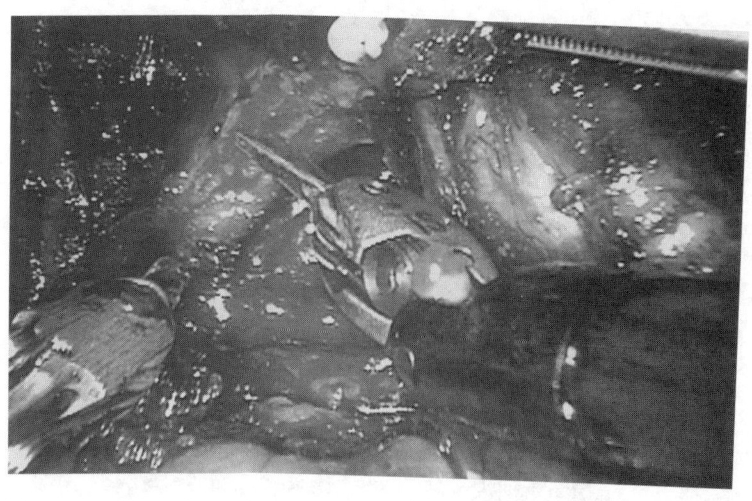

FIGURE 9 Dissection of left neurovascular bundle with bipolar forcep and articulated scissor.

vessels from the base to the apex. Once the correct plane is entered, most of the dissection occurs in a relatively avascular plane, and the neurovascular bundles can be teased away from the prostate easily.

J. Division of the Urethra, Separation of Specimen and Intraoperative Apical Biopsies

The urethra is divided at the apex of the prostate, subsequent to the division of the dorsal vein, with the help of articulated robotic scissor (Figure 10). The division of the posterior striated sphincter should be done carefully. Once the urethra is transected, parietal margin biopsies are obtained from the apex, base, and the area of the neurovascular bundles with the help of articulated scissor. The 3-D vision allows us to take precise periurethral biopsies without sacrificing any length of urethra. These biopsies are sent for frozen section, and if any are positive (a rare occurrence in our experience), then additional biopsies are taken from the appropriate site. This helps in lowering positive margin rates at the apex.

K. Vesicourethral Anastomosis

We prepare a special suture known as the MVAC (as in Menon, van Velthoven, Ahlering and Clayman) stitch by tying the tails of a 6 inches dyed and a 6 inch undyed 3-0 monocryl suture on a 17-mm round body (RB 1) needle (Ethicon), to make a single 12 inch suture with a bulky knot in the center and a needle at

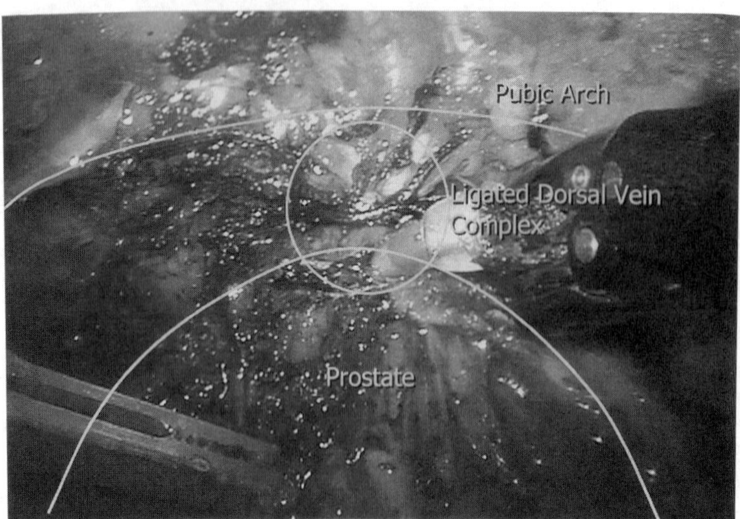

FIGURE 10   Division of Urethra.

either end. We use a slight modification of a technique recently published by van Velthoven et al [30]. Vesicourethral anastomosis is started by using the needle with the dyed end from the outside-in at the 5 o'clock position of the bladder neck and inside-out from the urethra at the corresponding site. We apply a continuous suture in a clockwise fashion, taking three throws in the bladder and two in the urethra, without attempting to snug the bladder down. At this point, the surgeon places the long-tip forceps in the bladder neck and pushes the bladder neck to the urethra. Because there is a wide plate of urethra and bladder, the stitches do not pull out in most instances. The suture is then continued until the 9 o'clock position, where it is turned in toward the bladder (Connel) and run until the 12 o'clock position. At this point, the assistant holds this suture taut, pulling cranially. The anastomosis is continued with the undyed end of the suture, passing it outside-in on the urethra at the 4 o'clock position, then inside-out on the bladder neck (Figure 11). The suture is then run counterclockwise until the dyed end of the suture is reached. The needles are cut off and both ends are tied together (Figure 12). Even if the bladder neck is wide, it can be anastomosed to the urethra using this parachute technique. We have had to refashion the bladder neck in only 5 patients. This approach has allowed us to complete the vesicourethral anastomosis with a single intracorporeal knot. The mean anastomotic time has been 14 min (range 8–20 min) over the last 200 cases. An indwelling 18 F Foley catheter is

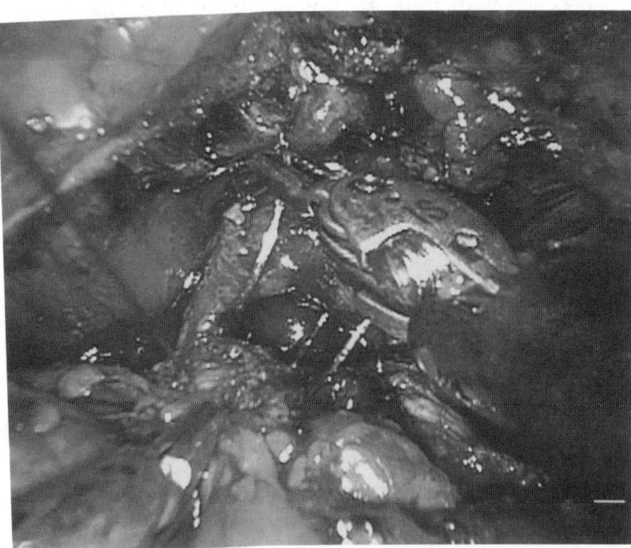

FIGURE 11   Near completion of vesicourethral anastomosis (final anterior sutures are being placed).

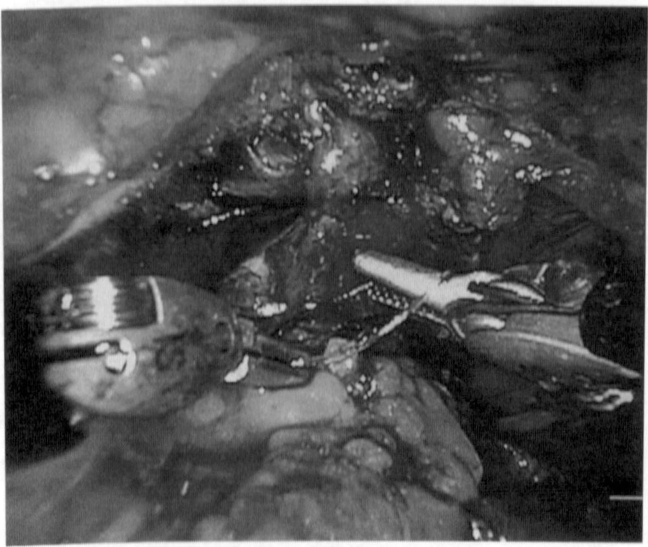

Figure 12 Both dyed and undyed sutures are tied in midline after placement of sutures to ensure water-tight anastomosis.

inserted and leakage is checked with an instillation of 200 cc of saline. In most instances there is no leakage, so no drain is needed.

POSTOPERATIVE CARE

Patients are generally discharged from the hospital within 24 hours. They return to the office between 4 days and 7 days after surgery for a cystogram. If there is no extravasation, the Foley catheter is removed. If extravasation is noted, then the catheter remains in place an additional 7 days and is removed without additional imaging.

RESULTS

We have performed 480 cases of robotic radical prostatectomy, of which 450 have been done utilizing the Vattikuti Institute Prostatectomy technique. The mean operating time (Veress needle to closure) of the last 200 cases operated on by Menon was 160 minutes, and the mean blood loss was 153 cc. Of this, about 40 min was spent in placing the ports, lysing any adhesions, retrieving the specimen, and closing the port sites. Thus, the actual robotic dissection time was 120 min. Pelic lymphadenectomy took 18 min on average. Patients with a history of previous abdominal surgery required lysis of adhesions. No patient required an intraoperative blood transfusion; no one donated autologous blood and none received erythropoietin. The average postoperative hematocrit was 39, compared to a discharge hematocrit of 32 for most open series. Ninety-three percent of the patients were discharged within 24 hours, and 40 patients elected to go home within 6 hours of surgery.

COMPLICATIONS

There were 4 intraoperative complications. Two rectal injuries were closed uneventfully. One unrecognized bowel injury occurred probably during the lysis of adhesions in a patient who had 2 previous exploratory laparotomies for bowel obstruction. This patient was reexplored with a laparotomy. One patient had a delayed bleed from a partial transaction of an aberrant obturator artery. Nine patients developed postoperative complications within 30 days of surgery. One patient developed a painful hematoma at a da Vinci port-site. Early in the series, 3 patients were readmitted for evaluation of abdominal distension. All 4 patients improved with conservative treatment. Two patients developed an incisional hernia at the site of specimen retrieval. One patient developed a deep-vein thrombosis despite prophylaxis and required systemic anticoagulation. Two patients were cystoscoped for evacuation of small clots. Delayed complications (1–12 months) were seen in 8 patients. Six patients required urethral dilation or an internal urethrotomy at 3–12 months after surgery. One additional patient has developed a recurrence of an umbilical hernia, and one patient presented with clot retention 4 weeks after catheter removal. Thus 429 of 450 (95.3%) VIP patients have had no intraoperative, postoperative, or delayed complications.

FUNCTIONAL RESULTS

Total continence, defined as using no pad, was achieved in 96% of our patients at a follow-up of 6 months, with a median time of 42 days [15–18]. Based on validated third party questionnaires (EPIC), 82% of preoperatively potent patients who were younger than 60 years had a return of some sexual activity and 64% had sexual intercourse at a follow-up of 6 months. Of patients over 60 years of age, 75% had some sexual activity and 38% had sexual intercourse [18–20].

COMPARISON OF VIP TO LAPAROSCOPIC RADICAL PROSTATECTOMY AND CONVENTIONAL RADICAL PROSTATECTOMY

Laparoscopic technique provides 4 degrees of movements compared to robotic surgery, which provides 6 degrees of freedom. Additionally, current laparoscopic displays do not provide 3-Dimensional orientation; they also lack tactile feedback. The instruments are not ergonomically suitable for the very difficult operations such as an LRP [21–22]. In the earlier experience of laparoscopic radical prostatectomy (LRP), the greatest time was spent creating the urethrovesical anastomosis; which takes double the time than actually removing of the prostate [4]; although in recent series of LRPs this time has been reduced significantly [23–25].

Many of these disadvantages can be overcome with robotic technology. The da Vinci surgical system is a master-slave robotic system. The assistance of this robot allows a surgeon to perform complex laparoscopic procedures. The features of the robot that make it superior include: 3-D visualization with a 10x magnification; wristed instrumentation (with intuitive- and finger-controlled movements); ergonomic manipulation of the robotic instruments without fatigue; and a comfortable seat for the surgeon [26–27]. We believe the superior view provided by the da Vinci system allows for a successful identification of the correct tissue planes. In addition, the improved coordination provided by the system allows one to perform a more anatomic dissection. The vesicourethral anastomosis, with robotic assistance, was performed in a range of 20–30 minutes in our earlier experience; now this time has dropped to 10–20 minutes [28]. The other significant advantage of the VIP technique is the minimal blood loss, thus requiring no transfusion [29].

A prospective comparison of 30 cases each of the robotic anatomical prostatectomy (RAP) and conventional radical prostatectomy evaluated the safety and efficacy of the technique [16]. This comparison was conducted during the initial phase of the development of the technique, and RAP was found to be safe and feasible (although longer surgical times were required), with less blood loss, decreased pain, decreased analgesia, and shorter hospital stays [16]. An analysis of 200 cases revealed a mean operating time of 160 minutes, as previously mentioned [18]; however, in our more recent cases, this time has further decreased, now ranging from 70–130 minutes. It was also appreciated that there is no difference in terms of oncological completeness, positive margin rates, and surgical outcomes. Surgical outcomes, here, are measured in terms of an excellent anastomosis, preservation of neurovascular bundles, and a superb cosmetic benefit. The preservation of neurovascular bundles and a perfect anastomosis translates into a return of erectile function and the achievement of earlier continence [28].

COMMENTS

Minimally invasive surgical techniques have received positive attention both from surgeons and patients. This increased attention is secondary to the many benefits, including the potential for decreased postoperative discomfort, minimal disfigurement, and a quicker recovery in comparison to conventional surgery. Although cost has been a major concern, rapid recuperation has provided the impetus to continue to offer these procedures for the patient. In robotic surgery, the surgeon operates utilizing 3-D vision and efficient and ergonomic movements; the surgeon also has the added advantage of tactile sensation. However, in conventional laparoscopy, the operator does not have the advantage of 3-D vision or tactile feedback. Additionally, there remain restricted movements because of nonarticulating laparoscopic instruments. The robot was designed to incorporate open surgical maneuvers into laparoscopic surgery. Robotic laparoscopic radical prostatectomy, in the field of urology, is the most complex operation, and it is a perfect example of ablative and reconstructive surgery.

The goals of surgery in the management of prostate cancer are many, but the most important remains the need to cure. The goals of performing a radical prostatectomy are to remove the cancer, maintain continence, and maintain potency [3]. The performance of laparoscopic radical prostatectomy is well established and effective. Treating prostate cancer effectively, which can be defined more on the basis of the complete removal of the prostate, excision of nodes and, positive margin rates is still a concern to some. In this aspect of surgery, both robotic (VIP) and laparoscopic (LRP) are fairly well established. When evaluating the outcomes of continence, the VIP technique reflects better outcomes than open surgery, as the time to continence is shorter. Patients are also likely to regain potency faster than open surgery, as neurovascular bundles are protected under vision, although long term data evaluation is necessary [28]. The time for vesicourethral anastomosis has been decreased to less than fifteen minutes in 90% of VIP cases. This is due to the excellent anatomical dissection, great visualization, precision, accuracy, and dexterity due to the scaling and filtering of hand movements for the robot. With the VIP approach, anastomotic leaks are usually extraperitoneal and remain confined to this space. This eliminates morbidity of urinary leakage into the peritoneal cavity.

The results are outstanding in terms of oncological cure, continence, potency preservation, and quality of life outcomes [18,28,29]. Without any doubt, laparoscopy is an exciting and revolutionary subspecialty being rapidly accepted in the field of urology. The robotic assistance is making it much more feasible especially for the complex urological procedures, which require ablative and reconstructive operation. This thought process may seem extreme; however, this will certainly help reduce the learning curve and assist open-surgery surgeons to adopt this new technology. At this point, the cost of new technology, initial technical training, instrumentation, and marginally longer operating times are still issues with most of the centers.

FUTURE HORIZONS

The VIP has made its way into the management of localized cancer of the prostate. The robot facilitates the flawless execution of complex surgical maneuvers, particularly during the dissection of the neurovascular bundles and anastomosis, which are often considered difficult steps. The robotic assistance is truly the way of the future, which has been amply presented by the authors at their center.

These newer developments are opening up many exciting opportunities for the various fields in urology, i.e., reconstructive urology, and complete remote-surgical interventions. However, telementoring and remote-controlled robotic surgery would necessitate many more developments. Nevertheless, this future is not very far off, especially when considering that the precision and maneuverability of these machines can be well utilized in the day to day urological procedures in most developed centers, as well as help provide mentoring at peripheral centers. Further developments are required in a robotic system, such as providing viable force feedback and utilizing more instruments.

CONCLUSION

Advances in surgical technique, technology, and the surgeon's skill have allowed the use of robotic assisted radical prostatectomy to be an option in the management of organ-confined prostate cancer. The goals of the VIP technique are to cure cancer, preserve urinary continence, preserve potency, and decrease morbidity; other benefits of this technique are minimally invasive surgery and excellent cosmesis. At this juncture, VIP is nearly equal to traditional retropubic prostatec-tomy with certain outstanding advantages. However, long-term data for the follow up of cancer control is essential. Undoubtedly this is a tremendous development in the field of laparoscopy for the management of localized prostate carcinoma. This is also opening new areas for training, including tele-surgery and telementor-ing at distant sites; however, one should cautiously watch these developments.

REFERENCES

1. Young HH. The early diagnosis and radical cure of carcinoma of the Prostate: being a study of 40 cases and presentation of radical operation, which was carried out in four cases. Bull Johns Hopkins Hosp 1905; 16:315–321.
2. Millin T. Retropubic urinary surgery. Baltimore: Williams & Wilkins, 1947.
3. Walsh PC. Anatomic radical prostatectomy: evolution of the surgical technique. J Urol 1998; 160:2418–2424.
4. Schuessler WW, Kavoussi LR, Clayman RV, Schulam PG. Laparoscopic radical prostatetectomy: initial case report. J Urol 1992; 147:246A.
5. Guillonneau B, Vallancien G. Laparoscopic radical prostatectomy: the Montsouris technique. J Urol 2000; 163:1643–1649.
6. Olsson LE, Salomon LE, Nadu A, Hoznek A, Cicco A, Saint F, Chopin D, Abbou CC. Prospective patient-reported continence after laparoscopic radical prostatectomy. Urology 2001 Oct; 58(4):570–572.

7. Rassweiler J, Sentker L, Seemann O, Hatzinger M, Rumpelt HJ. Laparoscopic radical prostatectomy with the Heilbronn technique: an analysis of the first 180 cases. J Urol 2001 Dec; 166(6):2101–2108.

8. Turk I, Deger S, Winkelmann B, Schonberger B, Loening SA. Laparoscopic radical prostatectomy. Technical aspects and experience with 125 cases. Eur Urol 2001 Jul; 40(1):46–52.

9. Gill IS, Zippe CD. Laparoscopic radical prostatectomy: technique. Urol Clin North Am 2001 May; 28(2):423–436.

10. Guillonneau B, Cathelineau X, Doublet JD, Vallancien G. Laparoscopic radical prostatectomy: the lessons learned. J Endourology 2001 May; 15(4):441–445.

11. Guillonneau B, Rozet F, Cathelineau X, Lay F, Barret E, Doublet JD, Baumert H, Vallancien G. Perioperative complications of laparoscopic radical prostatectomy: the Montsouris 3-year experience. J Urol 2002 Jan; 167(1):51–56.

12. Kavoussi LR. Laparoscopic radical prostatectomy: irrational exuberance?. Urology 2001 Oct; 58(4):503–505.

13. Abbou CC, Hoznek A, Salomon L, Olsson LE, Lobontiu A, Saint F, Cicco A, Antiphon P, Chopin D. Laparoscopic radical prostatectomy with remote controlled robot. J Urol 2001 Jun; 165:1964–1966.

14. Binder J, Kramer W. Robotically assisted laparoscopic radical prostatectomy. BJU 2001 Mar; 87(4):408–410.

15. Menon M, Shrivastava A, Tewari A, Sarle R, Hemal A, Peabody JO, Vallancien G. Laparoscopic and robot-assisted radical prostatectomy: establishment of a structured program and preliminary analysis of outcomes. J Urol 2002 Sep; 168(3):945–949.

16. Menon M, Tewari A, Baize B, Guillonneau B, Vallancien G. Prospective comparison of radical retropubic prostatectomy and robot-assisted anatomic prostatectomy: the Vattikuti Urology Institute experience. Urology 2002 Nov; 60(5):864–868.

17. Tewari A, Peabody J, Sarle R, Balakrishnan G, Hemal A, Shrivastava A, Menon M. Technique of da Vinci robot-assisted anatomic radical prostatectomy. Urology 2002 Oct; 60(4):569–572.

18. Menon M, Tewari A. Robotic radical prostatectomy and the Vattikuti Urology Institute technique: an interim analysis of results and technical points. Urology 2003 Apr; 61(4, Suppl 1):15–20.

19. Menon M, Tewari A. Vattikuti Institute prostatectomy: surgical technique and current results. Curr Urol Rep 2003 Apr; 4(2):119–123.

20. Menon M, Shrivastava A, Sarle R, Hemal A, Tewari A. Vattikuti Institute Prostatectomy (VIP)—A single team experience. Journal of Endourology 2003; 17(9): 785–790.

21. Rassweiler J, Frede T. Geometry of laparoscopy, telesurgery, training and telementoring. Urologe A 2002 Mar; 41(2):131–143.

22. Gettman MT, Blute ML, Peschel R, Bartsch G. Current status of robotics in urologic laparoscopy. Eur Urol 2003 Feb; 43(2):106–112.

23. Pasticier G, Rietbergen JB, Guillonneau B, Fromont G, Menon M, Vallancien G. Robotically assisted laparoscopic radical prostatectomy: feasibility study in men. Eur Urol 2001 Jul; 40(1):70–74.

24. Hoznek A, Antiphon P, Borkowski T, Gettman MT, Katz R, Salomon L, Zaki S, de la Taille A, Abbou CC. Assessment of surgical technique and perioperative morbidity

associated with extraperitoneal versus transperitoneal laparoscopic radical prostatectomy. Urology 2003 Mar; 61(3):617–622.

25. Guillonneau B, el-Fettouh H, Baumert H, Cathelineau X, Doublet JD, Fromont G, Vallancien G. Laparoscopic radical prostatectomy: oncological evaluation after 1,000 cases at Montsouris Institute. J Urol 2003 Apr; 169(4):1261–1266.

26. Hemal AK, Menon M. Laparoscopy, robot, telesurgery and urology: Future Perspective. J Postgrad Med 2002; 48:39–41.

27. Samadi DB, Nadu A, Olson E, Hoznek A, Salomon L, Saint F, Abbou C. Robot-assisted laparoscopic radical prostatectomy—initial experience in eleven patients. J Urol 2002 Apr; 167(4, Suppl):390(1445).

28. Tewari A, Peabody JO, Fischer M, Sarle R, Vallancien G, Delmas V, Hassan M, Bansal A, Hemal AK, Guillonneau B, Menon M. An operative and anatomic study to help in nerve sparing during laparoscopic and robotic radical prostatectomy. European Urology 2003; 299:1–12.

29. Menon M. Robotic radical retropubic prostatectomy. BJU Int 2003 Feb; 91(3): 175–176.

30. Van Velthoven RF, Ahlering TE, Peltier A, Skarecky DW, Clayman RV. Technique for laparoscopic running urethrovesical anastomosis: The single knot method. Urology 2003; 61:699–702.

EDITORIAL COMMENTARY

David B. Samadi

Assistant Professor of Urology at Columbia Presbyterian Medical Center, New York, New York, USA

This manuscript, "The VIP approach to the treatment of localized cancer of prostate" by Dr. Mani Menon and Dr. A.K. Hemal is a superb review of the step-by-step approach to performing this operation safely and efficiently. From the work of Schuessler and colleagues in 1992 to Guillonneau, Vallancien, and Abbou in 1997 to VIP approach by Menon in 2004, one can conclude that one of the important characteristics in common are being brave and facing the challenge. However, the importance of practice and more practice should not be underestimated. One of the main reasons for the popularity of robotic or laparoscopic radical prostatectomy is achieving the main goals of traditional open surgery, specifically cancer-cure rate, continence, and potency. In addition, the patients have a much lower rate of transfusion and blood loss, faster recovery period, and shorter catheterization time; the authors have achieved these goals without a doubt.

While it is important to be able to use the da Vinci robot in order to gain some of the advantages that it has to offer, it is more important, initially, to master the laparoscopic skills. This is especially important for the upcoming young surgeons training in many centers of excellence across the country. The steep "learning curve" could be overcome by a faster eye, better hand coordination, and knowledge of basic laparoscopic skills and surgical anatomy. While traditional open surgeons depended mostly on tactile feedback to perform these cases, the new technology compensates for tactile loss through much-improved quality of vision and magnification.

The authors have clearly demonstrated the importance of a team, including surgical assistant, nurses, and anesthesiologists who understand this technically demanding procedure. There seems to be a learning curve not only for the surgeon alone but every member of his team. It is also important to select your patients initially and follow the same surgical steps in the first thirty to forty cases. Morbid obesity, multiple previous abdominal surgeries, laparoscopic hernia repair with or without placement of a mesh would be some of the initial contraindications in our hands [1].

After establishing pneumoperitoneum and port placement, a Keith needle is used in order to suspend the epiploic of sigmoid colon to the left abdominal wall, exposing the pouch of Douglas and thereby avoiding an extra trocar on the left side of the patient. I prefer a direct approach to the seminal vesicles and vas deferens and continue on a posterior dissection midline. This is time well spent because it makes the posterior bladder neck dissection much easier and reduces the chance of rectal injury. Facing the open space and delivering free seminal vesicles after the posterior bladder neck is incised, initially, is very reassuring to a surgeon [2].

In order to save time, we have been using a 0-degree lens throughout our laparoscopic and robotic cases, which has not been a major issue. The control of dorsal venous complex is similar to the VIP technique; however, I have been incising the pubo-prostatic ligament, which has not translated into a lower continence rate. This is especially important in a very small prostate or with interference by a large bony exuberant from pubic symphysis, and, therefore, exposes the dorsal complex better.

I find it easier, initially, to dissect the bladder neck in the midline for two reasons. Occasionally the lateral portion of the prostate is not as clearly seen as the authors have described and the chance of positive margin or interfering with the prostatic pedicle is higher. Secondly, the risk of bleeding is much lower starting medially and moving laterally. Again, for surgeons that are just starting to perform these cases, safety and outcome is extremely important. Survival of the patient and the surgeon in a safe and timely fashion is very critical in today's competitive environment. Therefore, delivering the catheter through the anterior cystostomy could indicate the plane for the posterior dissection and visualize the ureteral orifices earlier.

The nerve sparing section of the surgery was well described in this chapter. There seems to be a magic triangle with the neurovascular bundle laterally, the rectum posteriorly, and the prostate anteromedially. The avascular plane can be seen at this junction and, as a result, the neurovascular bundle can be teased away from the base toward the apical portion of the prostate (interfacial nerve sparing technique). This also depends on stage and grade of tumor. We use extrafascial nerve sparing dissection on the side of positive biopsy and interfascial on the other side.

There are many ways to perform a watertight urethrovesical anastomosis. Whether it is an interrupted suture, VIP technique, or Abbou's technique is not as important as the comfort of the surgeon. I use one suture of 2-0 Vicryl on UR6 measuring 16 inches to perform the anastomosis as described by Hoznek et al. [3]. The median time in the past 80 cases has been 25 minutes. No bladder neck contractures have been seen within the past 18 months. The suture is made snug throughout the anastomosis by the assistant. The catheter is removed within 2–4 days after a cystogram [4]. We have seen less than 10% of patients in urinary retention requiring a recatheterization. Lately, more and more laparoscopic surgeons are using the two-suture running anastomotic technique described originally by R. F. Van Velthoven from Brussels, Belgium [5]. There are certainly advantages noted during this part of the operation using the da Vinci robot, as noted by the authors in this chapter.

In conclusion, robotic surgery is another modality to some of the challenges facing the field of prostate cancer. Ultimately, the goal for all different surgical modalities, whether open, laparoscopic, or robotic, is to cure the patient from his disease, maintain good urine control, and retain the ability for normal sexual function. If laparoscopy or robotic surgery can achieve this in addition to a much lower morbidity for our patients, this could certainly be a standard of care in the very near future. Many authors have claimed that this technique is as effective as traditional open surgery; however, further prospective analysis is necessary in order to confirm this claim. This chapter meets the Walsh targets of radical prostatectomy as (4 Cs); cancer control, continence, coitus (potency), and low complication.

From the oncological and functional point of view, a new surgical method, to be accepted as an alternative, must lead to results at least similar to those of the standard procedure in (4 Es) effectiveness, efficiency, equanimity (morbidity), and economy (costs & convalescence). This procedure meets these criteria, except for cost. Many more questions would be answered if, in the future, more studies use the International Continence Society's (ICS) men questionnaire, Health-related Quality of Life (SF36); pain analog scales; IIEF (Internation index of erectile functioning); or SHIM (Sexual Health Inventory for Men) in all open retropubic, perineal, and laparoscopic prostatectomy to compare each surgical treatment scientifically. The authors are to be congratulated for this manuscript and their achievements

REFERENCES

1. Brown JA, Dahl DM. Transperitoneal laparoscopic radical prostatectomy in patients after laparoscopic prosthetic mesh inguinal herniorrhaphy. Urology 2004; 63:380.

2. Hoznek A, Samadi DB, Salomon L, Abbou C, Olsson LE, Saint F, Chopin D. Laparoscopic radical prostatectomy. Curr Urol Rep 2002; 3:141.

3. Hoznek A, Salomon L, Rabii R, et al. Vesicourethral anastomosis during laparoscopic radical prostatectomy: the running suture method. J Endourol 2000; 14:749.

4. Nadu A, Salomon L, Hoznek A, et al. Early removal of the catheter after laparoscopic radical prostatectomy. J Urol 2001; 166:1662.

5. Van Velthoven RF, Ahlering TE, Peltier A, et al. Technique for laparoscopic running urethrovesical anastomosis: the single knot method. Urology 2003; 61:699.

EDITORIAL OVERVIEW

Kenneth B. Cummings

Menon's seminal contribution of employing the da Vinci TM System (Intuitive Surgical, Sunnyville, CA, USA) in the performance of radical prostatectomy is reflective of the competent, experienced open surgical oncologist bypassing conventional laparoscopy and embracing robotics. Conventional laparoscopic technique provides four degrees of movement, compared with robotic surgery, which provides six degrees of freedom. The assistance of this robot allows an open surgeon to perform complex laparoscopic procedures due to the robots three-dimensional visualization with 10-times magnification, wristed instrumentation (intuitive and finger-controlled movements), ergonomic manipulations of the robotic instruments without fatigue, and a comfortable seat for the surgeon [1]. The superior view provided by the daVinci system allows for successful identification of the correct tissue planes for dissection. The improved coordination provided by the system enables one to perform a more precise anatomic dissection.

The vesicourethral anastomosis performed with robotic assistance employs two 6-inch, dyed and undyed 3-0 monocryl sutures on a (RB-1) needle (Ethicon) to make a single 12-inch suture with a bulky knot in the center and a needle at either end. This is sutured according to the technique of van Velthoven et al. [2]. The operative time for this anastamosis has, with experience, been reduced to 10 to 20 minutes [3]. The authors compare their technique to open nonconcurrent radical retropubic prostatectomy (RRP) and find the return of continence to be shorter than or equal to that of open surgery. They believe that patients regain potency faster because the neurovascular bundles are protected due to superior vision with less traction [3]. They further contend outstanding oncologic results compared with open surgery [4].

Samadi's editorial comment reflects, I believe, the current generation of urologic oncologists who possess fellowship training in urologic oncology, as well as a fellowship in applied laparoscopy to urologic oncology. He appropriately recognizes the principals of appropriate cancer surgery and the necessary knowledge of surgical anatomy. Importantly, he does not under estimate the challenge or the reward of this minimally invasive technology. The surgeon's ''historic touch'' has been replaced by ''image enhancement.''

In principle, he implies that, currently, a ''team approach'' is a necessary prerequisite to permit the new technologies to flourish and become the standard of care in urologic oncology.

He appropriately acknowledges that the da Vinci TM system allows traditionally trained urologic oncologists to perform (without formal laparoscopic training) complex dissections and reconstructive suturing techniques. He underscores the importance of the surgeon's persistence, patience, practice, and appropriate patient selection, with mentoring as a prerequisite for success in this arena.

REFERENCES

1. Hemal AK, Menon M. Laparoscopy, robot, telesurgery and urology: future perspective. J Postgrad Med 2002; 48:39–41.
2. Van Velthoven RF, Ahlering TE, Peltier A, Skarecky DW, Clayman RV. Technique for laparoscopic running urethrovesical anastomosis: the single knot method. Urology 2003; 61:699–702.
3. Tewari A, Peabody JO, Fishcher M, Sarle R, Vallancien G, Delmas V, Hassan M, Bansal A, Hemal AK, Guillonneau B, Menon M. An operative and anatomic study to help in nerve sparing during laparoscopic and Robotic Radical Prostatatectomy. European Urology 2003; 299:1–12.
4. Menon M. Robotic radical retropubic prostatectomy. BJU Int 2003; 91(3):175–17.

5

Three-Dimensional Conformal Radiation Therapy: Practical Aspects, Therapeutic Ratio, and Future Directions

Parvesh Kumar
Professor and Chairman, Department of Radiation Oncology
University of Southern California Keck School of Medicine,
Los Angeles, CA, USA

INTRODUCTION

The American Cancer Society estimates that 230,110 new cases of prostate cancer will be diagnosed and 29,900 men are expected to die in the United States [1]. For patients with localized prostate cancer, treatment options range from observation, surgery, external beam radiation therapy (EBRT), and brachytherapy, to hormone therapy with or without radiation therapy (RT). Although EBRT has been a mainstay in the management of prostate cancer for the last 40 years, the delivery techniques for EBRT have radically changed during the past decade [2]. Specifically, the advent of three-dimensional conformal radiation therapy (3-DCRT) has radically changed the administration of EBRT; it has favorably altered the therapeutic ratio by improving the efficacy of EBRT and simultaneously decreasing the acute and late toxicity. This chapter will review the following as it pertains to 3-DCRT: Patient selection, technique, outcome, and toxicity. Furthermore, future directions in radiation therapy, such as intensity modulated radiation therapy (IMRT), will be briefly addressed as well.

Historical Perspective

The first technical advances in conformal RT were made by Takashima, Umegaki, Matsuda, and Abe in Japan as early as the 1960s [3–5]. Prostate cancer patients were treated with conformal RT in the late 1980s at the University of Michigan [6], Fox Chase Cancer Center (FCCC) [7–8] and Memorial Sloan-Kettering Cancer Center (MSKCC) [9]. In 1994, the National Cancer Institute (NCI) funded nine institutions to conduct a dose-escalation study and to develop a national quality assurance center. In the early 1990s in the United States, the next important advance was the commercial development of the ACQSIM CT scanner that was linked to a treatment planning system. Since then, the ACQSIM CT scanner (Phillips Medical Systems) has gone through several evolutions in software enhancement as well as design improvements, such as a large aperture size (85 cm) to accommodate patients in the "treatment position" with their immobilization devices. This system allows for easy reproducibility of the treatment position from localization of the tumor (simulation) to treatment on the linear accelerator. Other companies such as Uarian Medical Systems have also now developed their own CT-Simulators.

Patient Selection

The patient population eligible for 3-DCRT is fundamentally no different than those men who are candidates for conventional radiation therapy. In fact, given the lower toxicity profile of 3-DCRT as compared to conventional RT [10,11], conformal RT (CRT) may be even more suitable for such men as the very elderly than conventional RT. Generally, men eligible for definitive 3-DCRT are those presenting with nonmetastatic localized adenocarcinoma of the prostate. Obviously, the prognosis of these patients also depends upon the Gleason score and initial prostate-specific antigen (PSA) levels. Furthermore, men who are generally treated with definitive RT as compared to those who undergo radical prostatectomy tend to be older with significant medical comorbidities, which usually preclude surgery. Additionally, men who are radiated usually tend to have more advanced stage and unfavorable disease as compared to their counterparts, who undergo surgery [12–14]. These significant differences are important to remember when results between a surgically treated prostate cancer population are compared to men treated with definitive radiation therapy.

What Is 3-D Conformal Radiation Therapy?

Plainly put, three-dimensional conformal radiation therapy is the "shaping" of the radiation beam so that the tumor is given higher dose of radiation than the surrounding normal tissues. The "3-D" process minimizes the volume of surrounding critical organs that receive higher doses of radiation, thereby significantly reducing acute toxicity and late complications. Three-dimensional conformal radiation therapy is possible by better delineation of the target and surrounding normal tissues

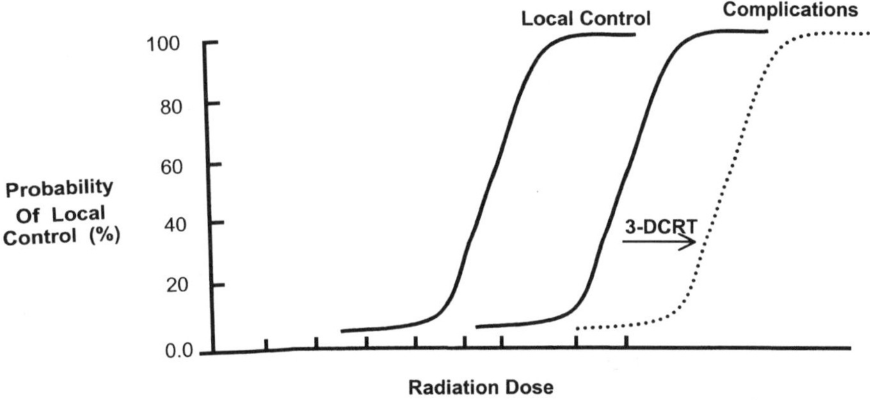

FIGURE 1 The two solid curves show the typical relationship between local control and complications for a given dose of radiation therapy. The dashed curve shows the effect of 3-DCRT as it pushes the complication curve more to the right in relationship to the local control curve, thereby reducing the likelihood of late sequalae for the same dose of radiation.

via computed tomographic scanning and immobilization of the patient; this allows reduced treatment margins around the prostate, thus decreasing the volume of surrounding critical organs that receive high doses of radiation. Furthermore, by lowering the dose to the surrounding critical organs such as the rectum and bladder, dose escalation to the prostate is also possible with the opportunity to improve local control, thereby improving the therapeutic ratio (Figure 1)

How is 3-D Conformal Radiation Therapy Given?

Three-dimensional conformal radiation therapy is administered in several major steps:

1. Patient Immobilization
2. Computed Tomographic (CT) Scanning
3. Dosimetric Planning including Conformal Beam Shaping
4. Simulation
5. Field Verification

First, patients are immobilized in the treatment position with a lower body cast. Patients must be positioned on the treatment table for their radiation treatment on 42–51 separate days. Placing the patient in a rigid posterior body cast improves the day-to-day set-up reproducibility. In a study done at Fox Chase Cancer Center [7], the day-to-day set-up error was a maximum of 1.5 cm for patients who were not immobilized. With cast immobilization, this maximum error was reduced to 7 mm. This meant that the extra margin that must be included in the treatment beam around the target to account for set-up error could be reduced from 1.5 cm to 0.7 cm, saving surrounding normal critical organs from radiation exposure while still assuring that the entire target is treated each day. In our department, patients are immobilized in a half-body alpha cradle from the waist to the knees (Figure 2).

Next, a CT scan is taken to localize the target (prostate and seminal vesicles) in three dimensions. Usually, CT slices of 3 mm thickness are obtained from the top of the sacroiliac joints through the bottom of the obturator foramen. The target and adjacent normal structures are contoured on each CT image to produce a three-dimensional reconstruction of the prostate, seminal vesicles, urinary bladder, and rectum (Figure 3).

Radiation target volumes are defined according to the International Commission on Radiation Units and Measurements #50 report [15]. The Gross Tumor Volume (GTV) is defined as all known gross disease indicated by the planning CT or any other information. The Clinical Target Volume (CTV) is defined as the GTV and any areas considered to potentially contain microscopic disease. In prostate cancer, the entire prostate is considered the CTV. Finally, the Planning Target Volume (PTV) is the CTV plus a surrounding margin to account for the variability of treatment setup and internal organ motion.

After the target and critical surrounding normal tissues have been identified on the CT scan, dosimetric planning is done to determine the shape and the number of beams. Multiple beams such as a 4 to 6 field arrangement are used to shape the radiation beams to conform to the contours of the target using a "beam's-eye view" (BEV) block design (Figure 4). The beam's-eye view is the view from the observer's perspective from the radiation source looking out along the radiation axis at the target included in that particular radiation portal. Treatment-planning computers with dosimetric algorithms are used to calculate the dose in three dimensions.

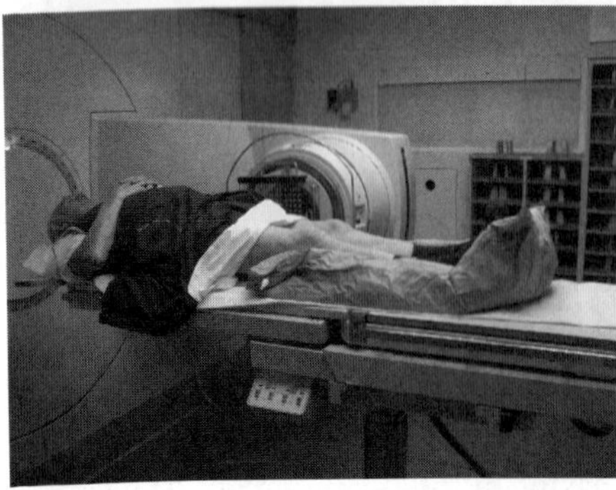

FIGURE 2 The patient is immobilized by a lower body alpha cradle during the radiotherapy treatments.

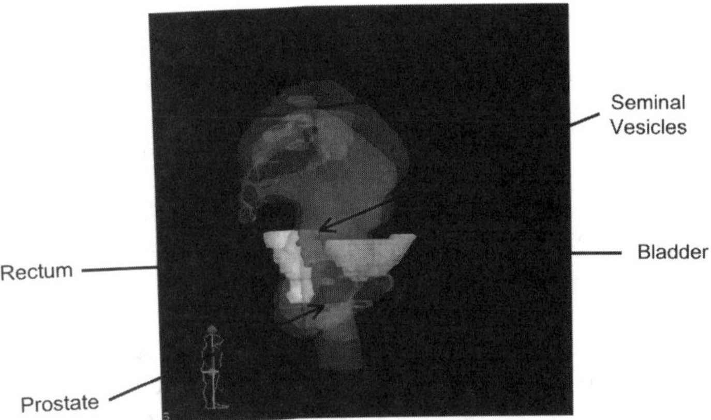

FIGURE 3 A computerized re-construction of the patient's inner anatomy shows the prostate gland, seminal vesicle and surrounding critical organs such as the rectum and bladder in the "treatment position" through a lateral view of the pelvis.

Dose-volume histograms (DVHs)—which are visual representations of the amount of radiation dosage that the volume of a target or a critical organ receives—are used to aid in the quantitative analysis of 3-DCRT treatment plans. Dose distributions for 3-DCRT are generated in a multiple planes, with the dose prescribed at the iso-center, typically normalized to the 100% isodose line.

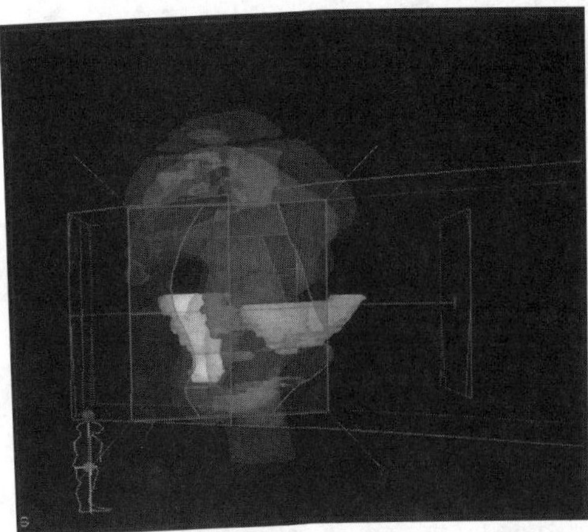

FIGURE 4 A "beam's eye view" shows the target (prostate and seminal vesicles) and the surrounding critical organs (rectum and the bladder) which will be shielded (grey shaded areas) during the radiotheraphy treatments.

The patient is then simulated in the same treatment position that he was originally imaged in for the CT scan. During simulation, the patient is filmed with the multiple conformal beams in place (Figure 5). Treatment field size and total radiation dose depend on pretreatment PSA level, Gleason score, and palpation T stage. For patients with high risk of nodal metastases (i.e., Gleason score ≥ 7, PSA ≥ 10, or T_3–T_4 disease), the pelvis is generally treated followed by a boost to the prostate and seminal vesicles. Generally, the pelvis is treated to a dose of 45 Gy at 1.8 Gy/fraction once daily. The superior border of the pelvic field is usually set at the level of the midsacroiliac joints and the inferior border at the bottom of the ischial tuberosities. Lateral borders on the anterior/posterior and posterior/anterior fields are set 1.5 to 2.0 cm lateral to the pelvic brim. For the lateral fields, the posterior border is set at the S2/S3 interspace. Anteriorly, the field edge is at the front edge of the pubic symphysis. For patients presenting with favorable disease, small fields encompassing only the prostate with or without seminal vesicles are used. If the seminal vesicles are considered to be at risk for subclinical involvement, they are generally treated to 54–59.4 Gy. The prostate is then boosted to doses in the range of *at least* 75.6 Gy or higher depending upon the patient's risk group and the institutute's protocols and/or philosophy. Multileaf collimation or individualized cerrobend blocks can be used to shape the treatment portal (Figure 6).

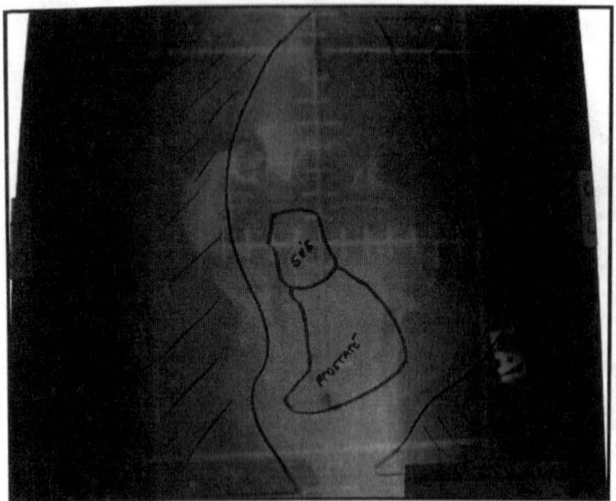

Figure 5   The "beam eye view" is then used to "simulate" the treatment field by digital reconstruction of the target (prostate and seminal vesicles) with appropriate shielding of the surrounding critical organs (i.e., posterior rectum, bowel and some anterior bladder). Barium is also inserted into the rectum for further anatomical confirmation as initially located on the planning CT scan.

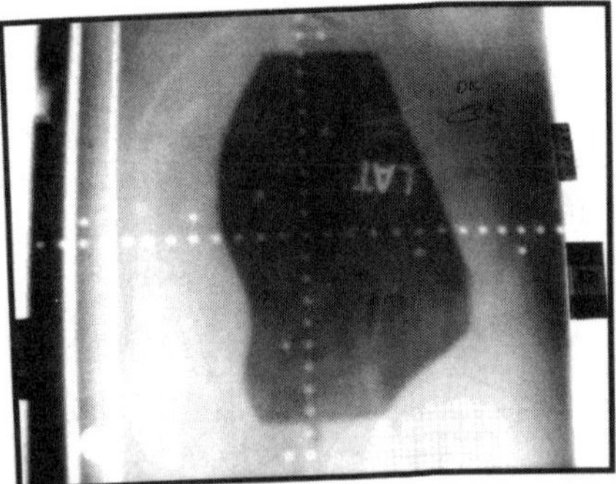

FIGURE 6 The "port film" shows the "dark area" which is the radiated region while the surrounding "light area" is shielded.

"Measuring Success"

With development of the prostate-specific antigen (PSA) test, not only have an increased number of men been diagnosed and subsequently treated for localized disease, but the way we measure the success of curative modalities has drastically changed. Biochemical control of disease as measured by posttreatment PSA levels has become the most rigorous way of measuring the efficacy of surgery or radiation therapy. Additionally, the pretreatment PSA level has been shown to be the strongest independent predictor of treatment outcome after both surgery and radiation [16–20].

Biochemical "no evidence of disease" (bNED) is defined by a non-rising posttreatment PSA level, while a rising posttreatment PSA level now predicts failure many years before disease becomes clinically detectable [21,22]. Routine use of PSA measurement entered clinical practice in the late 1980s. Initially, there was no standard definition of bNED control; biochemical cure after RT was variably defined and correlated with clinical progression and outcome. In a large series of 480 patients treated with conventional RT between January 1987 and December 1981, Horwitz et al. demonstrated that by merely changing the definition of biochemical control, statistically significant differences in outcome could be obtained ranging from 5% to 53% (p <001) [23].

In an effort to develop a unified definition of "PSA cure" following irradiation, a conference was convened by a committee of the Board of Directors of the American Society of Therapeutic Radiology and Oncology (ASTRO). The definition selected by the committee was to be applicable in clinical practice as well as in research trials, avoid the issue of the amount of baseline serum PSA that might be produced in the prostate gland following RT, be valid for comparing different methods of radiation delivery, and avoid requiring a specific single value for posttreatment nadir PSA, which is a notion fraught with statistical peril [23]. In March 1997, the committee published a consensus statement for the definition of PSA failure: three consecutive increases in posttreatment PSA after achieving a nadir [24]. The majority of series published in radiation literature now utilize this definition of bNED failure, thereby making comparisons of treatment efficacy more standard.

RESULTS

Comparison with Standard Radiation Therapy

Investigators from Washington University Medical Center compared their results of 3-DCRT to standard radiation therapy (SRT) alone during the same time period between January 1992 and December 1997. Perez et al [11]. reported their experience with a total of 277 patients, 146 who were treated with 3-DCRT and 131 who were treated with SRT alone for clinical stage T_{1C} or T_2 localized adenocarcinoma of the prostate. For patients undergoing 3-DCRT, 7 intercepting fields were used to deliver a dose of 68–73.8 Gy. Standard radiation therapy consisted of bilateral 120° rotational arcs, including portals with 2 cm margins around the prostate to deliver 68–70 Gy. Higher 5-year bNED survival was observed with 3-DCRT (91% for T_{1C} and 96% for T_2 tumor) compared to SRT (53% and 58%, respectively). In patients with Gleason scores of 5–7, the 5-year bNED survival rates were 96% with 3-DCRT compared to only 53% with SRT (p .01). In 111 patients with pretreatment PSA 10.0 ng/mL, treated with 3-DCRT, the 5-year bNED survival rate was 96% versus 65% in 94 patients treated with SRT (p .01). In patients with PSA of 10.1–20 ng/mL, the 5-year bNED survival rate for 26 patients treated with 3-DCRT was 88%, compared to only 40% for the 20 patients treated with SRT (p = .05). The corresponding values were 70% and 20% respectively for patients with PSA levels of >20 ng/mL. On multivaried analysis, the most important prognostic factor for biochemical control of disease were pretreatment PSA level (p = .023), nadir PSA (p = .001), and 3-DCRT technique (p = .003). Hence, and not all that unsurprisingly, the results with 3-DCRT compared to SRT in this nonrandomized report were superior. Furthermore, acute and late toxicity was also lower in the 3-DCRT group as compared to the SRT group. Moderate dysuria or urinating difficulties were reported by 2–5% of patients treated with 3-DCRT in contrast to 6–9% treated with SRT. The incidence of moderate loose stools/diarrhea was 3–5% in the 3-DCRT group compared to 8–19% in the SRT group. Late intestinal morbidity (proctitis) or rectal bleeding occurred in only 1.7% patients undergoing 3-DCRT in contrast to 8% in the SRT patients.

3-D CONFORMAL RADIATION THERAPY: LONG-TERM OUTCOME

Results of treatment with 3-DCRT with long-term follow-up of five years or longer are becoming available and demonstrate superior bNED control rates. Many single institutions such as University of Michigan [25], Fox Chase Cancer Center [26], Memorial Sloan-Kettering Cancer Center [27], University of California at San Francisco [28], Washington University [11], and MD Anderson [29] have reported their results using 3-DCRT. However, only those institutions with a large series of patients (i.e., $\geq$200) that have reported at least 5-year bNED results will be reviewed. Notably, University of Michigan, Fox Chase Cancer Center, and Memorial Sloan-Kettering Cancer Center have reported 5-year bNED outcome data with at least 200 patients in each series.

Fukunaga-Johnson et al [25]. reported the University of Michigan results treating patients with clinically localized prostate cancer using 3-DCRT (Table 1). A total of 707 patients were treated with 3-DCRT *alone* from January 1987 to June 1994; pretreatment PSA information was available for 649 patients. None of the patients were treated with hormone therapy. The median 3-D conformal dose in this study was 69 Gy (range of 49 to 80 Gy), although a few patients received greater than 72 Gy. Biochemical failure was defined as two consecutive PSA increases above 2 ng/mL or more if the nadir PSA was 2 ng/mL or less, two consecutive PSA increases over 2 ng/mL if the PSA nadir was more than 2 ng/mL, or whenever hormone therapy was initiated after RT. The 5-year bNED rate was 75% for the "favorable" subgroup (PSA $\leq$10, GS <7, and T_1–T_2 disease) of prostate cancer patients compared to 33% for the "unfavorable" subgroup (PSA >10, GS $\geq$7, or T_3–T_4 disease). The five-year actuarial rates of bNED were 88%, 72%, 43%, and 30%, respectively, for patients with pretreatment PSA values less than 4, 4 to 10, 10 to 20, and greater than 20 ng/mL. Only pre-RT PSA level >10 ng/mL (p = .0001), T-stage 3–4 (p = .0001), and Gleason score >7 (p = .0177) were independent predictors on multivariate analysis. A radiation dose response was not demonstrated, although few patients in this study received high doses. One criticism of this study was that their definition of biochemical failure can overestimate the rate of biochemical control. As expected, late toxicity was very low as graded according to the Radiation Therapy Oncology Group (RTOG) scale: 3% actuarial risk at 7 years of grade III/IV rectal complications and 1% actuarial risk at 7 years of grade III bladder toxicity with no grade IV morbidity.

The results from Fox Chase Cancer Center [26] describing the five-year outcome of their dose escalation study were reported by Hanks et al. (Table 1). A total of 232 were treated with 3-DCRT between June 1989 and October 1992, with median follow-up of 5 years. The median radiation dose to the prostate was 7158 cGy (range of 6316 to 7895 cGy). During this time, radiation dose to the

TABLE 1 Long-Term Outcome Following 3-DCRT from Selected Individual Institutional Series

Institutional/ Period	Patients, n	Hormone therapy	3-DCRT Dose, median (cGy)	Definition of biochemical failure	5-yr bNED rates	Late toxicity	Median follow-up interval
Univ of Michigan Jan 87'–June '94	707 (PSA available, n=649)	No	6900 (4900–8000)	(1) ↑ PSA × 2 over 2.0 ng/mL if nadir PSA ≤2.0 ng/mL (2) ↑ PSA × above 2.0 ng/mL if nadir PSA >2.0 ng/mL (3) If Hormone Rx post-RT	Favorable Group— 75% (PSA ≤10, GS ≤6, T_1–T_2) Unfavorable Group — 33% (PSA >10,GS ≥7, T_3–T_4) Pre-RT PSA (ng/mL) ≤4–88% >4, ≤10 – 72% >10,≤20 – 43% >20 – 30%	Rectal (Gr. III/IV)–3% Bladder (Gr. III)*–1% [*No Gr. IV toxicity]	36 Months
Fox Chase Cancer Center June 1989–Oct. 1992	232	No	7158 (6316–7895)	↑ PSA × 2 and nadir PSA >1.5 ng/mL	PSA ≤10 – 82% (n=96) PSA ≤10 – 19.9 – 55% (n=70) 70 Gy – 35% 76 Gy – 75% PSA ≥20 (n=66) 70 Gy – 10% 76 Gy – 32%	RTOG GI Gr. III/IV <1% LENT GU Gr. III/IV=4% Urinary Incontinence No TURP=0.6% ⊖ TURP=2%	5 Years
Memorial Sloan Kettering Cancer Center Oct. 1988–Dec. 1995	743 n=530 (no hormones)	Yes (n=59)	6480–8100	ASTRO Consensus	Favorable Group – 85% (PSA ≤10, T_1 – T_2, GS ≤6) [83% – no homones] Intermediate Group – 65% (↑ in 1 Feature) [61%–no hormones] Unfavorable Group–35% (↑ in ≥ 2 Features) [31%–no hormones]	Rectal Gr. III–0.8% Urinary Gr. III–1% Gr. IV–0%	3 yrs (1.7–6 yrs)

* Measured as biochemical control of PSA (ng/mL)

prostate was increased from 63 to 79 Gy. The definition of biochemical failure was 2 consecutive PSA increases and PSA >1.5 ng/mL. Stratified by initial PSA levels, dose responses were demonstrated for patients with pretreatment PSA values between 10 to 20 ng/mL and greater than 20 ng/mL, but not for PSA <10 ng/mL. Five-year bNED rates for patients with pretreatment PSA levels of less than 10 was 82%, and no dose-response relationship was noted. Five-year bNED rates for patients with pretreatment PSA levels between 10 to 20 ng/mL treated at 70 Gy was 35% versus 75% for the patients treated at 76 Gy (p = 0.02). For patients with pretreatment PSA levels greater than 20 ng/mL, 5-year bNED control was 10% at 70 Gy, versus 33% at 76 Gy (p = 0.02).

Multivariate analysis revealed that increasing dose (p = .0169), pretreatment PSA level (p = .0001), and Gleason Score 7–10 (p = .0001) were associated with bNED outcome. Only palpation T-stage predicted decreased rates of cause-specific (p = 0.002) and distant-metastases-free survival (p = 0.0004). The 5-year long-term complication rate was as follows: RTOG grade III/IV gastrointestinal (GI) toxicity <1%, late effects on normal tissue scale (LENT) grade III/IV genitourinary (GU) complication rate of 4%, and incontinence rate of 0.6% without a history of transuretheral resection of prostate (TURP) versus 2% with history of TURP. Late toxicity became potentially more significant as radiation doses were increased. Five-year rates of grades II and III/IV gastrointestinal toxicity were 33% and 8%, respectively, at doses of 75 to 76 Gy. When anterior rectal wall shielding was used to keep the dose below 72 Gy to the rectum, the five-year rates of grade II and III/IV gastrointestinal toxicity were reduced to 11% and 2%, respectively.

In a recent report, Hanks et al. updated the results of their 3-DCRT experience with 8–12 years follow-up In [30]. Biochemical failure was defined according to the ASTRO consensus definition. The bNED rate at 8 years for all patients treated with 3-DCRT 67–81 Gy) was 48% at 10 and 12 years of follow-up. For PSA levels between 0 and 9.9 ng/mL, and prostate cancer with unfavorable features (i.e., T2B/T3, and/or GS ≥ 7 and/or perineural invasion), the bNED rate was 62%; for PSA levels between 10 and 19.9 ng/mL with unfavorable features, it was only 44%; and for PSA ≥ 20 ng/mL, 14% of patients exhibited biochemical remission.

Zelefsky et al. reported the updated results of the Memorial Sloan-Kettering Cancer Center 3-DCRT dose escalation trial [27]. Seven hundred forty-three patients were treated as part of a phase I study where radiation dose increased from 64.8 to 81 Gy in increments of 5.4 Gy. The median follow-up was 3 years (range of 1.7–6 years). The ASTRO consensus definition was used to measure PSA failure. Of all patients who received 75.6 or 81 Gy, 90% achieved a posttreatment PSA nadir of 1 ng/mL or less compared with 76% and 56% of patients who received 70.2 and 64.8 Gy, respectively (p <.001). The 5-year actuarial

PSA relapse-free survival for patients with "favorable" prognostic indicators (stage T_1–T_2, pretreatment PSA $\leq$10.0 ng/mL and Gleason score $\leq$6) was 85%, compared to 65% for those with "intermediate" prognosis (one of the prognostic indicators with a higher value) and 35% for the group with "unfavorable" prognosis (two or more indicators with higher values) (p <0.001). Intermediate and poor prognosis patients treated with 75.6 Gy or more achieved improved bNED control rates (p <.05).

Posttreatment nadir PSA levels were correlated with biopsy findings 2.5 years after treatment to evaluate response. Of all patients (good and poor prognostic grouping) receiving 81 Gy, 7% (1 out of 15) had a positive biopsy, compared with 48% (12 out of 25) at 75.6 Gy, versus 45% (19 out of 42) at 70.2 Gy and 57% (13 out of 23) after 64.8 Gy (p <0.05). Using multivariate analysis, pretreatment PSA level ($\leq$ 10ng/mL, p <.001), T stage (<T_{2C}, p <.03), and radiation dose (>75.6 Gy, p<.001) were independent predictors of achieving nadir PSA levels of 1 ng/mL or less for 530 patients not treated with neoadjuvant hormones. The overall median time from treatment to this nadir response was 15 months, with 90% of such responses identified within 24 months after treatment. The 3-DCRT delivered at Memorial Sloan-Kettering Cancer Center was very well tolerated. The overall rate of significant grade III/IV late toxicities was only 1.9%. The rate of urinary grade III and IV late complications was 1% and 0%, respectively. The rate of late grade III rectal toxicity was 0.8%. The 5-year actuarial likelihood of chronic grade II GI and GU toxicity were 11% and 10%, respectively. However, the rate for late GI toxicity in patients receiving >75.6 Gy was 17%, compared to 6% in patients treated with $\leq$70.2 Gy (p <0.001). Similarly, the rates of late grade II GU toxicity were 13% and 8% for patients receiving >75.6 Gy versus $\leq$70.2 Gy, respectively (p=0.002).

In order to assess the impact of 3-DCRT on outcome of patients with high-risk prostate cancer, a multiinstitutional review was conducted by Fiveash et al [31]. Pooled results on 180 patients with Gleason Score 8–10 from Fox Chase Cancer Center, the University of Michigan, and the University of California, San Francisco, were analyzed (Table 2). The median radiation dose was 7162 cGy, with 30% of patients receiving <70 Gy, 37% receiving 70–75 Gy, 33% receiving >75 Gy; of significance, 27% of patients received neoadjuvant or adjuvant hormone therapy. The median follow-up was 3 years for patients in this study (range of 1.8–3.7 years). The 1997 ASTRO consensus definition was used to define freedom from PSA failure. The 5-year overall survival for all patients was 67.3%. The 5-year freedom from PSA failure was 62.5% for all patients and 79.3% in T_1–T_2 patients. Using a multivariate analysis, pretreatment PSA level and radiation dose were independent predictors of bNED control for patients with T_1–T_2 tumors. Patients treated with doses less than 70 Gy or with 70 to 75 Gy had 5-year bNED control rates of 65% and 88%, respectively (p = 0.02).

TABLE 2 Pooled Results After 3-DCRT for High Gleason Score Prostate Cancer

Institutional/ Period	Patients, n	Hormone therapy	3-DCRT Dose, Median (c/Gy)	Definition of biochemical failure	5-yr bNED Rates	Median follow-up interval
Pooled Analysis	n=180	Yes=27%	7162	ASTRO definition *PSA (ng/mL)* $\geq$4 <10 – 83% $\geq$10 <20 – 85% $\geq$20 – 43%	T_1–T_4 Tumors *PSA (ng/mL)* 4 <10 – 83% 10 <20 – 85% >20 – 43% T_1–T_2 Tumors–bNED 5 yrs *PSA (ng/mL)* <10 – 90% 10 – 20 [??019] >20 – 59% *RT Dose* <70 Gy – 65% 70–75 Gy – 88%	3.0 years (1.8–3.7)

TOXICITY

Comparison with Standard Radiation Therapy

In a randomized trial conducted at the Royal Marsden/Institute of Cancer Research, 225 patients were treated either with standard radiation therapy or with 3-DCRT to a dose of 64 Gy at 2 Gy per fraction [32]. The median follow-up interval was 3.6 years (range of 2 to 8 years). The risk of late gastrointestinal complications in the 111 patients treated with SRT was much higher as compared to the 114 patients treated with 3-DCRT. The risk of late grade II or higher rectal bleeding was 12% in patients treated with SRT, compared to only 3% in patients treated with 3-DCRT (p = .05). Additionally, the risk of late grade II or higher proctitis was also much higher in the SRT group as compared to the 3-DCRT group (15% versus 5%, respectively, p = .01). Several retrospective analysis from single institutions have also confirmed the results of this randomized trial; notably, that the risk of late sequela, especially gastrointestinal complications, is 3–4 fold higher with standard radiotherapy as compared to 3-DCRT [10,22].

Three-dimensional conformal radiation therapy treatments are extremely well tolerated. Acute grade III/IV toxicity is extremely rare doing 3-DCRT. In my own personal experience, the majority (≈50–60%) of patients will experience virtually no acute toxicity during 3-DCRT. Some patients will experience mild increased frequency or change in the quality of bowel or bladder habits not requiring any medical intervention, and an even smaller number will experience RTOG grade II GI/GU acute toxicity.

As noted previously, (Table 1) the risk of late sequela following 3-DCRT is extremely uncommon. The rate of gastrointestinal late grade III/IV toxicity varies from 0.8%, as reported by Memorial Sloan-Kettering Cancer Center, to 3% late rectal-complication rate (actuarial risk at 7 years), as reported by the University of Michigan. The rate of late grade III/IV GU late-toxicity rate varies from 1%, as reported by Memorial Sloan-Kettering Cancer Center, to 4%, as reported by Fox Chase Cancer Center. In these late reports, the rate of late grade IV toxicity is rare to nonexistent. These low rates of toxicities are not surprising given the capability to localize the prostate and seminal vesicles in relationship to the surrounding critical organs such as the rectum and the urinary bladder with the use of 3-DCRT.

In a report by Lee et al [33] of 257 patients treated at Fox Chase Cancer Center with 3-DCRT to minimum planning target volume doses of 71–75 Gy, the rate of late grade II rectal toxicity (usually consisting of rectal bleeding managed conservatively) was 16%, and the grade III late rectal-complication rate was 2%. The incidence of late grade II/III rectal morbidity increased as the dose at the isocenter of the prostate increased (p = .05). The actuarial rate at 18 months of late grade II/III rectal morbidity according to central axis dose was as follows: <74 Gy—7%, 74–76 Gy—16%, and >76 Gy—23% (p = .05). In order to address this increased late rectal-complication rate with increasing doses of radiation, a small rectal block was added to the lateral boost fields for the last 10 Gy. Calculations at Fox Chase Cancer Center determined that the addition of the lateral rectal block reduced the dose to a portion of the anterior rectal wall by 4 to 5 Gy. In patients receiving minimum planning target-volume doses of ≤ 76 Gy, the use of a lateral rectal block halved the incidence of late grade II/III actuarial toxicity from 18% without the blocks to 9% with the blocks (p = .003).

Michalski et al [34] reported on an RTOG prospective phase I dose-escalation trial (protocol 9406) with 3-DCRT for localized prostate cancer. Doses ranged from 68.4 Gy (level I) to 73.8 Gy (level II), and subsequently to 79.2 Gy (level III), with 1.8 Gy daily fractions. Patients were registered according to three stratification groups: Group 1 patients had clinically organ-confined disease (T_1-T_2) with a calculated risk of seminal vesicle (SV) invasion of $<15\%$; group 2 patients had clinical T_1-T_2 disease with a risk of SV invasion $\geq 15\%$; group 3 patients had clinical local extension of tumor beyond the prostate capsule (T_3). Between August 23, 1994, and July 2, 1997, 304 Group 1 and 2 cases were registered; 288 cases were analyzable for toxicity. Acute toxicity was low, with 53% and 54% of Group 1 patients having either no or grade 1 toxicity at dose levels I and II, respectively. Sixty-two percent of Group 2 patients had either none or grade 1 toxicity at either dose level. Few patients (0–3%) experienced a grade III acute bowel or bladder toxicity, and there were no acute grade IV or V toxicities. Late toxicity was very low in all patient groups. The majority (81% and 85%) had either no or mild grade I late toxicity at dose level I and II, respectively. A single late grade III bladder toxicity in a Group 2 patient treated to dose level II was recorded. There were no grade IV or V late effects in any patient. Compared to historical RTOG controls (trials 7506, 7706) at dose level I, no grade III or greater late effects were observed in Group I and Group 2 patients when 9.1 and 4.8 events were expected (p = 0.003 and p = 0.028), respectively. At dose level II, there were no grade III or greater toxicities in Group 1 patients and a single Grade III late toxicity in a Group 2 patient when 12.1 and 13.0 were expected (p = 0.0005 and p = 0.0003), respectively. This RTOG demonstrated that high doses of 3-DCRT can be delivered in a multiinstitutional setting with minimal toxicity.

In a study reported by Zelefsky et al [35], the rates of acute and late toxicities were analyzed in 96 patients following high doses (>75Gy) of 3-DCRT. Fifty patients received an initial dose of 75.6 Gy and the remaining 46 were dose-escalated to 81 Gy. Median follow-up for these cohorts of patients at 75.6 Gy and 81 Gy was 60 and 40 months, respectively. As expected, acute toxicity during high doses of 3-DCRT was very minimal. At the 75.6 Gy dose level, 84% of the patients experienced either no toxicity to only grade I rectal toxicity. Only 8 of 50 patients (16%) experienced acute grade II rectal toxicity at this dose level. Similarly, at the 81 Gy dose level, 18 of 46 (39%) and 20 of 46 (43%) of the patients experienced either no or only acute grade I rectal toxicities, respectively. Only 8 of 46 (17%) experienced grade II acute rectal toxicity at the 81 Gy dose level. No acute grade III or grade IV rectal toxicity was observed. Hence, acute rectal symptoms were absent or minimal (grade I) and necessitated no therapeutic intervention in 80 (83%) of the 96 patients. At the 75.6 Gy dose level, acute urinary effects included grade 0 in 8 (16%), grade I in 27 (54%), and grade II in 15 patients (30%). At the 81.0 Gy dose level, the acute urinary grade 0 toxicity was noted in 5 (11%), grade I in 21 (46%), and grade II in 20 patients (43%). No acute grade III or grade IV urinary toxicity was noted. Overall, 61 patients (64%) experienced no or grade I acute urinary symptoms.

Late rectal morbidity was absent or minimal (grade I) in 82 of the 96 patients (85%). Fourteen patients (15%) developed a late grade II rectal morbidity. In general, the grade II morbidity included rectal bleeding, which responded to conservative measures such as sitz baths and treatment with corticosteroid suppositories. The 5-year actuarial rates of late grade II rectal morbidity in patients who received 75.6 and 81.0 Gy were 16% and 15%, respectively (p = .59). Of the 14 patients who developed a late grade II rectal morbidity, 13 (93%) had subsequent resolution of their symptoms. No late grade III or higher rectal morbidities were observed. Late urinary morbidity was absent or minimal (grade I) in 86 of the 96 patients (90%). Nine patients (9%) developed a late grade II morbidity, which included chronic urinary frequency and urgency and necessitated the administration of nonsteroidal antiinflammatory medications, or α-blocking agents, for relief. The 5-year actuarial rates of chronic grade II urinary morbidity for patients who received 75.6 Gy and 81.0 Gy were 14% and 7%, respectively (p = .21). Of the nine patients who developed a grade II morbidity, seven (78%) had subsequent resolution of their symptoms. One patient treated with 81.0 Gy developed a grade III urethral stricture, which was relieved by dilatation.

Investigators from the University of California at San Francisco [36] and University of California Davis [37] have analyzed potency preservation rates after 3-DCRT. Generally, potency rates following 3-DCRT range from 60 to 65%. In a report by Chinn et al [35], the impact of 3-DCRT on potency rates in patients treated for clinically localized adenocarcinoma of the prostate was analyzed. Sixty patients reported having sexual function prior to 3-DCRT, including 47 who were fully potent and 13 who were marginally potent. Following 3-DCRT, 37 of 60 patients (62%) retained sexual function sufficient for intercourse. Of those with sexual function before radiation, 33 of 47 (70%) patients who were fully potent and 4 of 13 (31%) patients who were marginally potent maintained function sufficient for sexual intercourse (p <.01). Potency was retained in 6 of 15 (40%) patients with a history of major urologic surgical procedure (MUSP), and in 31 of 45 (69%) patients with no history of MUSP (p = .04). These investigators from University of California at San Francisco concluded that patients who received definitive 3-DCRT appear to maintain potency similar to patients treated with conventional radiotherapy treatments. However, patients who were marginally potent at presentation or had a history of MUSP appeared to be at increased risk for impotence following 3-DCRT. In a similar retrospective analysis from the University of California Davis, Wilder et al [37] retrospectively analyzed 52 patients presenting with "favorable" prostate cancer (T_{1B}–T_{2B}, N_0M_0, PSA <10, and Gleason Score ≤ 6) who were treated with 3-DCRT. One patient was not reviewable. The potency rate prior to radiation therapy was 69% ($n = 35/51$). The Kaplan-Meier estimates of potency preservation rates following 3-DCRT at 1, 2, and 3 years were 100%, 83%, and 63%, respectively. Three of seven patients who became impotent after 3-DCRT and used sildenafil (Viagra®) were successfully able to achieve erection sufficient for sexual intercourse.

Hence, 3-DCRT is indeed very well tolerated. Acute gastrointestinal and genitourinary toxicity during 3-DCRT is limited mostly to grade 0–I toxicity and is transient and self-limiting. The rates of late grade III GI and GU morbidity toxicity vary from 0% to 3% and from 0% to 4%, respectively. Severe (grade IV) late gastrointestinal or genitourinary complications following 3-DCRT are extremely rare.

INTENSITY MODULATED RADIATION THERAPY

What Is Intensity Modulated Radiation Therapy?

Intensity modulated radiation therapy (IMRT) represents a forward leap in the evolution of 3-DCRT: different intensities of radiation dosages can now be delivered within the same radiation field and with the same benefits as 3-DCRT, such as sparing critical surrounding structures, but with the added advantage of delivering much higher doses of radiation without the attendant increase in acute or late normal tissue toxicity. Technically, IMRT is a form of conformal therapy in which the radiation fluence of the beam can be varied by the use of multiple subfields given by using inverse treatment planning. Each beam is divided into multiple segments to modulate the dose. Hence, the resultant isodoses are highly conformal and can uniquely yield dose distributions that tightly hug the target and additionally limit the radiation doses to the surrounding critical organs. This is different from an unmodulated radiation beam where the fluence is constant, as in the case of 3-DCRT or conventional RT. Furthermore, unlike 3-DCRT, IMRT works backwards by choosing the desired dose to the target (prostate) and surrounding critical organs (e.g., rectum, bladder), and then determining the required number of beams and intensities that will achieve that dose distribution (i.e., inverse treatment planning). The target volume and surrounding critical organs are defined, and the upper and lower dose limits for the target and surrounding normal structures are selected. This is known as inverse treatment planning. With 3-DCRT, the maximum achievable dosage to the target is usually determined by the "tolerable" dosage delivered to the surrounding critical organs. Hence, IMRT is different from 3-DCRT in two fundamental ways: (1) The beam fluence varies across the IMRT beam versus being constant across the 3-DCRT beam; (2) Inverse treatment planning is used with IMRT.

Several institutions have reported their experience using IMRT for prostate cancer. Recently, Zelefsky et al [38] updated their experience using 3-DCRT and IMRT for 1100 patients with the clinical stages T_{1C}–T_3 prostate cancer treated between October 1988 and December 1998. As noted previously, radiation doses were escalated from 64.8 Gy to 86.5 Gy at 5.4 Gy intervals using 3D-CRT and IMRT. Three-DCRT was administered in 810 patients to doses between 64.8 to 75.6 Gy, as well as an initial 61 patients who received 81 Gy. The subsequent 289 patients received 81 and 86.4 Gy using IMRT. Treatment was given with 15 mV x-rays in daily fractions of 1.8 Gy. A total of 427 patients (39%) with a large volume prostate were given a 3-month course of neoadjuvant complete androgen deprivation to decrease the size of the gland. Median follow-up was 60 months (range 24 to 142) and 339 patients (31%) were followed 7 years or longer. Combined median follow-up for the high-dose group that received 75.6 Gy or greater was 69 months. Late toxicity was scored according to the RTOG morbidity grading scale. Biochemical PSA failure was defined according to the ASTRO consensus report. At five years, the PSA relapse-free survival rate in patients at favorable, intermediate, and unfavorable risk groups (as defined previously) was 85%, 58%, and 38%, respectively (p <0.001). Radiation dose was the most powerful variable impacting PSA relapse-free survival in each prognostic risk group. The 5-year actuarial PSA relapse-free survival rate for patients at favorable risk who received 64.8 to 70.2 Gy was 77% compared to 90% for those treated with 75.6 to 86.4 Gy (p = 0.05). The corresponding rates were 50% versus 70% in intermediate risk cases (p = 0.001), and 21% versus 47% in unfavorable risk cases (p = 0.002). Only 4 of 41 patients (10%) who received 81 Gy had a positive biopsy 2.5 years or longer after treatment compared with 27 of 119 (23%) after 75.6 Gy, 23 of 68 (34%) after 70.2 Gy, and 13 of 24 (54%) after 64.8 Gy. Treatment with IMRT significantly decreased the incidence of late grade II rectal toxicity as the 3-year actuarial incidence in 189 cases treated to 81 Gy was 2% compared with 14% in 61 patients treated to the same dose of 3-DCRT (p = 0.005). Intensity modulated radiation therapy did not affect the incidence of late urinary toxicity. These investigators concluded that IMRT is associated with minimal late rectal and bladder toxicity, and, hence, represents the treatment delivery approach with the most favorable risk-to-benefit ratio.

Investigators from the Cleveland Clinic also reported their initial results with the use of short course IMRT for localized prostate cancer and confirmed the low toxicity associated with this approach. Kupelian et al [39] reported their results with 51 patients who treated with IMRT between October 1998 and May 1999 to a dose of 70.0 Gy at 2.5 Gy delivered in 28 fractions over five and a half weeks. These investigators considered hypofractionated dose schedule to be equivalent to 78 Gy with a standard radiation therapy treatment schedule at 1.8 Gy per fraction. The median follow-up for this cohort of 51 patients was 18 months (range 11 to 26 months). In this series, only 1 patient experienced grade I late urinary toxicity. Furthermore, only 4 patients experienced late grade I rectal toxicity. No grade II or grade III late urinary or rectal complications have occurred. The actuarial rectal-bleeding rate observed at 18 months was 7%. Hence, paralleling the experience of the investigators from Memorial Sloan-Kettering Cancer Center, the investigators from the Cleveland Clinic further confirmed the extremely low rates of late GI or GU toxicities observed with fairly high doses of IMRT.

Although the acute and late toxicity associated with IMRT appears to be more favorable as compared to 3-DCRT in the context of even higher doses of radiation therapy, long-term results are still pending to determine if higher doses of radiation therapy for patients with intermediate- and high-risk disease will translate into better PSA bNED rates in the future.

OTHER TECHNOLOGIES

Although this chapter has focused mostly on photon beam–based external beam radiotherapy treatments using either 3-D conformal radiation therapy or intensity modulated radiation therapy, other ionizing beam technologies, such as particulate beam-based neutrons or protons have also been used to treat prostate cancer.

Neutrons

Neutrons have been used in the treatment of cancer since the 1930s. In the 1970s, RTOG protocol 77–04 randomized 91 patients with T_3–T_4, N_0–N_1, and M_0 disease to photon-alone treatment versus mixed photon/neutron treatment [40]. Among the 78 patients who were eligible for analysis, clinical local control at 10 years was 58% for the photon-alone treatment group versus 70% for the mixed photon/neutron treatment group (p = 0.03). Overall survival was also significantly different between the two arms: At 10 years, overall survival was 29% for the photon-alone group compared with 46% for the mixed photon/neutron arm (p = 0.04).

Based on this promising RTOG trial, the Neutron Therapy Collaborative Working Group was established to further assess neutrons in the treatment of prostate cancer [41]. One hundred seventy-eight patients with T_3–T_4, N_0–N_1, M_0, as well as high-grade T_2 disease, were randomized to receive either photon beam therapy alone (7,000–7,020 cGy) or neutron beam therapy alone (2,040 ncGy). For the 172 reviewable patients, the local regional failure was 47% for the photon arm versus 21% for the neutron arm (p = 0.0007) at ten years [40].

Survival at 10 years was 36% for the neutron group compared to 43% for the photon group (p = 0.80). However, incidence of severe grade IV late complications was higher in the neutron arm (11% versus 3%, p = 0.04). Based on this collaborative group trial, as well as the inherent high relative biological effectiveness (RBE) of neutrons compared to photons (i.e., × 2.6 for fractionated doses) [42] usually resulting in higher normal tissue toxicity, the use of neutrons to treat prostate cancer continues to be investigated.

Protons

The proton beam is very unique because of the "Bragg peak" [43]. The dose deposited by a beam of monoenergetic protons increases slowly with depth but reaches a sharp maximum near the end of the particles' range at the Bragg peak. The beam has sharp edges, with little side-scatter, and the dose falls to zero after the Bragg peak, at the end of the particles' range. The possibility of precisely confining the high-dose region to the tumor volume while minimizing the dose to surrounding normal tissue is an obvious attraction for the use of the proton beam in prostate cancer.

Investigators at Loma Linda University Medical Center have been treating prostate cancer patients with protons since the early 1990s. Slater et al [44] reported the Loma Linda University Medical Center experience with protons. Between 1991 and 1995, 643 patients received conformal proton boost treatment with or without photons. Patients at significant risk for subclinical involvement of regional nodes received 45 Gy in 25 fractions to the pelvis with photons followed by a prostate boost of 30 Cobalt Gray Equivalent (CGE) using 225–250 MeV protons in 15 fractions. For patients whose pelvic lymph nodes were thought to be at low risk for subclinical involvement, protons only were used for the entire treatment. These patients received lateral opposed proton fields that treated the prostate and seminal vesicles to a dose of 74 CGE in 37 fractions. The overall clinical disease-free survival was 89% at 5 years. The overall bNED rate at 5 years was 79%. Biochemical NED control rates at five years for patients with pretreatment PSA levels of less than 4, 4 to 10, 10–20, and more than 20 ng/mL were 100%, 89%, 72%, and 53%, respectively. Patients in whom the posttreatment PSA nadir was below 0.5 ng/mL did significantly better than those whose nadir values were between 0.51–1.0 or >1.0 ng/mL: the corresponding 5-year disease-free survival rates were 91%, 79%, and 40%, respectively. Late grade II gastrointestinal toxicity was the most common complication, occurring in 21% of patients. Only 5% of patients experienced late grade II genitourinary toxicity, and two patients developed late grade III toxicity. No late grade III to V gastrointestinal toxicity occurred.

Investigators at Massachusetts General Hospital conducted a prospective phase III trial in 202 patients with T_3–T_4, N_0–N_2, M_0 who were randomized to either photons only (5,040 cGy to the pelvis followed by a 1,680 cGy photon boost to the prostate) or mixed photon/ proton treatment (5,040 cGy to the pelvis with a 2,520 CGE proton boost to the prostate) [45]. Among the 189 patients completing the randomized trial, no significant differences in overall, disease-free, and cause-specific survival were observed between the two treatment arms. However, among patients with Gleason score 7–10 tumors, a statistically significant difference in clinical local control was observed between the mixed photon/ proton arm (84%) and the photon only arm (19%) at 8 years, (p = 0.0014). Furthermore, the rates of chronic grade I/II rectal bleeding was higher in the mixed-beam arm (32%) as compared to the photon-only arm (12%, p = .0002). Higher rates of urethral strictures were also observed in the mixed-beam arm (19% versus 8%, p = .07). Although the results from Loma Linda Medical Center have been very promising, the current high cost associated with the clinical use of protons may restrict the widespread adoption of this technology.

CONCLUSIONS

In summary, 3-DCRT results from single institutional series indicate fairly high bNED control rates for favorable (T_1-T_2, PSA $\leq$6 ng/mL, Gleason score $\leq$6) prostate cancer in the range of 75–85% at 5 years. For intermediate-risk disease, the long-term bNED control rates vary from 35% to 75% depending on the radiation dose or the use of neoadjuvant hormone therapy. With high doses of 3-DCRT (>76 Gy), the bNED rates for these men with intermediate-risk disease approaches 75% at 5 years. In patients with high-risk disease, the bNED rates approach $\approx$35% at 5 years with high doses of 3-DCRT. Dose-response data from Fox Chase Cancer Center [25] and dose comparison data from Memorial Sloan-Kettering Cancer Center [26] and M.D. Anderson Cancer Center [28] demonstrate a dose response for patients treated with high doses (>73 Gy) using 3-DCRT most strongly in the subgroup of patients with pretreatment PSA <10 ng/mL with unfavorable risk features (i.e., T_{2B}–T_3 disease, Gleason score 7–10 and/or perineal invasion) and those between PSA levels of 10 and 20 ng/mL. However, other strategies clearly are needed for those men presenting with high-risk disease, in whom a dose-response relationship has not been shown, and more dose may not result in more cure.

Future Directions

Several single institutions have now reported long-term outcomes following 3-DCRT and clearly show this approach to be superior to standard radiation therapy. However, prospective multiinstitutional data confirming the experience of single institutional series is currently lacking. Hence, efficacy outcome from the RTOG 3-DCRT dose-escalation trial (protocol 9406) will be crucial to confirming the results from single institutional series so that high doses of 3-DCRT become the standard of treatment in the community setting.

In addition to computed tomography (CT), there is also growing interest in incorporating complementary information available from other imaging modalities, such as magnetic resonance imaging (MRI), magnetic resonance spectroscopic imaging (MRSI), single photon emission computed tomography (SPECT), and positron emission tomography (PET) in 3-DCRT and IMRT planning. An example of a novel approach in the use of functional imaging would be defining the hypoxic region in the prostate gland by PET scanning and guide IMRT treatment to deliver super doses of radiation. Given the rapid pace of changes in current technologies, such novel approaches are not too far away in the distant future.

Other attempts to enhance the therapeutic ratio by adding hormone therapy to radiation therapy have not improved the survival outcome for men presenting with prostate cancer. In a prospective randomized trial conducted by the Radiation Therapy Oncology Group (RTOG) (protocol 86–10), the updated 8-year survival outcome was not different in patients with locally advanced disease receiving radiation therapy alone versus neoadjuvant hormone therapy and radiation therapy (44% versus 54%, p = 0.10) [46].

Similarly, in another trial (protocol 85–31), RTOG is testing the benefit of adjuvant hormone therapy (gosereoin acetate 3.6 mg/m^2 to be continued indefinitely or until progression of disease) versus radiation alone [47]. In this very large trial of 945 men, no improvement in long-term overall survival at 80 years was noted between radiotherapy alone compared to radiotherapy and adjuvant androgen suppression (47% versus 49%, respectively, p = .36). Another RTOG trial (protocol 9202) [48] also failed to confirm a survival benefit for adjuvant total androgen suppression in locally advanced prostate cancer. In this trial, patients were treated with neoadjuvant (2 months) and concurrent (2 months) hormone therapy followed by no further therapy or 2 years of additional adjuvant goserelin alone. Five-year overall survival was not different between the adjuvant hormone therapy arm compared to the no adjuvant therapy arm (78% versus 79%, respectively). Only the European Organization for Research and Treatment of Cancer (EORTC) trial (protocol 22863) has shown any benefit to the use of hormonal therapy [49]. In this trial, men with locally advanced prostate cancer were randomized to either radiation therapy alone or radiation therapy with 3 years of goserelin. At a median follow-up of 45 months, the 5-year survival was 79% in the radiation therapy and hormone therapy arm compared to 62% in the radiation therapy-only arm (p = .001).

Given the intermediate-to-poor results achieved thus far with either radiation therapy alone or in combination with hormone therapy in men with intermediate- or high-risk disease, other strategies are needed to improve local control and survival outcome for these men. Since long-term cure rates cannot be achieved without first

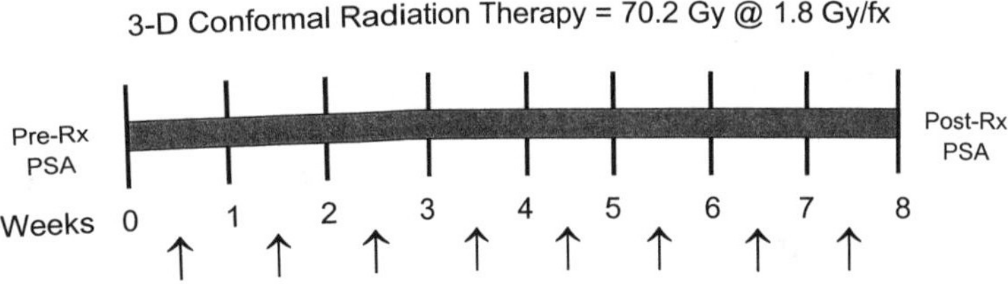

FIGURE 7 Schema of the completed phase I trial testing the use of concurrent weekly Docetaxel and 3-DCRT.

controlling local disease, a strategy that can enhance the local effects of RT is very appealing. Kumar and colleagues recently completed phase I trial testing the novel strategy of combining concurrent chemotherapy with radiation therapy as a radio-sensitizer in patients with high-risk prostate cancer [50,51]. In this I trial (Figure 7), concurrent weekly docetaxel with 3-DCRT was given to determine its maximally tolerated dose. Between January 2000 and August 2002, 22 men completed the chemoradiction therapy protocol at weekly docetaxel dose levels of 8, 12, 16, 20 and 25 mg/m². The dose-limiting toxicity was grade III diarrhea which occurred at the 25 mg/mL docetaxel weekly dose level. The MD was of weekly docetaxel was determined to be 20 mg/mL. Overall, the regimen was very well tolerated as 7 (32%) and 15 (68%) patients did not experience any diarrhea or dysuria. The results from this phase I trial will form one of the many pieces of new therapeutic strategies that will be necessary if new paradigms for the curative treatment of unfavorable prostate cancer are to be found.

REFERENCES

1. Jemal A, Tiwari RC, Murray T, Ghafoor A, Samels A, Ward E, Feuer EJ, Thun MJ. Cancer Statistics, 2004. CA Cancer J Clin 2004; 54:8–29.
2. Hanks GE, Hanlon AL, Epstein B, Horwitz EM. Dose Response in Prostate Cancer with 8-12 Years' Follow-up. Int. J. Radiation Oncology Biol. Phys. 2002; 54(2): 427–435.
3. Umegaki Y. Dose distribution in the moving field radiotherapy. Nippon Acta Radiol 1960; 20:2191–1209.
4. Takahashi S. Conformation radiotherapy. Acta Radiol Suppl 1965; 1:142.
5. Nishidai T, Nagata Y, Takahashi M, Abe M, Yamoaka N, Ishihara K, Kubo Y, Kazusa C. CT simulator: a new 3-D planning and simulating system for radiotherapy. Part 1: description of system. Int Radiat Oncol Biol Phys 1990; 18:499–504.

6. Sandler HM, Perez-Tamayo C, Ten Haken RK, Lichter AS. Dose escalation for stage C (T_3) prostate cancer: minimal rectal toxicity observed using conformal therapy. Radiother Oncol 1992; 23:53–54.

7. Soffen EM, Hanks GE, Hwang CC, Chu JCH. Conformal static field therapy for volume low-grade prostate cancer with rigid immobilization. Int J Radiat Oncol Biol Phys 1991; 20:141–146.

8. Hanks GE, Schultheiss TE, Hanlon AL, Hunt M, Lee WR, Epstein BE, Coia LR. Dose escalation in the conformal treatment of prostate cancer: optimization is made possible by understanding the dose responses for control of cancer and late morbidity. Int J Radial Oncol Biol Phys 1996; 36:197.

9. Liebel SA, Heimann R, Kutcher GJ, Zelefsky MJ, Burman CB, Melain E, Orazem JP, Mohan R, Losasso TS, Lo YC. Three-dimensional conformal radiation therapy in locally advanced carcinoma of the prostate: preliminary results of a Phase I dose-escalation study. Int J Radiat Oncol Biol Phys 1993; 28:55–65.

10. Schultheiss TE, Hanks GE, Hunt MA, Lee WR. Incidence of and factors related to late complications in conformal and conventional radiation treatment of cancer of the prostate. Int J Radial Oncol Biol Phys 1995; 32:643–649.

11. Perez CA, Michalski JM, Purdy JA, Wasserman TH, Williams K, Lockett ML. Three-dimensional conformal therapy or standard irradiation in localized carcinoma of prostate: preliminary results of a nonrandomized comparison. Int J Radial Oncol Biol Phys 2000; 47:629–637.

12. Kupelian P, Levin H, Zippe C, Klein E. External beam radiotherapy versus radical prostatectomy for localized prostate cancer: A single institution experience. J Urol 1996; 1555:556A.

13. Paulson D, Lin G, Hinshaw W, Stephani S. Radical surgery versus radiotherapy for adenocarcinoma of the prostate. Urol 1982; 128:502–504.

14. Keyser D, Kupelian PA, Zippe CD, Levin HS, Klein EA. Stage T_1-T_2 prostate cancer with pretreatment prostate-specific antigen level (10 ng/mL: Radiation therapy or surgery? Int J Radial Oncol Biol Phys 1997; 38(4):723–729.

15. International Commission on Radiation Units and Measurements: prescribing, recording, and reporting photon beam therapy, ICRU Report 50. International Commission on Radiation Units and Measurements. Bethesda. MD, 1993:3–16.

16. Zagars GK, von Eschenbach AC. Prostate-specific antigen: An important marker for prostate cancer treated by external beam radiotherapy. Cancer 1993; 72:538–548.

17. Vicini FA, Horwitz EM, Gonzalez J, Martinez AA. Treatment options for localized prostate cancer based upon pretreatment serum prostate specific antigen levels. J Urol 1997; 158:319–325.

18. Lee WR, Hanks GE, Schultheiss TE, Corn BW, Hunt MA. Localized prostate cancer treated by external-beam radiotherapy alone: serum prostate-specific antigen-driven outcome analysis. J Clin Oncol 1995; 13:464–469.

19. Schellhammer PF, el-Mahdi AM, Kuban DA, Wright GL Jr. Prostate-specific antigen after radiation therapy. Prognosis by pretreatment level and posttreatment nadir. Urol Clin N Am 1997; 24:407–414.

20. Zagars GK, Pollack A, Eschenbach AC. Prognostic factors for clinically localized prostate carcinoma: analysis of 938 patients irradiated in the prostate specific antigen era. Cancer 1997; 79:1370–1380.

21. Lee WR, Hanks GE, Hanlon A. Increasing prostate-specific antigen profile following definitive radiation therapy for localized prostate cancer: clinical observations. J Clin Oncol 1997; 15:230–238.

22. Sandler HM, Dunn RL, McLaughlin PW, Hayman JA, Sullivan MA, Taylor JMG. Overall survival after prostate-specific-antigen-detected recurrence following conformal radiation therapy. Int J Radial Oncol Biol Phys 2000; 48(3):629–633.

23. Horwitz EM, Vicini FA, Ziaja EL, Gonzalez J, Dmuchowski CF, Stromberg JS, Brabbins DS, Hollander J, Chen PY, Martinez AA. Assessing the variability of outcome for patients treated with localized prostate irradiation using different definitions of biochemical control. Int J Radiat Oncol Biol Phys 1996; 36:565–571.

24. American Society for Therapeutic Radiology and Oncology Consensus Panel. Consensus statement: Guidelines for PSA following radiation therapy. Int J Radiat Oncol Biol Phys 1997; 37:1035–1041.

25. Fukunaga-Johnson N, Sandler HM, McLaughlin PW, Strawderman MS, Grijalva KH, Kish KE, Lichter AS. Results of 3D conformal radiotherapy in the treatment of localized prostate cancer. Int J Radiat Oncol Biol Phys 1997; 38:311–317.

26. Hanks GE, Hanlon AL, Schultheiss TE, Pinover WH, Movsas Z, Epstein BE, Hunt MA. Dose escalation with 3-D conformal treatment: five-year outcomes, treatment optimization and future directions. Int J Radiat Oncol Biol Phys 1998; 41:501–510.

27. Zelefsky MJ, Leibel SA, Gaudin PB, Kutcher GJ, Fleshner N, Venkatramen ES, Reuter VE, Fair WR, Ling CC, Fuks Z. Dose escalation with three-dimensional conformal radiation therapy affects the outcome in prostate cancer. Int J Radiat Oncol Biol Phys 1998; 41:491–500.

28. Roach M, Meehan S, Kroll S, Weil M, Ryu J, Small EJ, Margolis LW, Presti J, Carroll PC, Phillips TL. Radiotherapy for high grade clinically localized adenocarcinoma of the prostate. J Urol 1996; 156:1719–1723.

29. Pollack A, Zagars GK. External beam radiotherapy dose response of prostate cancer. IntJ Radiat Oncol Biol Phys 1997; 39:1011–1018.

30. Hanks GE, Hanlon AL, Epstein B. EM Horwitz. Dose response in prostate cancer with 8–12 years follow-up. Int J Radiat Oncol Biol Phys 2001; 51(3, Supplement 1): 138–139.

31. Fivesh JB, Hanks G, Roach M, Wang S, Vigneault E, McLaughlin PW, Sandler HM. 3-D conformal radiation therapy (3-DCRT) for high-grade prostate cancer: A multi-institutional review. Int J Radiat Oncol Biol Phys 2000; 47(2):335–342.

32. Dearnaley DP, Khoo VS, Norman AR, Meyer L, Nahum A, Tait D, Yarnold J, Horwich A. Comparison of radiation side effects of conformal and conventional radiotherapy in prostate cancer: a randomized trial. The Royal Marsden NHS Trust/ Institute of Cancer Research. Lancet 1999; 353:267–372.

33. Lee WR, Hanks GE, Hanlon AL, Schultheiss TE, Hunt MA. Lateral rectal shielding reduces late rectal morbidity following high-dose three-dimensional conformal radiation therapy for clinically localized prostate cancer: further evidence for a significant dose effect. Int J Radiat Oncol Biol Phys 1996; 35:251–257.

34. Michalski JM, Purdy JA, Winter K, Roach M III, Vijayakumar S, Sandler HM, Markoe AM, Ritter MA, Russell KJ, Sailer S, Harms WB, Perez CA, Wilder RB, Hanks GB, Lax JD. Preliminary report of toxicity following 3D radiation therapy

for prostate cancer on 3DOG/RTOG 9406. Int J Radiat Oncol Biol Phys 2000; 46(2): 391–402.

35. Zelefsky MJ, Fuks Z, Wolfe T, Kutcher GJ, Burman C, Ling CC, Venkatraman ES, Leibel SA. Locally advanced prostatic cancer: long-term toxicity outcome after three-dimensional conformal radiation therapy—a dose-escalation study. Radiology 1998; 209:169–174.

36. Chinn DM, Holland J, Crownover RL, Roach M. III. Potency following high-dose three-dimensional conformal radiotherapy and the impact of prior major urologic surgical procedures in patients treated for prostate cancer. Int J Radiat Oncol Biol Phys 1995; 33(1):15–22.

37. Wilder RB, Chou R, Ryu JK, Stern RL, Wong MS, Ji M, Roach M III, White RD. Potency preservation after three-dimensional conformal radiotherapy for prostate cancer: preliminary results. Am J Clin Oncol August 2000; 23(4):330–333.

38. Zelefsky MJ, Fuks ZVI, Lee M, Lombardi D, Ling CC, Reuter VE, Venkatraman ES, Leibel SA. High-dose radiation delivered by intensity-modulated conformal radiotherapy improves the outcome of localized prostate cancer. J Urol 2001; 166(3): 876–881.

39. Kupelian PA, Reddy CA, Klein EA, Willoughby TR. Short-course intensity-modulated radiotherapy (70 Gy at 2.5 Gy per fraction) for localized prostate cancer: preliminary results on late toxicity and quality of life. Int. J Radiat Oncol Biol Phys 2001; 51(4):988–993.

40. Laramore GE, Krall JM, Thomas FJ, Russell KJ, Maor MH, Hendrickson FR, Motz KL, Griffin TW, Davis LW. Fast-neutron radiotherapy for locally advanced prostate cancer. final report of a Radiation Therapy Oncology Group randomized clinical trial. Am J Clin Oncol 1993; 16:164–167.

41. Russell KJ, Pakak TJ, Burnison CM, Maor MH, Taylor ME, Davis LW, Laramore GE. Fast-neutron radiotherapy versus photon radiotherapy for locally-advanced adenocarcinoma of the prostate: final report on a randomized clinical trial of the Neutron Therapy Collaborative Working Group. Int J Radiat Oncol Biol Phys 1999; 45:168.

42. Hall EJ. Radiobiology for the Radiologist: Linear Energy Transfer and Relative Biological Effectiveness. 4th Edition. Philadelphia: J.B. Lippincott Company, 1994: 153–164.

43. Hall EJ. New Radiation Modalities. 4th Edition. Philadelphia: J.B Lippincott Company, 1994:231–244.

44. Slater JD, Yonemoto LT, Rossi CJ, Reyes-Molyneux NJ, Bush DA, Antoine JE, Loredo LN, Schulte RW, Teichman SL, Slater JM. Conformal proton therapy for prostate carcinoma. Int J Radiat Oncol Biol Phys 1998; 42:299–304.

45. Shipley WU, Verhey LJ, Munzenrider JE, Suit HD, Urie MM, McMarus PL, Young RH, Shipley JW, Zietman AL, Biggs PJ. Advanced prostate cancer: the results of a randomized comparative trial if high-dose irradiation boosting with conformal protons compared with conventional dose irradiation using photons alone. Int J Radiat Oncol Biol Phys 1995; 32:3–12.

46. Pilepich MV, Winter K, John MJ, Mesic JB, Sause W, Rubin P, Lawton C, Machtay M, Grignon D. Phase III radiation therapy oncology group (RTOG) trial 86–10 of

androgen deprivation adjuvant to definitive radiotherapy in locally advanced carcinoma of the prostate. Int J Radiat Oncol Biol Phys 2001; 50(5):1243–1252.

47. Lawton CA, Winter K, Murray K, Machtay M, Mesic JB, Hanks GE, Coughlin CT, Pilepich MV. Updated results of the phase III radiation therapy oncology group (RTOG) trial 85–31 evaluating the potential benefit of androgen suppression following standard radiation therapy for unfavorable prognosis carcinoma of the prostate. Int J Radiat Oncol Biol Phys 2001; 49(4):937–946.

48. Hanks GE, Lu JD, Machtay M, Venkatesan M, Pinover WH, Byhardt RW, Rosenthal SA. RTOG Protocol 92–02: a phase III trial of the use of long term androgen suppression following neoadjuvant hormonal cytoreduction and radiotherapy in locally advanced carcinoma of the prostate. Int J Radiat Oncol Biol Phys 2000; 48(3): 112.

49. Bolla M, Gonzales D, Warde P, Dubois JB, Mirimarolb RO, Storme G, Bernier J, Kuten A, Sternberg C, Gil T, Collette L, Pierast M. Improved survival in patients with locally advanced prostate cancer treated with radiotherapy and goserelin. N Engl J Med 1997; 337:295–300.

50. DiPaola R, Kumar P, Hait W, Weiss R. State-of-the-art prostate cancer treatment and research. A report from the Cancer Institute of New Jersey. New Jersey Medicine, 2001:23–33.

51. Kumar P, Perrotti M, Weiss R, Todd M, Goodin S, Cummings K, DiPaola RS, Phase I Trial of Weekly Docetaxel with concurrent Three-Dimensional Conformal Radiation Therapy in the Treatment of Unfavorable Localized Adenocarcinoma of the Prostate Journal of Clinical Oncology, 2004; 22:1909–1915.

EDITORIAL COMMENTARY

Mark Shaves

Assistant Professor, Department of Radiation Oncology, Eastern Virginia Medical School, Norfolk, VA, USA

Paul F. Schellhammer

Professor of Urology, Department of Urology, Eastern Virginia Medical School, Norfolk, VA, USA

We wish to comment on the issues of target and dose, which are the cornerstones of radiation oncology. Like surgery, radiation oncology is a local therapy. In order to eradicate the tumor, the correct target must be determined and an appropriate dose must be delivered to that target. Make the target too small or the dose too low and a treatment failure results. Make the target too large or the dose too high and tumor control is achieved at the cost of unacceptable side effects. There is controversy and intriguing new data surrounding both of these issues in contemporary radiotherapeutic management of prostate cancer. Intensity-modulated radiation therapy (IMRT) challenges us further to precisely define the target while delivering increasingly higher doses with acceptable toxicity

TARGET

There is controversy surrounding the role of elective pelvic lymph node irradiation in patients with prostate cancer. This was first prospectively evaluated in Radiation Therapy Oncology Group 77–06 [1] 445 patients with clinical stage A2 or B (Jewitt) and no clinical or pathologic evidence of pelvic lymph node involvement were randomized to receive either 4500 to 5000 centigray (cGy) of pelvic nodal irradiation followed by a 2000 cGy boost to the prostate or 6500 cGy to the prostate only. There was no benefit for elective pelvic irradiation in local control, freedom from distant metastases, disease-free survival or overall survival. Criticisms of this study include the rather low dose used, clinical definition of failure, and, most importantly, the patient population analyzed had a low-risk of occult lymph node involvement. Recently, RTOG 9413 evaluated elective pelvic nodal irradiation in clinically staged patients with greater than 15% risk of involved lymph nodes [2]. Over 1300 patients were randomized to receive either 50.4 Gy (1 Gy = 100 cGy) to the pelvis plus a 19.8 Gy prostate boost or 70.2 Gy to the prostate alone. All patients were also randomized to receive total androgen suppression (TAS), either neoadjuvant and concurrent or adjuvant. Preliminary results showed a significant improvement in 4-year progression-free survival (56% vs. 46%) when elective pelvic irradiation was compared with prostate-only irradiation among patients also receiving neoadjuvant and concurrent TAS. An overall survival benefit was not demonstrated and continued follow up for this critical endpoint is planned. This study more accurately reflects contemporary practice with its widespread use of androgen deprivation therapy (ADT), higher dose, clinical vs. surgical staging, and largely biochemical determination of disease progression.

Including the seminal vesicles in the radiation treatment volume results in an additional dose being delivered to the rectum [3]. Therefore, eliminating seminal vesicle irradiation in patients at low risk for involvement is important to minimize rectal toxicity. Roach et al. derived an empirical equation to estimate the risk of seminal vesicle involvement based on clinical factors [4]. This is an excellent tool to guide target volume selection and has been adopted into the RTOG 9406 dose escalation trial. Using pathologic review of prostatectomy specimens, Kestin demonstrated that only the proximal 2 cm of the seminal vesicles needs to be included in the treated volume in nearly all patients at risk of involvement, and this limitation should further reduce rectal dose [5].

DOSE

Dose reporting between different institutions may vary somewhat, depending on how dose is defined. Published values of delivered dose may be specified to a point in the middle of the prostate or to the whole gland. The distinction is important, since a reported difference of 200 to 350 cGy may actually reflect the same delivered dose. This is a semantic issue that causes confusion among nonradiation oncologists seeking to compare studies. Considering that the whole gland is at risk, a dose to a target volume encompassing the prostate is more meaningful than a dose to a point.

As reviewed by the author, patients with intermediate- and high-risk prostate cancer have been shown to benefit from dose escalation. Conventional doses of radiation therapy (68 to 70 Gy) may, however, be inadequate, even for those with favorable risk disease—generally recognized as T1-2A, Gleason 2–6, and PSA < 10. Zietman and colleagues analyzed the long-term outcome of over 1000 patients with localized prostate cancer who received conventional dose radiation therapy [6]. 50.4 Gy was given to the pelvis followed by a boost to 68.4 Gy to the prostate. Using a strict definition of biochemical failure, 65% of patients with T1–2, well-to-moderately differentiated tumors were disease free at 5 years and only 47% remained so at 10 years. Using the American Society of Therapeutic Radiology and Oncology (ASTRO) consensus criteria for biochemical failure, Catton et al. reviewed the outcome of 706 patients treated with conventional dose radiation therapy for localized prostate cancer [7]. The biochemical relapse-free rate (bNED) of the favorable risk patients was 73% at 5 years. Several series have evaluated the use of high-dose three-dimensional conformal radiation therapy (3DCRT) or IMRT for favorable risk patients. Hanks and others at Fox Chase Cancer Center showed a 12% difference in 5-year bNED rate favoring doses above 72.5 Gy [8]. The difference did not achieve statistical significance, likely due to the fact that very few patients received < 70 Gy. Pollack and colleagues recently reported updated results of a randomized trial comparing 70 Gy with 78 Gy for T1-3 patients. There was no difference in freedom from clinical or biochemical failure between the two doses for patients with PSA ≤ 10. However, Zelefsky demonstrated a statistically significant improvement in 5-year PSA relapse-free survival (90% vs. 77%) for favorable risk group patients who received ≥ 75.6 Gy compared with those who were treated with 64.8 to 70.2 Gy[10].

Taken together, these studies provide evidence that some patients characterized as low risk by current prognostic indicators may benefit from doses as high as 75.6 Gy to the whole prostate (or stated differently, 78 Gy to isocenter).

IMRT

Intensity-modulated radiation therapy represents an important advance beyond 3DCRT. Its major advantage lies in the ability to conform does more closely to the target volume, thus decreasing dose to surrounding normal tissues. In a recent update of IMRT for prostate cancer at Memorial Sloan-Kettering Cancer, Grade 2 or higher rectal toxicity was seen in only 4% of 772 patients [11]. As does delivery becomes increasingly conformal, however, it naturally follows that margins around the target become smaller and dose gradients around the tumor become steeper. The cost of overzealous protection of adjacent organs may be a "marginal miss," where tumor lies just outside of the area receiving the full intended radiation does. Even with strict immobilization of the patient, there will be daily variation of patient position and internal prostate motion that must be accounted for in planning. In an analysis of rigidly immobilized patients receiving six-field conformal radiation therapy, investigators at the University of California, San Francisco, found a median patient position variability between simulation and treatment of 4 mm [12]. Using serial computed Tomography (CT) images, Beard and colleagues demonstrated that positional differences of the prostate and seminal vesicles exist between the treatment planning session and actual treatment delivery. In the anterior–posterior axis, these exceeded 5 mm in approximately 20% of the patients [13]. Ten Haken et al, also observed an average of 5 mm of prostate movement due to differential filling of the rectum and bladder in 50 patients [14]. Respiration, valsalva, and pelvic floor contraction/relaxation all give rise to moment to moment changes in prostate position. As margins become tighter, it becomes necessary to localize the position of the prostate on a daily basis using such techniques as transabdominal ultrasound targeting [15] or implanted radiopaque seed markers [16] in order to accurately deliver dose to the target. In essence, new technology (real-time imaging) is needed to support new technology. This translates into increased time requirements for radiation oncology personnel and increased costs to the patient. As pointed out by Glatstein, there are also practical and theoretical concerns about increased second malignancies with IMRT [17]. More data with long term follow-up of patients treated with IMRT will be necessary to see whether this technology delivers on its promise of increased tumor control and decreased toxicity.

The discussion of treatment options for localized prostate cancer requires a thorough review of surgical and irradiation therapy against the background of an ever-evolving playing field. Therefore, considering the local therapeutic options of radiation and surgery, it is reasonable to assess their current status and future potential. Over the past decade, prostate cancer has been diagnosed in patients who are younger and more fit, the tumors have been smaller than in the past, and, therefore, outcomes are more favorable. Surgeons have made great strides to better understand pelvic anatomy and have developed more precise techniques of dissection that have been honed with the experience of hundreds and even thousands of procedures. Therefore, the main objective of surgery, namely removal of all cancer, both by virtue of reduced prostate cancer volume and operative precision, is more likely. Surgery offers the significant advantage of removal of billions of cancer cells in a three-hour procedure and provides pathologic staging information regarding extracapsular extension, seminal vesicle invasion, and lymph node involvement information, which might direct further therapy. Surgery, however, is a strictly anatomical treatment strategy. In the field of radiation therapy, the acceleration of improvements has indeed been impressive and has the potential to exceed the gains that have been realized by surgery. The physical, chemical, and biological interactions that radiation physicists and biologists are investigating may provide an expanded potential of treatment applications. While both surgery and radiation strive to achieve complete local tumor control, the sine qua non for the long-term success of local treatment, they both await advances in systemic therapies to achieve long term cure.

Lastly, in the sphere of randomized trials, oncology certainly has led the charge and has developed, enrolled, completed, and analyzed an impressive array of randomized studies. These efforts have been both from academic centers and the community. Randomized Controlled Trials address selection, confound, attrition, and detection bias—the four horsemen of subjectivity when treatment is based on retrospective or historical data. The conduct of clinical trials is laborious and at times, intrusive. However, they provide the real advantage of replacing treatment based on "hunches" with evidence-based recommendations.

REFERENCES

1. Asbell SO, Krall JM, Pilepich MV, Baerwald H, Sause WT, Hanks GE, Perez CA. Elective pelvic irradiation in stage A2, B carcinoma of the prostate: analysis of RTOG 77-06. Int J Radiat Oncol Biol Phys 1988; 15:1307–1316.
2. Roach M, Lu JD, Lawton C, Hsu IC, Machtay M, Seider MJ, Rotman M, Jones C, Asbell SO, Valicenti RK, Han S, Thomas CR, Shipley WS. A phase III trial comparing whole-pelvic to prostate-only radiotherapy and neoadjuvant to adjuvant total androgen suppression: preliminary analysis of RTOG 9413. Int J Radiat Oncol Biol Phys 2001; 51(suppl 1):3.
3. Diaz A, Roach M, Marquez C, Coleman L, Pickett B, Wolfe JS, Carroll P, Narayan P. Indications for and the significance of seminal vesicle irradiation during 3D conformal radiotherapy for localized prostate cancer. Int J Radiat Oncol Biol Phys 1994; 30:323–329.
4. Roach M. Equations for predicting the pathologic stage of men with localized prostate cancer using the preoperative prostate-specific antigen (PSA) and Gleason score. J Urol 1993; 150:1923–1924.
5. Kestin LL, Goldstein NS, Vicini FA, Yan D, Korman HJ, Martinez AA. Treatment of prostate cancer with radiotherapy: should the entire seminal vesicles be included in the CTV. Int J Radiat Oncol Biol Phys 2001; 51(suppl 1):138.
6. Zietman AL, Coen JJ, Dallow KC, Shipley WU. The treatment of prostate cancer by conventional radiation therapy: an analysis of long-term outcome. Int J Radiat Oncol Biol Phys 1995; 32:287–292.
7. Catton C, Gospodarowicz M, Mui J, Panzarella T, Milosevic M, McLean M, Catton P, Warde P. Clinical and biochemical outcome of conventional dose radiotherapy for localized prostate cancer. Canadian J Urol 2002; 9:1444–1452.
8. Hanks GE, Hanlon AL, Pinover WH, Horwitz EM, Price RA, Schultheiss T. Dose selection for prostate cancer patients based on dose comparison and dose response studies. Int J Radiat Oncol Biol Phys 2000; 46:823–832.

9. Pollack A, Zagars GK, Starkschall G, Antolak JA, Lee JJ, Huang E, von Eschenbach AC, Kuban DA, Rosen I. Prostate cancer radiation dose response: results of the M.D. Anderson Phase III randomized trial. Int J Radia Oncol Biol Phys 2002; 50: 1097–1105.

10. Zelefsky MJ, Fuks Z, Hunt M, Lee HJ, Lombardi D, Ling C, Reuter VE, Venkatraman ES, Leibel SA. High-dose radiation delivered by intensity-modulated conformal radiotherapy improves the outcome of localized prostate cancer. J Urol 2001; 166: 876–881.

11. Zelefsky MJ, Fuks Z, Leibel SA. Intensity-modulated radiation therapy for prostate cancer. Semin Radiat Oncol 2002; 12:229–237.

12. Rosenthal SA, Roach M, Goldsmith BJ, Doggett E, Pickett B, Hae-Sook Y, Soffen EM, Stern RL, Ryu JK. Immobilization improves the reproducibility of patient positioning during six-field conformal radiation therapy for prostate cancer. Int J Radiat Oncol Biol Phys 1993; 27:921–926.

13. Beard CJ, Kijewski P, Bussiere M, Gelman R, Gladstone D, Shaffer K, Plunkett M, Costello P, Coleman CN. Analysis of prostate and seminal vesicle motion: implications for treatment planning. Int J Radiat Oncol Biol Phys 1996; 34:451–458.

14. Ten Haken RK, Forman JD, Heimburger DK, Gerhardsson A, McShan DL, Perez-Tamayo C, Schoeppel SL, Lichter AS. Treatment planning issues related to prostate movement in response to differential filling of the rectum and bladder. Int J Radiat Oncol Biol Phys 1991; 20:1317–1324.

15. Lattanzi J, McNeeley S, Donnelly S, Palacio E, Hanlon A, Schultheiss TE, Hanks GE. Ultrasound-based stereotactic guidance in prostate cancer- quantification of organ motion and set-up errors in external beam radiation therapy. Comput Aided Surg 2000; 5:289–295.

16. Litzenberg D, Dawson LA, Sandler H, Sanda MG, McShan DL, Ten Haken RK, Lam KL, Brock KK, Balter JM. Daily prostate targeting using implanted radiopaque markers. Int J Radiat Oncol Biol Phys 2002; 52:699–703.

17. Glatstein E. Intensity-modulated radiation therapy: the inverse, the converse, and the perverse. Semin Radiat Oncol 2002; 12:272–281.

EDITORIAL OVERVIEW

Kenneth B. Cummings

Kumar has provided a thoughtful review of three-dementional (3D) conformal radiation therapy (3DCRT). The March 1997 ASTRO consensus statement for definition of PSA failure includes: three consecutive increases in posttreatment PSA after achieving a nadir, which has been a step forward in making comparisons of treatment efficacy [1].

Data presented for 3DCRT demonstrate superior outcomes compared to standard radiation therapy. It appears evident that higher doses are tolerated with acceptable toxicity and higher doses appear to be associated with improved five-year biochemical–no evidence of disease (bNED) [2–4].

A major problem in assessing therapeutic efficacy of 3DCRT is the absence of pathological staging. There has been an inherent bias to treat the higher-risk patient (prognostically less-favorable disease or comorbid conditions) with radiation therapy. Despite PSA observations, long-term disease-specific survival is still perceived as best achieved by anatomic radical prostatectomy.

Shaves and Schellhammer place many of the issues of radiation vs. surgical treatment into perspective by considering "target and dose." In the surgically treated patient, if the target "prostate and seminal vesicle" is extirpated while the disease is confined, cure is the expectation. The absent prostate likely accounts for the long-term disease-specific survival in surgical series compared to radiation-treated patients. This is in contrast with the radiated prostate, in which the retained viable stem cells give rise to a recurrent cancer years later or the target dose has been inappropriate to achieve durable control of the original cancer.

Intensity-modulated radiation therapy (IMRT) attempts to precisely define the target delivering increasingly higher doses with acceptable toxicity to surrounding normal tissues. IMRT likely represents an important advance beyond 3DCRT, in which the major advantage lies in the ability to more closely conform the dose to the target volume. Early data from IMRT show promising therapeutic efficacy with acceptable toxicity [5,6].

More data with long-term follow-up of patients treated with IMRT will be necessary to see whether the technology delivers on its promise of increased tumor control and decreased toxicity.

REFERENCES

1. American Society for Therapeutic Radiology and Oncology Consensus Panel. Consensus statement: Guidelines for PSA following radiation therapy. Int J Radiat Oncol Biol Phys 1997; 37:1035–1041.
2. Fukunaga-Johnson N, Sandler HM, McLaughlin PW, Strawderman MS, Grijalva KH, Kish KE, Lichter AS. Results of 3D conformal radiotherapy in the treatment of localized prostate cancer. Int J Radiat Oncol Biol Phys 1997; 38:311–317.
3. Hanks GE, Hanlon AL, Schulteiss TE, et al. Dose escalation with 3D conformal treatment: five-year outcomes, treatment optimization and future directions. Int J Radiat Oncol Biol Phys 1998; 41:501–510.
4. Zelefsky MJ, Leibel SA, Gaudin PB, et al. Dose escalation with three-dimensional conformal radiation therapy affects the outcome in prostate cancer. Int J Radiat Oncol Biol Phys 1998; 41:491–500.
5. Zelefsky MJ, Fuks Z, Hunt M, Lee HJ, Lombardi D, Ling C, Reuter VE, Venkatraman ES, Leibel SA. High-dose radiation delivered by intensity-modulated conformal radiotherapy improves the outcome of localized prostate cancer. J Urol 2001; 166:876–881.
6. Zelefsky MJ, Fuks Z, Leibel SA. Intensity-modulated radiation therapy for prostate cancer. Semin Radiat Oncol 2002; 12:229–237.

6

Modern Prostate Brachytherapy

Haakon Ragde
The Haakon Ragde Foundation for Advanced
Cancer Studies, Seattle, Washington, USA

This chapter will provide an overview of prostate brachytherapy using permanent radioactive sources such as Iodine-125 and Palladium-103. The discussion will include patient selection, conformal planning, intraoperative seed placement, postimplant dosimetry evaluation, and long-term outcome.

INTRODUCTION

Traditionally, radical prostatectomy and external beam radiotherapy have been the preferred treatments for clinically localized prostate cancer. Over the last several years, however, interest in brachytherapy, or radioactive seed implantation, has been growing. Brachytherapy either temporarily or permanently places sealed radioactive sources into the prostate. It has been estimated that the number of American prostate cancer patients treated with permanent brachytherapy has numbered 40,000.

Likely reasons for the increased interest in brachytherapy:

- The major advantage of brachytherapy is its ability to deliver a curative radiation dose to a confined volume, i.e., the prostate, yet spare normal tissue because of rapid dose fall-off. As such, brachytherapy fulfills a major goal of radiation treatment.

- Prostate brachytherapy is a minimally invasive procedure that provides excellent long-term outcome results with minimal morbidity [1].
- Prostate brachytherapy is well tolerated by older patients in less-than-favorable medical condition.

Approximately 80% of all prostate implants today are "permanent" implants, meaning that sealed sources containing either radioactive Iodine-125 or Palladium-103 are inserted into the prostate and left in place. Iodine-125, with a half-life of 60 days, delivers approximately 99% of the dose within 12 months, and Palladium-103, with a half-life of 17 days, accomplishes the same within 6 months.

Over the last few years, the development of temporary (removable) implants in association with external beam therapy has arisen. High activity Iridium-192 is inserted through catheters, which have been temporarily placed in the prostate. These catheters are left in the prostate for the duration of the implant and then removed. While in the prostate, a robot assists in moving the radioactive sources into predetermined "dwell" positions for specified lengths of time. It is not possible to deliver the total dose in a single session, so several administrations are required. Compared to permanent prostate brachytherapy, a one-time outpatient procedure, the temporary method is more costly and is more labor-intensive. Additionally, the procedure requires hospitalization, calls for significant analgesia, and requires the patient be bed-bound for extended periods of time. To date, only a few institutions have published outcome data on temporary Iridium-192 implants, and none of these publications offers long-term follow-up regarding tumor-control rates and morbidity [2].

HISTORY OF PROSTATE BRACHYTHERAPY

Attempts to cure prostate cancer by radioactive isotopes go back to the early part of the last century, when radioactive Radium was inserted into the urethra [3]. Despite the early start, prostate brachytherapy generated only passing interest until low-energy sources became available on a commercial basis. This change occurred in the early 1960s, when three such isotopes became available for clinical investigation at Memorial Hospital (now Memorial Sloan-Kettering Cancer Center) in New York [4]. The early isotopes, all with energies around 30 kv, were Xenon-133, Cesium-131, and Iodine-125, which were embedded in sealed miniature titanium cylinders.

Whitmore and Hilaris launched a study treating prostate cancer with the new Iodine-125 radioisotope [5]. Their technique required open surgery to expose the prostate, a staging pelvic lymph node dissection, and free-hand insertion of the implant needles using the operator's finger, placed in the rectum, gauging the needle depth.

The intent was to deliver a significantly higher radiation dose to the prostate than was possible with external beam therapy while, at the same time, to limit the radiation to adjacent normal tissue such as the bladder and rectum. The prescribed dose of radiation was based on a nomogram derived from external beam radiation therapy and early brachytherapy planning concepts. Compared to surgery and external beam radiation, the procedure appeared ingeniously simple. It was also associated with fewer side effects, such as incontinence and impotence.

However, the free-hand implant technique frequently resulted in uneven seed arrays and inconsistent dose distributions. An overabundance of seeds in some parts of the prostate often led to serious complications, while the often sublethal radiation of areas with too few seeds left the cancer cells unaffected and resulted in a high rate of local failure. To compound the problems, implantation was often attempted in patients with advanced disease, in whom cure was highly unlikely. The erratic patient selection, the inability to control seed spacing and doses, and the unacceptable local control and late-complication rates, coupled with advances in surgical procedures and advent of megavoltage radiation, all contributed to loss of interest in prostate brachytherapy [6–11].

In 1983, Dr. H.H. Holm and his associates in Copenhagen provided the technical and intellectual foundation for a new beginning of prostate brachytherapy [12]. Employing transrectal ultrasound to guide placement of the radioactive sources, Holm and his team inserted seed-bearing needles transperineally into the prostate. They injected the seeds at preplanned sites in the gland, thereby achieving a uniform three-dimensional distribution.

Dr. Holm's implant technique was introduced to the United States by Dr. Ragde, who performed the first such procedure in Seattle, Washington in 1985. By 1987, Dr. Ragde and Dr. Blasko had developed a modification of Dr. Holm's implant procedure that resulted in evenly distributed seed configurations in the prostate with minimal attendant normal-tissue complications. Since then, several authors have published various modifications of this basic technique.

PATIENT SELECTION

Prostate brachytherapy, like surgery, is a locally directed treatment. Cure by an implant alone is contingent on whether the cancer is organ confined. Investigators have yet to produce a reliable method for accurately computing pathological stage on a pretreatment basis, though increasing evidence suggests that a collation of clinical stage, Gleason score, and pretreatment PSA level may identify patients at risk for extracapsular extension of the disease [13,14]. Of the three clinical variables, pretreatment PSA has been shown to be the strongest predictor of posttherapy PSA failure, followed by the biopsy Gleason score, and, finally, clinical stage [15]. In borderline cases, the number of positive biopsies, evidence of perineural invasion, and positive base biopsies with risk for seminal vesicle invasion may be added to the equation to strengthen the prediction [16–18]. The fundamental principle of risk stratification rests on the premise that it may identify prostate cancer patients who will not have a good chance of cure from single-modality treatments.

Patients whose tumors are likely to be organ confined (stage T1–T2a, Gleason score less than 7, and PSA less than 11 ng/mL) can be treated with a seed implant as monotherapy. Patients suspect for extracapsular extension of the disease (stage T2b and higher, Gleason score 7 and above, and PSA over 10 ng/mL), are generally treated with a 45 Gy dose of external beam therapy to the pelvis first followed by a seed implant (combination therapy). Because seed radiation is minimally penetrating, tumoricidal radiation from seeds alone is confined to about 5 mm beyond the margin of the prostate (except posteriorly). Because of this confinement, it seems reasonable to pretreat the prostate and extraprostatic tissue with external beam radiation in patients at risk for extraprostatic disease extension [18]. Since the external beam radiation is delivered to small fields with blocking of sensitive normal structures, it is well tolerated (Ragde H, Grado GL, Smith LG III, personal experience). Table 1 shows a general guideline for recommending brachytherapy alone or brachytherapy in combination with external beam irradiation.

Patients who have undergone prior transurethral prostate resection (TURP) and were then treated to a uniform (Quimby-type) implant have been shown to incur a higher risk for postimplant urinary incontinence and stricture formation (Ragde H, Grado GL, Smith LG III, personal experience). If the TURP defect is not unduly large and irregular, such patients may be treated using the Manchester (Paterson-Parker) loading technique, where the central radiation dose is reduced by placing the majority of the seeds at the periphery of the prostate (Ragde H, Grado GL, Smith LG III, personal experience). Even then, such patients, if they wish to have their prostate cancer treated with seed implantation, should be counseled regarding the risks of urinary complications.

Patients with significant lower urinary-tract obstruction are generally poor candidates for prostate brachytherapy. If the obstruction is due to lateral-lobe

TABLE 1   Selecting Therapy According to Patient Factors

	Monotherapy	Combination therapy
Nodule	None or Small	Large or Multiple
Gleason Score	2–6	7–10
PSA	≤10 ng/mL	>10 ng/mL
Biopsy	Unilateral Disease	Bilateral Disease or Locally Extensive

intrusion, the obstruction may be remedied by neoadjuvant hormonal downsizing prior to radiation. Patients with median bar/lobe enlargement are best treated with a transurethral incision of the prostate (TUIP) with a period of healing before radiation begins.

NEOADJUVANT/ADJUVANT ANDROGEN WITHDRAWAL

Compelling clinical and experimental evidence suggest that neoadjuvant/adjuvant androgen deprivation combined with external beam radiation will show improvement in outcome compared to radiation treatment alone [19–21]. An additive or synergistic effect has been postulated as the reason. Although brachytherapy plus or minus androgen withdrawal has not yet been put to clinical trial, it should follow the same basic biological principles as external beam therapy. However, for patients with low risk prostate cancer, the addition of androgen withdrawal would probably offer little advantage, and the side-effects and cost of the treatment are both substantial.

SALVAGE BRACHYTHERAPY

A large body of evidence shows that, based on routine PSA-monitoring of patients with clinically localized prostate cancer treated with conventional external beam therapy, many patients will experience biochemical failure [22–24]. Early experience suggests that salvage brachytherapy can benefit a wide range of patients treated with both curative and palliative intent. In a retrospective study, 79 patients with biopsy-proven localized recurrent prostate cancer, previously treated with either external beam radiation therapy or Iodine-125 brachytherapy, received either Iodine-125 or Palladium-103 brachytherapy salvage. The actuarial biochemical disease-free survival of patients who achieved a PSA nadir of less than 0.5 ng/mL was 77% and 56% at 3 and 5 years respectively [25].

CONFORMAL PLANNING

Radiation dose planning is regarded as the most important component for a successful brachytherapy procedure. Its purpose is to implant the individual patient's prostate volume with a radiation dose that will achieve maximum tumoricidal response with minimal side-effects.

INITIAL VOLUME STUDY

Planning begins with a transrectal ultrasound (TRUS) volume study with the patient in a dorsal lithotomy position, similar to the position used during the actual implantation. The study provides serial transverse images of the gland at

5-mm increments. The target domain is determined on each of the transverse images by inscribing a 5-mm margin onto the periphery of the prostate, except at the posterior boundary. The volume study also helps determine if the pubic arch will block needle access to the anterior and anterolateral part of the prostate. For patients with significant pubic arch overlap, androgen suppression therapy can be used to reduce the size of the gland, thereby reducing the degree of arch blockage.

The transverse TRUS images are then entered into a treatment-planning computer to determine the optimal seed configuration and seed activity that will deliver the minimum prescribed dose to the periphery of the prostate while sparing uninvolved normal structures. The software is interactive and allows for virtual placement of seeds within the prostate with an instant display of the resulting isodose curves over transverse-, sagittal-, and coronal-image planes. Dose prescription is generally based on the minimum peripheral dose (MPD), defined as the lowest dose that covers the periphery of the gland. Regardless of the tumor volume, an MPD of 144 Gy is considered the optimal dose for Iodine-125 and 120 Gy for Palladium-103.

The planning process may produce a variety of seed arrangements for a given application. The conventional approach for evaluating a treatment plan involves visually inspecting the isodose surfaces of the different planes. With this approach, the radiation oncologist and physicist can determine the isodose level that best covers the target, yet is favorable to the neighboring normal structures.

Calculation and analysis of the distribution of dose within the prostate volume is becoming a principal aspect of brachytherapy physics. Dose-volume

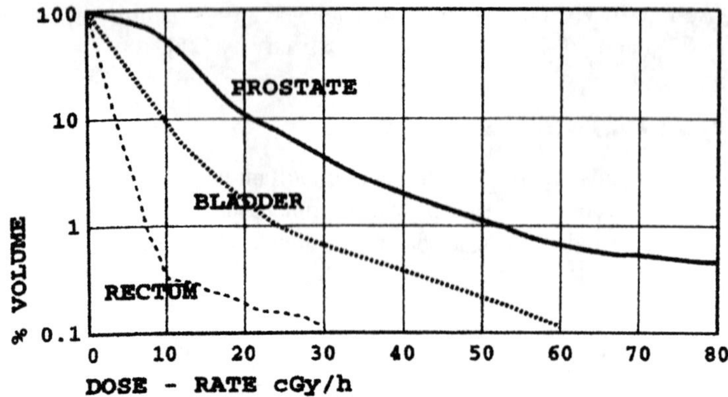

FIGURE 1 Cumulative dose-volume histogram of a permanent prostate implant with curves for prostate, bladder, and rectum.

histograms, describing dose variation within the prostate or other structures by specifying the volume irradiated at a certain dose level, have become a cornerstone in radio-biological or tumor-control probability assessments. They are also useful for answering questions about dose uniformity and about the extent to which normal tissues are irradiated. The dose-volume histogram may be used to further evaluate several treatment plans before selecting the final plan. Figure 1 shows a relative dose-volume histogram for a permanent prostate implant with the curves for the prostate, bladder, and rectum. The graph displays the dose delivered on the abscissa and the volume receiving "at least" that dose on the ordinate. As expected, the curve shows large volumes receiving low doses and small volumes receiving high doses.

IODINE-125 OR PALLADIUM-103?

The seeds of the two radioisotopes are physically similar, and both produce a low level of radiation outside of the patient. The differences between them are dose rate at the time of implantation, activity level per seed, and half-life (Table 2). In treating poorly differentiated tumors and presumably rapidly proliferating tumors, some investigators believe the 7 cGy/hr initial dose rate of Iodine-125 may be less effective than Palladium-103 which has an initial dose rate of 22 cGy/hr [26]. The higher dose-rate concept has been supported by mathematical models using cell lines, but to date there is no clinical proof from human trials to document tumoricidal differences between the two isotopes. The currently recommended doses for the two isotopes in monotherapy and in combination with external beam therapy are shown in (Table 3).

SOURCE LOADING APPROACHES

Several loading systems are available. The Manchester System, also known as the Paterson-Parker System, and the Quimby System, or some derivative of these systems, are the ones generally used in prostate brachytherapy. In the Manchester System, the majority of the seeds are kept toward the periphery of the gland with

TABLE 2   Comparison of Iodine-125 and Palladium-103

	Size (mm)	Half-life	Energy	Half-value layer
I-125	0.8 × 4.5	60 days	28 KeV	2cm Tissue
Pd-103	0.8 × 4.5	17 days	21 KeV	1.6cm Tissue

I-125: Iodine-125
Pd-103: Palladium-103

TABLE 3 Implant Doses for Monotherapy and Combination Therapy

Treatment	Isotope	Dose
Monotherapy	Iodine-125	144 Gy
	Palladium-103	115GY
Combination Therapy	Iodine-125	108 Gy + 45 Gy EBT
	Palladium-103	90 Gy + 45 Gy EBT

* EBT, external-beam therapy

the goal of delivering a *uniform* dose to the implant volume, where *uniform* means the prescribed dose plus/minus 10%.

In the Quimby System, the seeds are distributed in a uniform fashion throughout the prostate. The uniform loading results in an inhomogenous dose distribution, delivering a higher dose to the center of the implant than to the periphery. Regions of high dose, as long as they remain small and isolated, have no clinical significance in the intact prostate; however, recent practice leans toward minimizing urinary morbidity by deleting seeds adjacent to the urethra.

Either of these systems can be used for larger volume glands, but the uniform-type distribution may be more practical with smaller glands. In smaller glands, lower activity seeds without any spacing may be more effective than the more common one-centimeter seed-center-to-seed-center spacing.

INTRA-OPERATIVE SEED PLACEMENT

The implant procedure can generally be completed in 30–45 minutes. The anesthetized patient is placed in the dorsal lithotomy position with the hips flexed as much as possible. This positioning permits maximal width of the pubic arch and improved access to anterior portions of the gland. The two body halves are evenly balanced so that the cephalad extension of a notional line perpendicular to the perineum bisects the body (Figure 2).

A Foley catheter is inserted and left indwelling, and the bladder is filled with dilute contrast media. The indwelling catheter serves several functions. Besides helping to delineate the base of the prostate, the catheter is readily visualized on the midsagittal ultrasound image and can be tracked. Visualization of the catheter reduces needle insertion and seed deposition into the urethra. Additionally, the Foley catheter helps to stabilize prostate gland movement.

The perineum is prepped and draped and the scrotum elevated onto the abdominal wall with a plastic adhesive. An inactive gold seed marker is placed

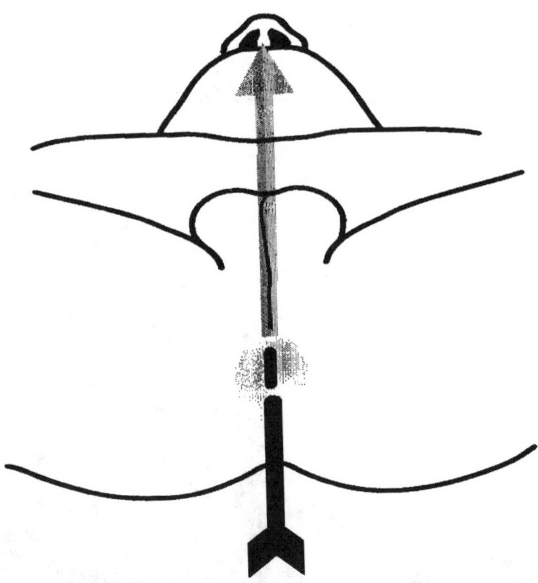

FIGURE 2 Schematic representation of body-halves symmetry in patients positioned for a transperineal prostate implant.

at the prostate apex. The marker seed is readily visualized on fluoroscopy and is the most accurate means of identifying the inferior margin of the gland.

A C-arm fluoroscope is centered over the prostate to visualize the area from the lower part of the bladder to the apical gold seed marker at the apex (Figure 3). A biplanar, multifrequency ultrasound probe is inserted into the rectum perpendicular to the perineum and at a slightly downward angle to best approach the posterior margin of the prostate. The probe is supported by a table-mounted, multipositional cradle system containing a stepper unit that allows advancement and retraction of the ultrasound probe in 5-mm increments. A template is then attached to the cradle system. There should be a space between the template and perineum to facilitate manual manipulation of the implant needles when this is required.

The volume study is repeated to make certain no significant changes in prostate volume and shape have occurred since the original volume study was performed. It has been our experience that in the absence of androgen ablation therapy, significant changes in volume and shape of the prostate are uncommon.

The prostate is a very mobile and pliable organ, and real-time ultrasound and fluoroscopic monitoring of the needle insertion and seed placement are critical. Any deviation or internal distortion of the gland should be recognized and

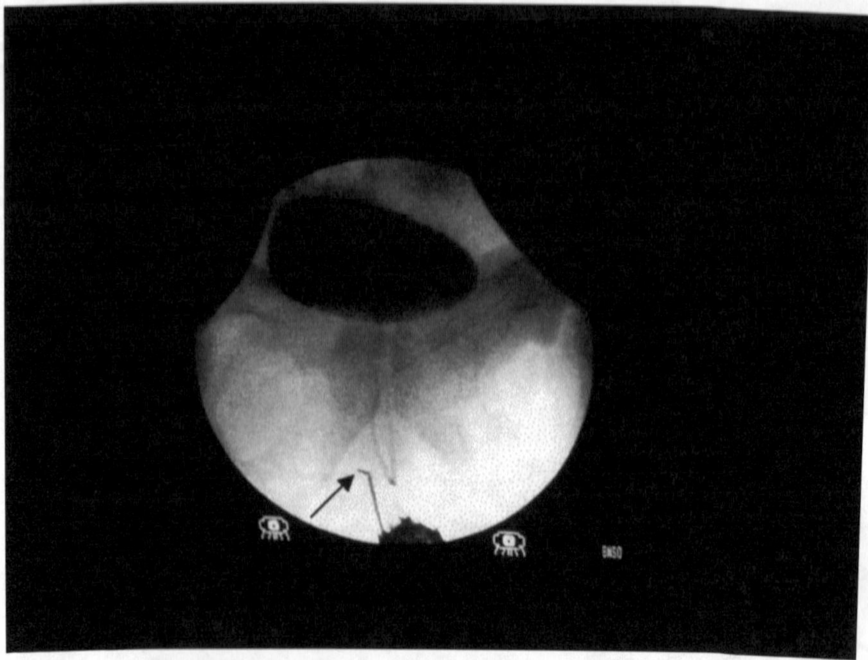

FIGURE 3   X-ray showing prostate base delineated by contrast media in the bladder and an implant needle ejecting a marker seed (*arrow*) at the prostate apex.

corrected. Glandular movements can be minimized using stabilizing needles. The implant needles are inserted one row at a time; usually four or five rows cover the prostate. Within each row, central needles are inserted first. Subsequent placements are made in an alternating left to right pattern. This technique helps prevent lateral or rotational movements of the prostate.

The implant begins with the most anterior row and ends with the most posterior row. Although needles can be easily repositioned, the goal should be to position them accurately at the first try. Trauma from repeat sticks can cause bleeding and excessive swelling of the gland. Reducing the needle sticks will also reduce seed displacement.

After satisfactory placement of a row of needles, as checked by both ultrasound (transverse and saggital views), and by fluoroscopy, the seeds are placed into the gland using a Mick applicator. As each seed is placed, it is visualized using real-time fluoroscopy to ensure distribution and spacing in accordance with the treatment plan.

Attention to the fluoroscopic and ultrasound images during needle insertion is critical. The physician must recognize and immediately adjust for the effects of cephalad movement, internal distortion, and rotation of the prostate. Sometimes the Mick applicator will fail to inject a seed at its intended site, or a seed will move laterally after leaving the rigid confines of a needle. The aberration can be readily detected on fluoroscopy, allowing for immediate correction and adjustment of the seed array.

When all the seeds have been placed, the resulting ultrasound images are sorted through for potential "cold spots" that have developed due to unavoidable prostate movement and distortions to needle insertions. Additional seeds may be placed at this time. The Foley catheter is removed; the patient is generally discharged within two hours after the procedure. Discharge medication usually includes an alpha-blocker and an oral antibiotic.

POST-IMPLANT QUALITY CONTROL

Dosimetric evaluation of the implant is performed on every patient within 24 hours postimplant using three-dimensional CT-based analysis. The 3-mm CT slices of the prostate, with the seeds visualized as bone densities, verify that the prostate has been implanted and that normal tissue structures are out of the high-dose radiation volume. The images are entered into a planning computer where the three-dimensional display of prostate slices and seeds are computer analyzed and overlaid with isodose contour margins to prepare for the construction of a dose-volume histogram. The dose-volume histogram permits detailed and accurate evaluation of the implant quality, and is particularly valuable in detecting consistent errors in implantation.

FOLLOW-UP

The patients are generally evaluated every three-to-six months the first year, and yearly thereafter. The follow-up includes clinical evaluation and serum PSA determination. Some investigators advocate postimplant biopsies, though the biopsy significance is questionable considering faulty sampling, timing of the biopsy, and expertise of the pathologist. Since postimplant biopsies are usually triggered by PSA elevation, which does not distinguish between local, regional, or distal disease, biopsies become mandatory when considering salvage therapy.

OUTCOME EVALUATION

Trial design for drug approval traditionally requires survival as an endpoint. With the lengthy natural history of prostate cancer even in advanced disease, such an endpoint would prove impractical. It is now generally accepted that serum PSA can accurately predict subsequent disease progression, and that the antigen may serve as a surrogate marker for disease-free survival after treatment.

When serum PSA was first introduced into clinical practice, it was unknown how to use this tumor marker to manage patients. Recognizing that a rising PSA level could be used as an early indication of treatment failure, physicians developed different end-points to signify failure. The end points have varied over time, though, and one of the hang-ups has been the mindset of some that the same PSA end point denoting therapy failure should be used for radical prostatectomy, external beam radiation, and brachytherapy. This reasoning is faulty because each of the procedures leaves a different potential for PSA production. If we assume that PSA is produced both by malignant and benign prostate cells, the PSA production will vary according to the volume of each type remaining after treatment. Consequently, if all prostate tissue, both healthy and malignant, has been removed surgically, the PSA value should rapidly approach zero; today most surgical series use a threshold PSA >0.2 ng/mL as evidence of treatment failure. Settling on a PSA end point to denote radiation failure has been more difficult, at least in the short term. Ideally, an analysis of PSA magnitude after a full course of external beam radiation, brachytherapy, and a combination of external beam radiation and brachytherapy, should have its own criteria for PSA-determined failure. This has not proven practical, and, today, radiation centers are increasingly favoring the failure definition proposed by the American Society for Therapeutic Radiology and Oncology (ASTRO), with the aim of establishing postradiation PSA standards to facilitate objective efficacy comparisons among treatment series [27]. The definition requires 3 consecutive PSA rises after reaching a nadir, with the date of failure fixed at the midpoint between the nadir and the first ascent in the rising PSA sequence. The interval between the PSA increases was not specified in the failure criteria, nor was the PSA nadir taken into account.

At our centers, where postimplant PSA levels are measured about every 6 months, we have accepted the ASTRO recommendation with the following reservations:

- The PSA nadir (which is typically not reached until 6 months and may take as long as 24 months) must reach a value of PSA <1.0 ng/mL.
- No PSA or biopsy event is taken into account before 18 months postimplant.
- The value of the third elevation in the rising PSA sequence must be above 0.5 ng/mL. Fail time is where the sequence curve crosses the 0.5 ng/mL plane.

Nonmalignant PSA rises, frequently referred to as "PSA bumps," may occur 12 to 30 months after the implant. While no credible explanation for the bumps exists, it is of interest that drugs that suppress inflammation may cause a drop in the PSA level in men with a bump. It is important to distinguish the innocuous bumps from true recurrence so as not to institute therapy unnecessarily. To a patient, posttreatment PSA rises may suggest that the treatment failed, so it is

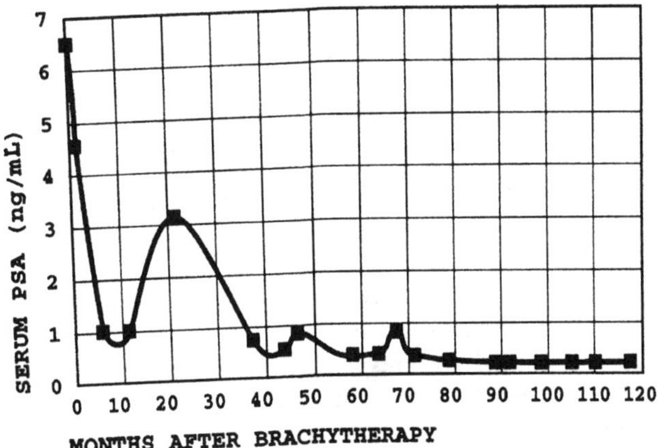

FIGURE 4 Graph showing "PSA bump" followed by a PSA decline to PSA (0.5 ng/mL)

important to apprise patients of the possibility of PSA bumps. Figure 4 shows a typical PSA bump, and Figure 5 shows a PSA failure.

RESULTS OF PROSTATE BRACHYTHERAPY

Introduction

This report presents the 13-year disease-free survival results of 769 consecutive prostate cancer patients treated solely with permanent implants.

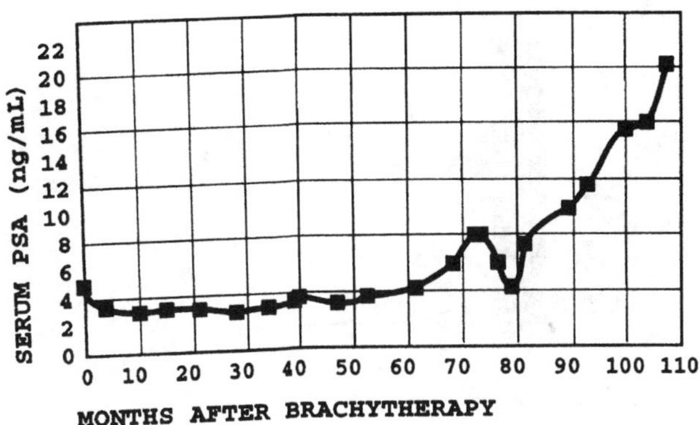

FIGURE 5 PSA versts time graph showing treatment failure. PSA not only fails to reach the desired nadir of PSA (0.5 ng/mL), but also continues to elevate.

Materials and Methods

Seven hundred sixty-nine patients with stage T1–T3, low-to-high Gleason score prostate cancer underwent prostate implants with Iodine-125 or Palladium-103 between January 1, 1987, and January 1, 1997. Median age was 69 years (range 43–92).

The patients were divided into two risk groups, 1 (low-risk for extraprostatic disease) and 2 (high-risk for extraprostatic disease). Group placements were based mainly on clinical stage and Gleason score. In general, pretreatment PSA was not a factor in group assignment. Figure 6, Figure 7, and Figure 8 show clinical stage, Gleason score, and PSA-level distributions in the low- and high-risk groups.

Group 1 consisted of 542 low-risk patients treated with Iodine-125 alone. Group 2 comprised 227 high-risk patients treated with Palladium-103 alone. None of the patients was pathologically staged, and none received androgen withdrawal therapy.

Disease-free survival end points included positive biopsies 18 or more months postimplant evidence of metastatic disease and biochemical (PSA) progression. As seen in Table 4, the vast majority of treatment failures were biochemical. A total of 4,731 PSA determinations were performed on the 769 patients. Cumulative survival functions were calculated by the Kaplan and Meier method. Implant quality was assessed on most patients by isodose surfaces, and dose-

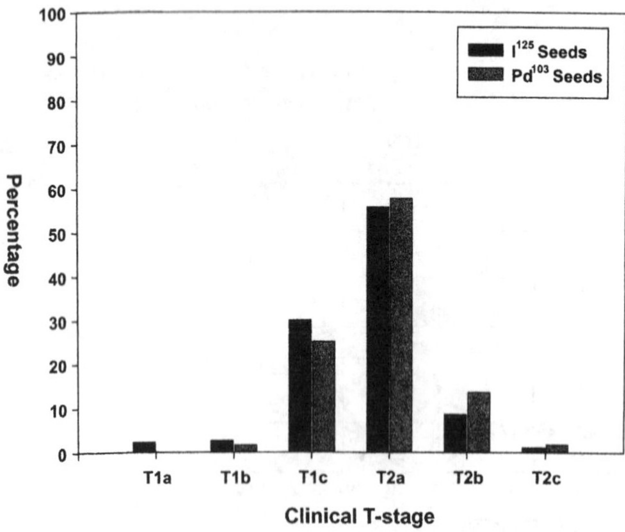

FIGURE 6 Clinical T-stage distribution for the I-125 (Group 1) and the Pd-103 (Group 2) treatment cohorts.

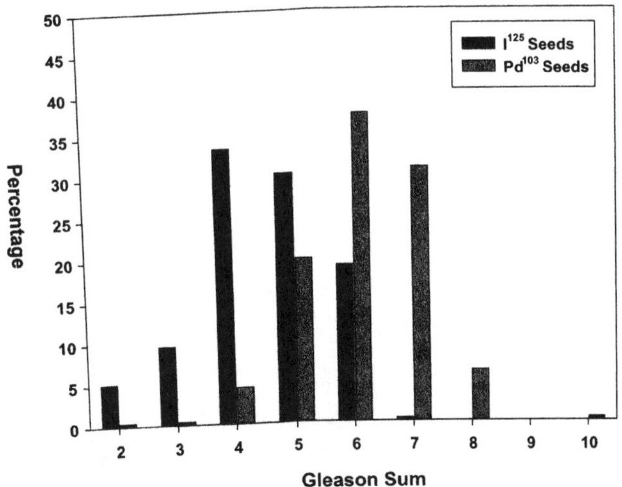

FIGURE 7   Gleason score distribution for the I-125 (Group 1) and the Pd-103 (Group 2) treatment cohorts.

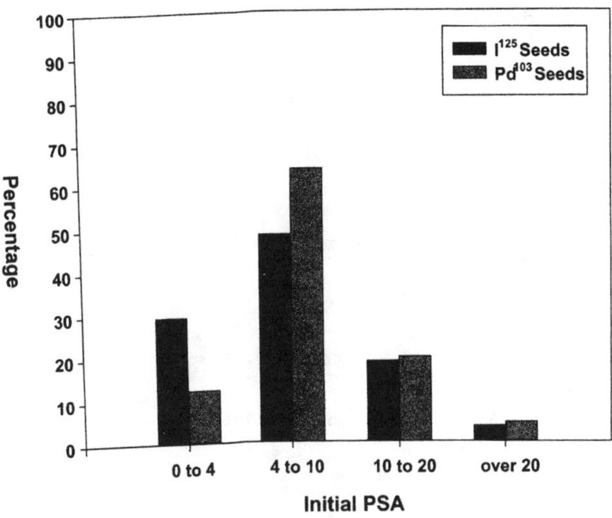

FIGURE 8   Pretreatment PSA distribution for the I-125 (Group 1) and the Pd-103 (Group 2) treatment cohorts.

TABLE 4   Treatment Failure Distribution: 619 Evaluated Patients

	Bone scan	Biopsy	PSA
3 Years	0.3%	1.6%	13.3%
5 Years	0.7%	2.5%	17.1%
10 Years	0.7%	2.4%	19.6%
13 Years	0.7%	2.6%	19.7%

Treatment failure distribution of the entire study cohort

volume histograms constructed from CT images obtained within 24 hours of the implant.

The patients were usually evaluated every three-to-six months the first year, and annually thereafter. The follow-up included clinical evaluation and serum PSA determinations. Additional studies were performed as dictated by the patient's symptoms and signs.

Results

One hundred fifty patients were excluded from our results—13 by death from noncancerous causes within 18 months postimplant and 137 with incomplete PSA

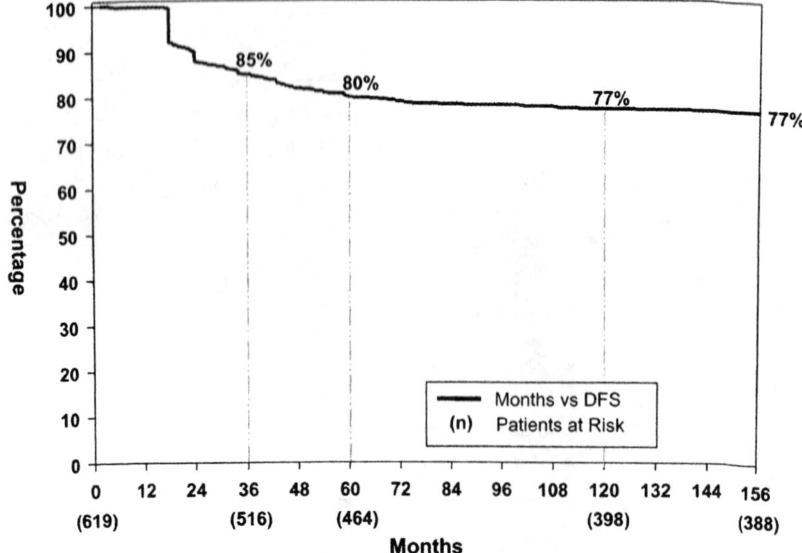

FIGURE 9   Disease-free survival versus years from implant for the entire cohort. The number of patients at risk for failure is shown in parentheses at the end of each plot line.

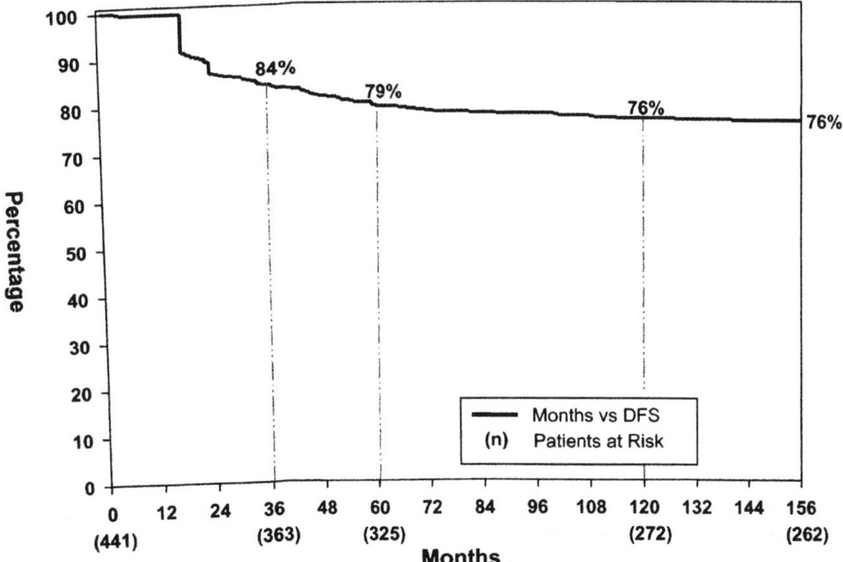

FIGURE 10   Disease-free survival versus years from implant for the Iodine-125 treated group. The number of patients at risk for failure is shown in parentheses at the end of each plot line.

follow-up*. This left 619 patients with a median posttreatment follow-up time of 71 months (range 19–156) for evaluation. (*Over 50% of this patient cohort resided outside Washington or lived in foreign countries.)

The disease-free survival rates of all 619 patients at 5, 10, and 13 years were 80%, 77%, and 77%, respectively. The 5, 10, and 13-year disease-free survival rates of the 441 Iodine-125 treated patients (Group 1) were 79%, 76%, and 76%, respectively; and the rates for the Palladium-103 treated patients (Group 2) were 82%, 80%, and 80%, respectively. Figure 9, Figure 10, and Figure 11 portray these results graphically.

MORBIDITY

The recent emphasis on quality-of-life issues after treatment for prostate cancer has led to increased scrutiny of complications. As with radical prostatectomy, morbidity data for seed implants are both limited and conflicting. Differences between treatment series are partly explained by several factors: retrospective crude statistics with small number of patients and short follow-up, variation in patient selection, treatment and implant techniques, and the treating physician's experience with seed implantation.

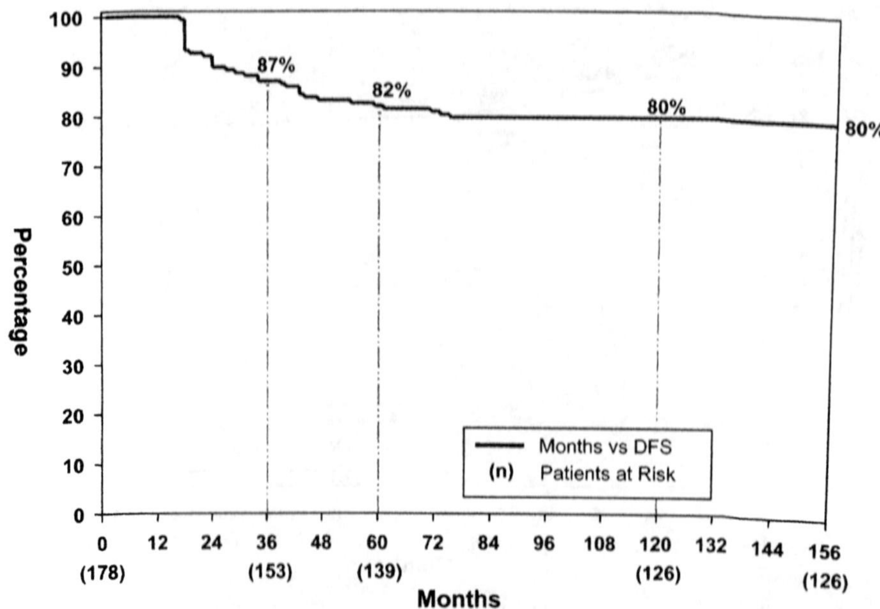

FIGURE 11   Disease-free survival versus years from implant for the Palladium-103 treated group. The number of patients at risk for failure is shown in parentheses at the end of each plot line.

Our combined clinical experience with over 7,000 patients treated at our centers in Seattle, Washington, and Scottsdale, Arizona, reveals that most patients experience some degree of irritative and/or obstructive urinary tract symptoms due to ongoing radiation. The symptoms usually begin 1–2 weeks after implant and persist in varying degrees for a couple of weeks to months. The symptoms are usually mild and short-lasting, but, even so, may be a bother to patients anticipating rapid return to pretreatment health.

If symptoms occur immediately after the implant procedure, the condition is likely due to mechanical trauma from the implant needles. (Large glands, which require a greater number of needle punctures and seeds, are subjected to more trauma from needle punctures than small glands). Postimplant urinary retention is, to a large extent, related to significant obstructive symptoms prior to implantation.

Approximately 5% of patients require intermittent or indwelling catheterization (Ragde H, Grado GL, Smith LG III, personal experience). It is our experience that even protracted urinary retention will improve over time. A suprapubic tube may be needed, or even a transurethral incision (TUIP). A transurethral resection of the prostate (TURP), on the other hand, should be avoided in patients who have undergone a uniform-(Quimby) type implant, because such patients are at high risk of incomplete healing, which leads to incontinence and stricture formation (Ragde H, Grado GL, Smith LG III, personal experience).

Acute proctitis, manifested by frequent blood-tinged bowel movements, is infrequent in our experience. When it occurs, it is generally mild and does not often require treatment. If treatment becomes necessary, the condition is usually corrected with local therapy.

Long-term symptoms of proctitis are generally mild and characterized by intermittent rectal bleeding. Patients with these symptoms should be examined to rule out nonradiation causes. Patients should be strongly advised against biopsy and fulguration of the hyper-vascular rectal wall overlying the prostate. It is a totally unnecessary procedure that may lead to a urethrorectal fistula and either a temporary or permanent bowel/urinary divershon (Ragde H, Grado GL, Smith LG III, personal experience; Gillenwater JY, personal communication).

Significant urinary incontinence is singularly rare in patients who have not had prior TURPs, and there appears to be no obvious difference in incontinence risk between patients treated with monotherapy and patients receiving brachytherapy and external beam irradiation (Ragde H, Grado GL, Smith LG III, personal experience). Over 20% of patients with a TURP history and a uniform-type implantation may experience incontinence, mainly of the stress type (Ragde H, Grado GL, Smith LG III, personal experience). A TURP postimplant in such patients may raise the incontinence rate to about 80%, and, therefore, should be avoided (Ragde H, Grado GL, Smith LG III, personal experience).

Postimplant patients generally have a bloody ejaculate and experience burning on ejaculation; these symptoms may last for several weeks. In the months or years that follow the implant, the ejaculate volume will generally recede, at times to nothing. This situation occurs in about 25% of implanted patients (Ragde H, Grado GL, Smith LG III, personal experience).

Published results of potency maintenance after prostate brachytherapy varies. In our experience, erectile dysfunction increased with age and averaged 30% for all ages (Ragde H, Grado GL, Smith LG III, personal experience). Patients younger than 60 years of age, who claimed sexual proficiency prior to the implant, generally maintained that competence after the procedure. Some patients experienced temporary difficulties. Overall, fewer than 10% of patients between 60 and 70 years of age who claimed to be sexually functional prior to the implant lost that ability after the implant. Some of the patients claiming dysfunction have benefited from treatment with Sildenafil. We would reasonably predict that a higher erectile dysfunction rate would result from the combination of age and radiation injury than would result from age alone.

DISCUSSION

Clinically localized prostate cancer can be managed by potentially curative treatments or by using palliative approaches. Curative treatments include radical prostatectomy, external beam radiotherapy, and brachytherapy. Palliative approaches include immediate- or delayed-hormone therapy, often referred to as "watchful waiting." Characteristically, advocates for watchful waiting, maintain that the protracted natural history of prostate cancer and competing acute causes of death outweigh the lethal consequences of the malignancy. They therefore question the necessity of both surgical and radiotherapeutic intervention.

As for curative treatments, there is a lack of consensus among physicians regarding which treatment offers the most practical and effective route of control. Despite the widely recognized need for a head-to-head outcome comparison between patients managed with surgery, external beam irradiation, and brachytherapy, prospective randomized clinical trials have never materialized. Even if such trials were started today, it would be two or three decades before results would be available. Whether patients would choose to participate in a randomized trial is also a question, as most men and their families want to make informed treatment choices. In the absence of randomized clinical trials, well-designed retrospective comparative studies will continue to be the basis for treatment selection.

The advantage of brachytherapy resides in the ability to deliver high doses of radiation to a confined target volume with little or no radiation damage to the adjacent normal tissue. Brachytherapy results that are being reported today, such as the 13-year results described here, demonstrate a high rate of long-term biochemical and clinical tumor control with minimal attendant morbidity.

Some physicians contend that all clinically localized prostate cancers ought to be treated with a combination of seed implantation and external beam therapy, and back up the contention with excellent long-term disease-free survival results [28]. However, at least as practiced today, a majority of physicians believe that until clinical trials prove otherwise, the combination therapy is probably not indicated when treating low-risk disease. Not only would the addition of external beam therapy subject patients to increased morbidity, it would also dramatically raise the cost of treatment. For example, of the 769 patients referred to in this chapter, the extra cost of adding 45 Gy conventional external beam therapy would approach $8,000,000, and close to double that if 3-D conformal radiotherapy was used.

CONCLUSIONS

Modern prostate brachytherapy with permanent implants is a minimally invasive outpatient procedure that offers a viable alternative to surgery and external beam radiation therapy. Long-term studies of prostate cancer patients treated with prostate brachytherapy have provided dramatic and convincing evidence of excellent cancer control and of a favorable side-effect profile. The result being that patient and physician preferences are increasingly favoring brachytherapy [29].

REFERENCES

1. Ragde H, Grado GL, Nadir B, Elgamal AA. Modern prostate Brachytherapy CA. A Cancer Journal for Clinicians 2000; 50(6):380–393.

2. Brindel JS, Martinez A, Schray M. et al. Pelvic lymphadenectomy and transperineal interstitial implantation of Ir-192 combined with external beam radiotherapy for the bulky stage C prostatic carcinoma. Int J Radiat Oncol Biol Phys 1989; 17:1063–1066.

3. Pasteau O. The radium treatment of cancer of the prostate. Arch Roentgen Ray 1914; 18:396–410.

4. Hilaris BS. History of brachytherapy. In Nag S, Ed. Principles and Practice of Brachytherapy. Armonk. NY: Futura Publishing Company, Inc., 1997:13–26.

5. Whitmore WFJr, Hilaris B, Grabstald H. Retro-pubic implantation of iodine-125 in the treatment of prostatic cancer. J Urol. 1972; 108:918–920.

6. Elkin D, Kim J, Constable WC. Anatomic localization of radioactive gold seeds of the prostate by computer-aided tomography. Comput Tomogr 1981; 5:89–93.

7. Gore RM, Moss AA. Value of computer tomography in interstitial 125-Iodine brachytherapy of prostate carcinoma. Radiology 1983; 146:453–458.

8. Kuban D, el-Mahdi A, Schellhammer P. I-125 interstitial implantation for prostate cancer. Cancer 1989; 63:2415–2420.

9. Fuks Z, Leibel S, Wallner K, et al. The effect of local control on metastatic dissemination of carcinoma of the prostate: long-term results in patients treated with I-125 implantation. Int J Radiat Oncol Biol Phys 1991; 21:537–547.

10. Young HH. The cure of cancer of the prostate by radical perineal prostectomy (prostato-seminal vesiculectomy): history, literature, and statistics of Young's operation. J Urol 1945; 53:188.

11. Bagshaw MA, Kaplan HS, Sagerman RH. Linear accelerator super-voltage radiotherapy. VII Carcinoma of the prostate. Radiology 1965; 85:121–129.

12. Holm HH, Juul N, Pedersen JF, et al. Transperineal 125-iodine seed implantation in prostatic cancer guided by transrectal ultrasonography. J Urol. 1983; 130:283–286.

13. Partin AW, Kattan MW, Subong ENP, et al. Combination of prostate-specific antigen, clinical stage, and Gleason score to predict pathological stage of localized prostate cancer: a multi-institutional update. JAMA 1997; 277:1445–1451.

14. D'Amico AV, Whittington R, Malkowicz SB, et al. A multivariate analysis of clinical and pathological factors which predict for prostate-specific antigen failure after radical prostatectomy for prostate cancer. J Urol 1995; 154:131–138.

15. Partin AW, Yoo J, Carter B, et al. The use of prostate specific antigen, clinical stage, and Gleason score to predict pathological stage in men with prostate cancer. J Urol 1993; 150:110.

16. Conrad S, Graefen M, Pichlmeier U, et al. Systematic sextant biopsies enhance the accuracy of predicting lymph node metastasis in prostate cancer. J Urol 1997; 157: 1672–1677.

17. Wills M, Sauvageot J, Epstein JI. Ability of sextant biopsies to predict radical prostatectomy (RP) stage. J Urol 1997; 157:295.

18. Bostwick DG. Gleason grade of prostate needle biopsies: correlation with grade in 316 matched prostatectomies. Am J Surg Pathol 1994; 18:796.

19. Shearer RJ, Davies JH, Gelister JS, et al. Hormonal cytoreduction and radiotherapy for carcinoma of the prostate. Br J Urol 1992; 69(5):521–524.

20. Laverdiere J, Gomez JL, Cusan L, et al. Beneficial effect of combination hormonal therapy administered prior to and following external beam radiation therapy in localized prostate cancer. Int J Radiat Oncol Biol Phys 1997; 37(2):247–252.

21. Zietman AL, Prince EA, Nakfoor BM, et al. Androgen deprivation and radiation therapy: sequencing studies using the Shionogi in vivo tumor system. Int J Radiat Oncol Biol Phys 1997; 38(5):1067–1070.

22. Kaplan ID, Cox RS, Bagshaw MA. Prostate specific antigen after external beam radiotherapy for prostate cancer: follow-up. J Urol 1993; 149:519–522.

23. Lai PP, Perez CA, Lockett MA. Prognostic significance of pelvic recurrence and distant metastases in prostate carcinoma following definitive radiotherapy. Int J Radiat Oncol Biol Phys 1992; 24:423–430.

24. Holzman M, Carlton C, Scardino PT. The frequency and morbidity of local tumor recurrence after definitive radiotherapy for stage C prostate cancer. J Urol 1991; 146:1578–1582.

25. Grado GL, Collins JM, Krieghauser JC, et al. Salvage brachytherapy for localized prostate cancer after radiotherapy failure. Urology 1999; 53(1):2–10.

26. Ling C, Li W, Anderson L. The relative biological effectiveness of I-125 and Pd-103. Int J Radiat Oncol Biol Phys 1995; 32:373–378.

27. Anonymous. Consensts statement: guidelines for PSA following radiation therapy. American Society for Therapeutic Radiation and Oncology Consensus Panel. Int J Radiat Oncol Biol Phys 1997; 37(5):1035–1041.

28. Critz F, Tarlton R, Holladay D. Prostate-specific antigen–monitored combination radiotherapy for patients with prostate cancer. Cancer 1995; 75:2383–2391.

29. Hudson R. Brachytherapy treatments increasing among Medicare population. Health Policy Brief of the American Urological Association September 1999; IX(9):1.

EDITORIAL COMMENTARY

Molly Gabel

Department of Radiation Oncology, Robert Wood Johnson Medical School, The University of Medicine and Dentistry of New Jersey, The Cancer Institute of New Jersey, New Brunswick, New Jersey, USA

Drs. Ragde, Grado, and Smith have provided an excellent review of the selection criteria, techniques, and outcomes for prostate brachytherapy. It is clear from their discussion that patients at low risk for extracapsular spread may benefit from this more convenient and less costly treatment technique.

Their cohort of patients, treated from 1987 through 1997, have a median follow-up of less than six years, with a range of 1 to 13 years. Although this may allow accurate estimates of toxicity, the median follow-up is too brief to accurately compare local control and survival rates to surgical and standard radiotherapy approaches.

However, in Vijverberg and colleague's study of 46 patients undergoing prostate implant [1], all patients underwent posttreatment prostate biopsy. At four years, the negative biopsy rate was 50%, indicating tumoricidal doses were successfully delivered at the widely accepted brachytherapy dose of 160 Gy to the prostate.

Wallner et al. evaluated three-year outcomes in 92 patients undergoing implant [2], and found 46% suffered irritative urinary symptoms, with 14% experiencing long-term urinary symptoms of grade 2 or more. Despite variation in patient risk factors, their three-year freedom from progression rate was 63%, which is comparable to surgical and external beam radiation series. They also noted an inverse relationship between toxicities and physician experience in transperineal brachytherapy.

Zelefsky et al. performed an elegant study comparing 137 patients treated with standard three-dimensional (3D) conformal radiotherapy (3DCRT) with 145 patients undergoing transperineal implant (TPI) [3]. While their 5-year PSA freedom-from-relapse rates were comparable (88% for the 3DCRT and 82% for the TPI groups), the toxicity profile differed greatly. For 3DCRT and TPI, respectively, they found that acute urinary symptoms were 8% vs. 31%, urinary strictures were 2% vs. 12% and erectile dysfunction was 43% vs. 53%. Of note, their reports of erectile dysfunction are some of the highest found in the brachytherapy literature, but correspond with rates found in the general radiation oncology and urology literature.

Crook et al. performed a meta-analysis in 2001 [4], reviewing 16 studies of prostate brachytherapy. They showed that although there was wide variation in tumor control and toxicity rates, patients at low risk (Gleason $<$ 7, PSA $<$ 10 and Stage $<$ T2b) fared comparably to those treated with radical prostatectomy. They also found that acute urinary toxicity was only reported in 1 to 14% of patients, long-term sequelae occurred in less than 5% of patients, and studies demonstrated excellent potency rates of greater than 86%. Despite these findings, they concluded that there was insufficient evidence to recommend prostate brachytherapy over standard treatments.

The reluctance of the general community to embrace prostate brachytherapy as a viable treatment option stems from two basic concerns: the paucity of biochemical and survival data exceeding ten years and the widely variable reports of potential increased toxicity, particularly with urinary symptoms, seen with implant. Wei et al., reporting a comprehensive quality-of-life study on patients undergoing surgery, external beam or brachytherapy [5], found the following: although patients in all three groups reported bothersome sexual dysfunction, those treated with brachytherapy reported the worst urinary, rectal, and erectile dysfunction rates. Other clinicians [6–8] confirmed that although acute low-grade urinary toxicity occurs in roughly 30% of patients treated with external beam radiotherapy, the risk of urinary obstruction, urinary stricture, and erectile dysfunction seemed higher in patients undergoing implant.

As clinicians await more mature brachytherapy prostate cancer control data, and as more patients present with early stage disease, it would be prudent to focus on the toxicity profiles of the various prostate cancer treatment options when counseling newly diagnosed patients. Inherent in this treatment decision is not only careful patient selection for brachytherapy but also careful selection of the clinicians performing the implant. Review of the literature shows wide-scattering outcomes with brachytherapy, with the majority of authors remarking that toxicity decreased with physician experience.

In our practice, we are encouraged by early results of brachytherapy, but remain cautious. After determining that a patient might be eligible for implant, and after counseling the patient on the relative toxicity profiles of his treatment options, we refer those interested in brachytherapy to institutions performing more than 50 brachytherapy cases per year. We also encourage patients to engage in a frank discussion with their radiation oncologist to learn the rates of urinary and erectile dysfunction at their institution.

REFERENCES

1. Vijverberg PL, Kurth KH, Blank LE, Dabhoiwala NF, de Reijke TH, Koedooder K. Treatment of localized prostatic carcinoma using the transrectal ultrasound guided transperineal implantation technique. Eur Urol 1992; 21(1):35–41.
2. Wallner K, Roy J, Harrison L. Tumor control and morbidity following transperineal iodine 125 implantation for stage T1/T2 prostatic carcinoma. J Clin Oncol 1996; 14(2):449–453.
3. Zelefsky MJ, Wallner KE, Ling CC, Raben A, Hollister T, Wolfe T, Grann A, Gaudin P, Fuks Z, Leibel SA. Comparison of the five-year outcome and morbidity of three-dimensional conformal radiotherapy versus transperineal permanent iodine-125 implantation for early-stage prostate cancer. J Clin Oncol 1999; 17(2):517–522.
4. Crook J, Lukka H, Klotz L, Bestic N, Johnston M. Systematic Overview of the evidence for brachytherapy in clinically localized prostate cancer. CMAJ 2001; 164(7): 975–981.
5. Wei JT, Dunn RL, Sandler HM, McLaughlin PW, Montie JE, Litwin MS, Nyquist L, Sanda MG. Comprehensive comparison of health-related quality of life after contemporary therapies for localized prostate cancer. J Clin Oncol 2002; 20(2):557–566.
6. Chou RH, Wilder RB, Ji M, Ryu JK, Leigh BR, Earle JD, Doggett RL, Kubo HD, Roach M, deVere White RW. Acute toxicity of three-dimensional conformal radiotherapy in prostate cancer patients eligible for implant monotherapy. Int J Radiat Oncol Biol Phys 2000; 47(1):115–119.
7. Nguyen LN, Pollack A, Zagars GK. Late effects after radiotherapy for prostate cancer in a randomized dose-response study: results of a self-assessment questionnaire. Urology 1998 Jun; 51(6).991–997.

8. Schultheiss TE, Hanks GE, Hunt MA, Lee WR. Incidence of and factors related to late complications in conformal and conventional radiation treatment of cancer of the prostate. Int J Radiat Oncol Biol Phys 1995; 32(3):643–649.

EDITORIAL COMMENTARY

Jay Y. Gillenwater

Professor of Urology at The Medical School, University of Virginia, Charlottesville, Virginia, USA

Drs. Ragde, Grado, and Smith provide a nice review of brachytherapy. Dr. Holm told me several years ago that, although he developed the technique of ultrasound-guided transperineal prostate brachytherapy, he stopped after the first 30 patients because of too many complications. It turned out that the dose of radiation being used was much too high. It was only in 2000 that Dr. Holm resumed using his brachytherapy technique.

The technique of TRUS-guided prostate brachytherapy with preplanning and template placement of preloaded needles was brought to the United States by Dr. Ragde after he visited Dr. Holm in Denmark in 1983. Dr. Ragde was joined by Dr. Blasko, and later by Dr. Grimm. Dr. Ragde performed the first ultrasound-guided prostate brachytherapy on November 12, 1985, with the assistance of Dr. Blasko. Drs. Ragde and Blasko performed the first closed temporary Iridium implant and the first 103 Palladium implant, both in 1987. Also in 1987, Dr. Ragde performed the first-ever transrectal ultrasound-guided biopsy gun prostate needle biopsy.

The two big advances that allowed this technique to develop were advances in ultrasound technology and in computerization, enabling calculations of radioactivity dosimetry to be done in a timely manner.

The selection of a low-risk group and a high-risk group was done arbitrarily. The assumption that the worst cancers would need supplemental external radiation was also somewhat arbitrary. Time has borne out the hypothesis that prostate cancers of higher grade and stage need more radiation. Fortunately for this type of treatment, the correct doses of radiation were chosen. It also needs to be said that many of the patients in the early study were understaged as far as Gleason scoring, as later reviewed by Drs. Bostwick and Schellhammer. Additionally, many of the early patients had high PSA readings; however, the significance of various PSA levels was not understood at that time.

The 13-year data looks good. Other institutions doing brachytherapy do not yet have follow-ups as long as this time frame, but data suggest prostate brachytherapy may be a good alternative to radical prostatectomy in certain patients. Still, when and whether to use androgen blockade as a radio sensitizer and exactly which patients will benefit from supplemental external radiotherapy need to be worked out. With recent changes in the techniques we are seeing fewer urethral and rectal complications. Studies on CT and MRI-guided techniques do not yet have follow-ups long enough for evaluation; however, they do show that radioactive seeds can certainly be implanted well using these techniques.

I think prostate brachytherapy offers a viable option for treating prostate cancer. Surgery remains the tried and true treatment, but experiences with brachytherapy look increasingly promising.

EDITORIAL OVERVIEW

Kenneth B. Cummings

Ragde and coworkers provide an excellent overview of the history of prostate brachytherapy, noting the initial enthusiasm in the early 1970s by Whitemore and Hilaris employing iodine-125 with open-surgical placement and pelvic lymphadenectomy [1]. However, as a consequence of patient selection, inability to control seed spacing and doses, unacceptable local control, and late complications, interest progressively waned in favor of improved/evolving megavoltage radiation [2] and evolving surgical technique [3]. In 1983, Dr. Holme and associates, in Copenhagen, were the first to guide placement of seed-bearing needles transperineally guided by transrectal ultrasound. Ragde introduced the technique into the United States in 1985.

Their experience is well documented and exhibits that patients at low risk (Gleason sum < 6 and PSA ≤ 10) may benefit from this minimally invasive therapy. It is less obvious that patients at higher risk (Gleason sum > 7, PSA > 10) gain an advantage with external beam therapy followed by seed placement as opposed to current external beam radiation therapy alone (either from a cost standpoint or therapeutic efficacy).

Gillenwater praises the innovations of Ragde and acknowledges the problems inherent in patient selection early in their series. The 13-year data and median follow-up make comparisons of local control and survival to surgical or standard radiotherapy outcomes too brief.

Gabel provides a thoughtful review of contemporary brachytherapy. Comparisons to outcomes from three-dimensional (3D) conformal radiation therapy (3DCRT), with respect to the toxicity profile, favored 3DCRT with respect to urinary symptoms, urinary strictures, and erectile dysfunction [4]. The reluctance of the general community to embrace prostate brachytherapy as a viable therapeutic alternative stems from two basic concerns: (a) the paucity of biochemical and survival data exceeding 10 years and (b) the widely variable reports of potential increased toxicity, particularly with urinary symptoms seen with implants.

Gabel comments further, identifying wide-scattering outcomes with brachytherapy, along with the observation that toxicity decreased with physician experience [5].

REFERENCES

1. Whitemore WFJr, Hilaris B, Grabstald H. Retro-pubic implantation of iodine 125 in the treatment of prostatic cancer. J Urol 1972; 108:918–920.
2. Bagshaw MA, Kaplan HS, Sagerman RH. Linear accelerator super-voltage radiotherapy. VII Carcinoma of the prostate. Radiology 1965; 85:121–129.
3. Walsh PC, Donker PJ. Impotence following radical prostatectomy: insight into etiology and prevention. J Urol 1982; 128:492–294.
4. Zelefsky MJ, Wallner KE, Ling CC, Raben A, Hollister T, Walfe T, Grann A, Gaudin P, Fuks Z, Leibel SA. Comparison of the five-year outcome and morbidity of three-dimensional conformal radiotherapy vs. transperineal permanent iodine-125 implantation for early stage prostate cancer. J Clin Oncol 1999 Feb; 17(2):517–522.
5. Wei JT, Dunn RL, Sandler HM, McLaughlin PW, Montie JE, Litwin MS, Nyquist L, Sanda MG. Comprehensive comparison of health-related quality of life after contemporary therapies for localized prostate cancer. J Clin Oncol 2002; 20(2):557–566.

7

Combined Modality Therapy With Brachytherapy and External Beam Irradiation in the Management of Localized Prostate Cancer

Richard G. Stock and Nelson N. Stone

Mount Sinai Medical Center, New York, NY, USA

INTRODUCTION

The impetus to combine permanent radioactive seed implantation of the prostate gland and external beam radiation therapy (EBRT) probably derives from two main sources. The first rational for using this combined modality therapy (CMT) comes from the experience of the retropubic prostate seed implant. Since this technique of implantation was implemented prior to the use of transrectal ultrasound and computer tomography (CT)-based technology, it relied on the free hand placement of seeds with an open exposure of the prostate. This technique resulted in poor seed distribution and inadequate dose coverage. The concept of combining this technique with external beam irradiation made sense because the external beam portals could be made large enough to ensure coverage of the entire prostate and potentially make up for cold spots created with the retropubic implant. One of the first reported uses of CMT was with the open retropubic technique [1]. The second rational for using CMT probably derived from a commonly used radiation therapy technique. This technique involves the use of large external beam ports to encompass the known tumor, as well as the organ at risk, draining lymphatics, and a brachytherapy boost to the tumor, usually using a temporary radioactive source implant. This technique is commonly used to treat gynecologic malignancies and head and neck tumors. This treatment allows the tumor to receive the highest dose with contributions from both the EBRT and the brachytherapy while the peritumor surrounding tissues and draining lymphatics receive prophylactic radiation form the EBRT.

This latter rationale would serve as the major force behind CMT in the modern ultrasound-guided transperineal age of prostate brachytherapy. In the late 1980s, as ultrasound-guided implants began to be used, data emerged from the radical prostatectomy series demonstrating higher-than-expected rates of extracapsular extension, positive margins, and nonorgan confined disease. In addition, the effect of disease-related prognostic factors such as stage, prostate specific antigen (PSA), and Gleason score on a pathologic stage began to be realized [2]. This lead to investigators using EBRT in combination with seed implant in higher-risk patients in hopes of better addressing extracapsular disease and eradicating the local disease [3,4].

PATIENT SELECTION

As the importance of prognostic factors in predicting pathologic stage and outcome became known, and as brachytherapy techniques were refined, the question of when and in whom to use EBRT with brachytherapy arose. The use of CMT for all patients or just in a select group is still a matter of debate. Certain practitioners advocate the use of CMT on all prostate cancer patients without regard to disease presentation [1,5]. Others have advocated the use of CMT only for patients with more advanced-presenting disease features and reserve brachytherapy alone for patients with low-risk features [3,4]. Much of the data used to select patients for CMT comes from pathologic studies of radical prostatectomy specimens, as well as reports on the use of implant alone to treat prostate cancer [2,6,7]. In the early years of the use of transperineal ultrasound-guided brachytherapy, there was little information available to guide physicians in selecting patients for brachytherapy. Initially, many centers treated patients with brachytherapy alone without regard to disease extent. As data became available highlighting the importance of PSA, tumor grade, and clinical stage in predicting both the risk of nonorgan confined disease and treatment outcome, patient selection for brachytherapy became more important. Stock and Stone analyzed patients treated with brachytherapy and defined a low-risk group of patients with PSA ≤ 10 ng/mL, Gleason score <7, and clinical stage $\leq$ T2a who had a significantly improved rate of biochemical control of 88% at 4 years, compared with 60% for patients with higher-risk features. The study suggested that patients with low-risk features can be adequately treated with implants alone and those with higher-risk features require more aggressive approaches, such as CMT [7]. An analysis by D'Amico et al. of 1872 men with localized prostate cancer also supported the finding that low-risk patients treated with brachytherapy alone did as well as those treated with EBRT or prostatectomy [8]. It also suggested that high-risk patients did poorly with all of the earlier-mentioned treatments. This data supports the use of CMT for these high-risk patients. Davis measured the amount of extracapsular extension of the cancer following prostatectomy and found that in low-risk patients, the maximal radial extension of disease outside the prostate was 2.1 mm (mean 0.13 mm). He concluded that doses generated by brachytherapy, which provides a 3–5-mm margin, would encompass the entire prostate and the cancer in 96% to 99% of low-risk patients [9]. This data supports the use of brachytherapy alone in low-risk patients.

In addition, Potters et al. performed a matched pair analysis comparing patients treated with implants alone with those treated with CMT. In low-risk patients, there was no significant difference in PSA failure rates between the two treatment groups. Patients with PSA $\leq$10 ng/mL had an 88% 5-year freedom from PSA failure rate with CMT compared to 88% with implant alone (p = 0.99). Low-risk patients (PSA $\leq$10 ng/mL, Gleason score $\leq$6, and stage T1–T2 disease) had a 5-year freedom from PSA failure rate of 91% with CMT versus 88.5% with implants alone (p = 0.86). In addition, no difference between treatment groups was found in higher-risk patients [10].

TECHNIQUES

Radioactive Seed Implant

There are many techniques available to perform prostate brachytherapy. Two major techniques are the preplanned and real-time ultrasound-guided techniques. The preplanned technique was first described by Holm using transrectal ultrasound to help plan seed distribution [11]. This technique was later refined by Ragde and Blasko [12]. It involves the generation of a preimplant ultrasound study with the patient in the treatment position. The exact needle and seed positions are then planned out on a grid with the help of planning software. The patient is then set-up in the operating room in order to replicate the preplanned position. Needles are deposited according to the preplan. In this technique, seeds are most often preloaded into needles that are then inserted into the prostate. In order to overcome some of the limitations of preplanning, such as difficulty replicating the preplan position, as well as changes in prostate shape and position that occur both before and during the implant, the real-time ultrasound-guided system was developed by Stock and Stone [13]. This system relies on a nomogram to determine the amount of activity to implant per prostate volume. Real-time ultrasound is used to guide needle and seed placement. This technique has been shown to achieve excellent dose distributions based on postimplant CT-based dosimetric analysis [14]. This method of implantation has recently been refined with the use of an intraoperative dosimetry system [15]. *Intraoperative dosimetry* is a method of replicating the delivered dose on a computer as the implant is performed, and modifying the dosage accordingly.

With this method, all of the planning is interactive and done at the time of the implant. First, a planimetry volume study is performed in the treatment position to determine the amount of activity to implant based on an activity per volume table [16]. The total number of seeds is determined by dividing the total activity by the activity per seed. 75% of the seeds are used for implanting peripheral needles and 25% are used to implant the interior needles.

Needle-based dosimetry is generated using the Variseed implant planning software. Implantation begins by inserting the needles into the periphery of the gland using the largest ultrasound transverse diameter cut as a guide. Needles are inserted one centimeter apart into the capsule. Once these peripheral needles have been placed, the first step of real-time planning is performed. The prostate is recontoured using 5 mm transverse ultrasound cuts from base to apex, and acquired by the planning system. An internal grid on the Variseed system is then superimposed on the grid positions of the acquired ultrasound images. A three-dimensional grid matrix with and x, y, and z-axis is created. The prostate volume contoured from the ultrasound images will lie within this matrix. The position of the needles is determined on the acquired ultrasound images by identifying the echo-bright markings of the implanted needles. The planning system assumes that the needles run straight and do not deviate. Needle positions can be identified using any of the transverse images and marked on the x − y-axis. From this point on, the implantation procedure proceeds by depositing seeds using the Mick applicator. Seeds are marked on the planning system along the needle track to correspond to the actual implant. The locations of the seeds in the planning matrix are determined manually by examining the path of the needle through the transverse-captured prostate images. Seeds can be placed on any of the 5-mm slices, or 2.5 mm above or below any slice of the prostate. Corresponding isodose lines can be visualized after seed placement.

The next step involves placing the internal needles and implanting the remaining 25% of the seeds. Using the largest transverse diameter image on the planning system, the positions of the interior needles and seeds are planned. Typically between 6 and 8 needles are inserted into the periphery such that they encompass the periphery of the base and apical slices and remain 0.5 to 1 cm from the urethra. If cold or hot areas within the prostate are discovered, then needle and seed positions in the interior can be modified. This is the step of the procedure that allows for optimization. In addition, seed positions in the interior can be optimized to limit dose to normal structures. Once the plan is finalized, the interior needles are inserted into the prostate and seeds deposited to match the plan as closely as possible.

A comparison of dosimetry results generated intraoperatively to CT-based dosimetry performed one month post-implant was performed in 70 patients, 37 I-125 alone and 33 partial Pd-103. This revealed a good correlation between intraoperative and post-implant results. The mean D90 results intraoperatively versus post-implant were 178 Gray (Gy) versus 188.5 Gy for Iodine (I)-125 implants and 98 Gy versus 98.5 Gy for partial Palladuim (Pd)-103 implants, respectively [17]. Real-time intraoperative dosimetry promises to be the best technique for performing prostate brachytherapy [18]. This system is particularly important when combining implants with EBRT, since the ability to precisely modulate delivered dose to the rectum and urethra can help decrease treatment related morbidity.

External Beam Radiation Therapy

Many different approaches and techniques have been used to deliver external beam irradiation in conjunction with brachytherapy. This includes the use of whole pelvic fields to include regional lymphatics, small pelvic fields, as well as conformal fields that treat the prostate and seminal vesicles with a small margin of surrounding normal tissue.

The use of pelvic fields in the radiotherapeutic management of prostate cancer is controversial [19]. The issue is particularly relevant to CMT, since CMT is primarily used in more high-risk prostate cancer in which the risk of lymph node metastasis is greater. Unfortunately, there is no consensus regarding this issue and there are no prospective data that show an advantage of whole pelvic EBRT over prostate only EBRT [19]. One approach advocates the use of lymph node dissections to assess high-risk prostate cancer patients. This approach has the advantage of selecting node positive patients and offering them sustained hormone therapy in addition to radiation. Radiation Therapy and Oncology Group (RTOG) 85–31 showed a significantly improved disease-free survival in patients receiving sustained hormone therapy plus radiation therapy versus radiation therapy alone [20]. In addition, in a study reported by Messing et al., androgen suppression plus prostatectomy showed improved survival over prostatectomy in node positive patients [21].

Although a number of techniques are available to deliver radiation therapy to the prostate or prostate and seminal vesicles, multiple field therapy using 3-D conformal techniques is preferred. This usually involves delivering radiation therapy to the prostate and seminal vesicles with a 1–2 cm margin of normal tissue. In this way, potential microscopic extracapsular extension of the disease will be included in the fields. One common technique is to use 6 converging fields, including right and left anterior obliques, right and left posterior obliques, and 2 lateral fields [22]. This technique is used to limit dosage to the rectum and bladder. Newer radiation therapy techniques are being developed including intensity modulated radiation therapy (IMRT) [23]. This technique allows the radiation beam to be further manipulated to provide a more conformal radiation field. This technology probably holds it greatest promise in the treatment of prostate cancer with EBRT alone. With the relatively low dose of EBRT used with CMT, the theoretical advantages of IMRT are less clear.

ISOTOPE SELECTION

The most common permanent radioactive isotopes used in prostate brachytherapy are I-125 and Pd-103; both have been used in CMT. The isotopes differ primarily in their dose rates and energies. I-125 has an energy of 28 kilovolts (keV) and a half-life of 60 days. Pd-103 has an energy of 22 keV and a half-life of 17 days. I-125 will deliver almost all of its radiation therapy in 8 months, while Pd-103 will deliver its radiation over 2 months. Due to the greater energy of I-125 over Pd-103, radiation emitted from I-125 will penetrate tissue to a greater depth than Pd-103. Pd-103's emitted radiation will be greater attenuated by tissue than I-125. This property is very relevant to CMT since radiation doses to normal tissues, such as the bladder and rectum, will come from both the isotope as well as the external beam irradiation. Critz et al. have described using CMT with I-125, performing the implant first then delivering EBRT soon after. In this technique, the prostate is irradiated simultaneously from the I-125 seeds and the external beam irradiation [1]. Others have used Pd-103, both given before and after EBRT [4,22]. The theoretical advantage of using Pd-103 over I-125 is the potentially lower rectal dose delivered by Pd-103, due to its greater tissue attenuation. Currently there are no data supporting the superiority of one isotope over the other in terms of efficacy or toxicity. The one study, which compared the two isotopes in both the CMT setting as well as brachytherapy alone, found no differences in outcomes or morbidity [24].

SEQUENCING

In CMT, the brachytherapy implant can be delivered either prior to or after the EBRT. There are theoretical and practical advantages and disadvantages of both sequences. The use of brachytherapy as a boost following EBRT has been advocated by certain investigators [3,4]. The theoretical advantage of this order of therapy is that the EBRT treats the larger volume of the prostate and surrounding normal tissues and will sterilize any potential extracapsular disease, as well as reduce the intraprostatic tumor volume. The implant is then used as the boost dose to destroy any residual tumor. In this way, there is no overlap in the delivery of radiation dose from the implant and the EBRT. In fact, there is a treatment break from the time the EBRT is complete to the time of the implant. Alternatively, the implant can be delivered first and followed by EBRT [1,22,25]. In this sequence, the implant is used to achieve the bulk of the tumor kill and the EBRT is used to destroy any extracapsular cells that were not eradicated by the implant and eradicate any remaining tumor cells in the prostate. Depending on which isotope is used, as well as when the EBRT is started, there can be simultaneous irradiation of the prostate and normal tissues by the implant and EBRT. This may be beneficial in terms of maximizing tumor control, but may also increase normal tissue morbidity. As with the isotope selection, there are no data available to demonstrate the superiority of one sequence or the other in terms of tumor control. In addition, there his no evidence that one sequence is associated with greater toxicity than the other. At Mount Sinai Hospital in New York, the implant is performed first using the isotope Pd-103. A 2-month break is then given to allow the Pd-103 to deliver its radiation. The EBRT is then delivered [6]. In this way, there is no overlap of delivered radiation from the implant and the EBRT. One of the major advantages of this sequence is that it allows for post-implant dosimetry to be performed prior to delivering the EBRT. The information obtained from the post-implant analysis will reveal the delivered dosage to the prostate as well as to the urethra, bladder, and rectum. The advantage is that the subsequent EBRT can now be altered in terms of fields, margins, and total dosage based on the findings of the post-implant analysis. An implant delivering a dosage much lower than planned amount can be supplemented by increasing the EBRT dosage. Lowering the total dosage of EBRT can compensate an implant that turns out to be hotter than planned. In addition, an implant that results in a high rectal dosage can be offset by decreasing the rectal margin of the EBRT.

RADIATION DOSE

The optimal dosage of both the EBRT and implant portion of CMT is not known. Early experience with CMT used EBRT doses of 4140 Centigray (cGy) to 4500 cGy [1,2,3]. These doses were based on the classic radiation oncology teaching that advocated a dose of 45Gy to sterilize microscopic disease. In addition, the use of combined EBRT and brachytherapy has historically been used most frequently to treat cervical cancer. In this treatment, doses of EBRT of 40–45 Gy typically have been given to the whole pelvis in combination with a low-dose rate temporary implant of the cervix, uterus, and paracervical tissues. Stock et al. tested the use of higher doses of EBRT in CMT. In a phase I/II trial, EBRT was delivered using 3-D conformal techniques to a dose of 5940 cGy. Implant doses of Pd-103 were escalated in a dose-escalation trial. The commonly used

Pd-103 dose for an implant alone was 115 Gy [13]. In this trial, a planned Pd-103 dose was escalated from 50% of a full dose (57.5 Gy) to 67% (77 Gy) to 75% (86Gy). Results from the trial revealed increased radiation proctitis with implant doses based on post-implant CT dosimetry >70 Gy and increased biochemical failure with doses <65 Gy. Based on these outcomes, implant doses with Pd-103 of 65–70 Gy were recommended with doses of 59.4 Gy of EBRT [22]. Other investigators who deliver doses of EBRT of 41–45 Gy have used implant doses for Pd-103 of 80–90 Gy and doses of 100–120 Gy for I-125 [1,2,3,25].

In 1999, National Institute of Standards and Technology (NIST) established a new dose-rate constant for Pd-103. This effectively changed the way dose is described. Based on these changes, the American Brachytherapy Society recommended that the current dose of Pd-103, which would be equivalent to the 90 Gy used in the past, with 45 Gy of EBRT is 100 Gy [26].

HORMONE THERAPY AND CMT

Hormone therapy in the form of an luteinizing hormone releasing hormone (LHRH) agonist and an antiandrogen has been used in conjunction with both EBRT and radical prostatectomy. It has been shown to decrease positive margin rates and prostate volume when given prior to surgery [27,28]. Prospective trials in patients with locally advanced prostate cancer have demonstrated improved outcomes with combined hormone therapy and EBRT alone [29,30,31]. The increased benefit of hormone therapy in combination with radiation therapy may result from cytoreduction of the tumor mass prior to the radiation, from apoptotic synergism, or both [30,32,33].

There are two potential benefits of using hormone therapy with CMT. The first is a technical benefit, in terms of hormone therapy's ability to cause gland shrinkage. A large prostate size makes the prostate implantation process more difficult. If the gland size is larger than 50 cc, interference from the pubic arch can interfere with the quality of the implant. An average volume reduction of 40% can be accomplished with 3 months of hormone therapy [34]. There is also an advantage in decreasing the prostate size in men who present with significant urinary symptoms from an enlarged prostate. The risk of developing significant outlet obstruction, urinary retention, and the need for subsequent transurethral resection of prostate (TURP) may be decreased with the use of hormone therapy [35].

The second potential benefit is in terms of cytoreduction. Hormone therapy has been shown to improve PSA control when used with brachytherapy. Lee demonstrated that 6 months of hormonal therapy with Pd-103 or I-125 implantation improved freedom from PSA failure at 5 years over implant alone (74% versus 46%, respectively [p = 0.001]) in high-risk prostate cancer patients (2 or more of the following: PSA >10 ng/mL, Gleason score ≥7, or stage ≥T2b) [36]. Whether hormone therapy is needed when high-dose radiation such as that delivered with CMT is used is unknown. Stock found that 9 months of a combined androgen blockade combined with 59.4 Gy of EBRT and Pd-103 brachytherapy resulted in a 4-year freedom from PSA failure rate of 74% in very high-risk prostate cancer patients (Median PSA 16 ng/mL, Gleason ≥7 in 77%, and positive seminal vesicle biopsies in 49%) [22].

RESULTS

Although there are no prospective data analyzing the effect of CMT on disease control, there does exist numerous single institutional retrospective reports. Although CMT has been used both solely for all patients as a treatment modality as well as selectively for advanced patients, it is important to report results by presenting disease characteristics. Overall disease-free survival rates are reported on mixed groups of patients (see Table 1). In general, these populations usually contain higher grade and PSA patients. Failure rates most often have been broken-out by presenting PSA, although investigators have also used grade and a combination of factors to break-out outcome rates. Some reports have used risk-group breakouts. Tables 2, 3 and 4 list freedom from PSA failure rates for low-, intermediate-, and high-risk groups based on available subgroup analyses. Of all the prognostic variables analyzed, it may be that grade has the greatest prognostic value. In an analysis by Stock of 132 high-risk patients treated with 9 months of hormone therapy, Pd-103 brachytherapy, and EBRT, Gleason score was the only variable that was found to be significantly prognostic. Patients with score of 8–10

TABLE 1 Overall Freedom from Prostate-Specific Antigen (PSA) Failure Following Combined Modality Therapy (CMT)

Author	No. Pts	Median FU	Rate	Time	PSA Failure definition
Ragde (39)	51	119 mos	76%	10 yrs	PSA >0.5 ng/mL
Critz (37)	689	48 mos	88%	5 yrs	PSA >0.2 ng/mL
Dattoli (38)	124	43 mos	79%	4 yrs	PSA >1.0 ng/mL
Potters (10)	108	45 mos	83.5%	5 yrs	ASTRO
Lederman (25)	348	44 mos	77%	6 yrs	PSA >1.0 ng/mL
Stock (40)	132	50 mos	86%	5 yrs	ASTRO

FU = follow up

Mos = months

Yrs = years

ASTRO = American Society of Therapeutic Radiology and Oncology

TABLE 2 Overall Freedom from Prostate-Specific Antigen (PSA) Failure (Low-Risk Patients)

Author	No. Pts	Prognositc group	Rate	Time	PSA Failure definition
Critz (37)	451	PSA 4.1–10	93%	5 yrs	PSA >0.2ng/mL
Dattoli (38)	60	PSA 4.1–10	80%	5 yrs	PSA >1.0ng/mL
Blasko (2)	NA	PSA 0–10	78%	8 yrs	PSA >1.0ng/mL
Lederman (25)	164	PSA <20, stage ≤T2b, Gleason score ≤6	88%	6 yrs	PSA >1.0ng/mL
Potters (10)	52	PSA ≤10, Gleason score ≤6, stage T1–T2	91%	5 yrs	ASTRO

NA = not available
Yrs = years
ASTRO = American Society of Therapeutic Radiology and Oncology

did significantly worse with freedom from PSA failure rates at 5-years, 76%, versus 85% for scores of 7 and 97% for scores ≤6 (p = 0.03) [40]. This data may reflect that those patients with high-grade tumors are those most likely to have microscopically disseminated disease at onset. Despite aggressive local therapy and control, these patients will still demonstrate a high PSA failure rate.

TREATMENT-RELATED MORBIDITY

The three main treatment-related morbidities are rectal toxicity, urinary complications, and erectile dysfunction. Urinary side effects from implantation are second-

TABLE 3 Overall Freedom from Prostate-Specific Antigen (PSA) Failure (Moderate-Risk Patients)

Author	No. Pts	Prognostic group	Rate	Time	PSA Failure definition
Critz (37)	144	PSA 10.1–20	75%	5 yrs	PSA >0.2ng/mL
Blasko (2)	NA	PSA 10–20	67%	8 yrs	PSA >1.0ng/mL
Dattoli (38)	29	PSA 10–20	75%	5 yrs	PSA >1.0ng/mL
Stock* (40)	44	PSA 10–20	92%	5 yrs	ASTRO
Lederman (25)	124	PSA ≥20, or Gleason score ≥7, or stage ≥T2c	5%	6 yrs	PSA >1.0ng/mL
Potters (10)	NA	PSA >10, or Gleason score >6, or Stage >T2	85%	5 yrs	ASTRO

NA = not available
Yrs = years
ASTRO = American Society of Therapeutic Radiology and Oncology
* Includes the use of hormone therapy.

TABLE 4 Overall Freedom from Prostate-Specific Antigen (PSA) Failure (High-Risk Patients)

Author	No. Pts	Prognostic group	Rate	Time	PSA Failure definition
Blasko (2)	NA	PSA >20	36%	8 yrs	PSA >1.0
Critz (37)	44	PSA >20	75%	5 yrs	PSA >0.2
Dattoli (38)	35	PSA >20	70%	5 yrs	PSA >1.0
Lederman (25)	59	(>1 feature: PSA ≥20, Gleason score ≥7, Stage ≥T2c)	51%	5 yrs	PSA >1.0
Potters (10)	NA	(>1 feature: PSA >10, Gleason score >6, Stage >T2)	74%	5 yrs	ASTRO
Stock* (40)	38	PSA >20	79%	5 yrs	ASTRO
Stock (40)	37	Gleason Score 8-10	76%	5 yrs	ASTRO

NA = not available
Yrs = years
ASTRO = American Society of Therapeutic Radiology and Oncology
* Includes the use of hormonal therapy.

ary to the edema, and bleeding is associated with the implantation procedure itself, as well as irritation caused by radiation-induced prostatitis and urethritis. One of the more serious complications seen after implantation is urinary retention. This side effect is most commonly seen in patients with predisposing urinary outflow compromise [35]. The cause is secondary to increased edema, and intra-prostatic bleeding secondary to needle sticks. There is currently no evidence to demonstrate that the addition of EBRT, either before or after seed implantation, increases the risk of urinary retention. Table 5 lists reported retention rates following CMT.

Morbidity from radiation can also take the form of late reactions, which can occur months to years after treatment. One of the more common late complica-

TABLE 5 Urinary Retention Rates Following Combined Modality Therapy (CMT)

Author	No. Pts	Modality	Rate
Datto li (3)	73	EBRT + Pd-103	7%
Kaye (41)	76	EBRT + I-125	5%
Zeitlin (5)	212	EBRT/I-125/Pd-103	1.5%

tions of CMT is radiation proctitis. Due to the proximity of the anterior rectal wall to the posterior aspect of the prostate, it is often difficult to spare the rectal wall radiation dosages and adequately treat the prostate to the prescribed dose. Radiation proctitis can range in severity from the most common, intermittent painless rectal bleeding, to the rarer ulceration and fistula formation. In general, proctitis rates following CMT appear to be higher then those associated with implant alone. Reported proctitis rates following implant alone have ranged from 1%–10% [42–45] Table 6 lists proctitis rates following CMT that range from 7%–21%. Other retrospective studies have shown that the addition of EBRT to brachytherapy does not increase the risk of proctitis [45,46].

Another complication of CMT is the development of erectile dysfunction. The exact mechanism of radiation-induced erectile dysfunction is not known. It is felt that vascular changes are a major component of this effect. Theoretically, any method that reduces radiation doses to the pelvic vessels and neurovascular bundles would reduce erectile dysfunction. Since implantation is associated with a rapid fall-off of radiation dosage from the seeds, it should deliver lower doses to the neurovascular bundles. The addition of EBRT to seed implantation would increase dosage to the neurovascular bundles and theoretically increase impotency over implant alone. The longest follow-up potency data comes from Stock et al., where 416 patients treated with implant alone had their potency status prospectively assessed prior to treatment and at regular follow-up periods. Overall, preservation of potency was 59% at 6 years [48]. There are limited data on the effect of CMT on potency. Dattoli reported a 77% potency preservation in 73 patients at 3 years [3]. Critz reported a 76% potency preservation rate in 239 patients at 5 years [1]. Zeitlin found that potency was preserved in 62% at 5 years in 239 patients treated with CMT [5]. Potters demonstrated that the addition of EBRT increased impotency over implant alone with a 56% 5-year preservation of potency rate compared to a 76% 5-year potency rate, respectively (p = 0.08) [49]. Merrick reported that the addition of EBRT to brachytherapy had a negative effect on potency with a 26% 6-year rate [50]. The addition of hormone therapy to CMT also seems to negatively effect potency preservation. Stock found that

TABLE 6 Proctitis Rates Following Combined Modality Therapy (CMT)

Author	Modality[AQ11]	No. Pts	Rate	Grade
Zeitlin (5)	EBRT + I-125/Pd-103	212	21.4%	NA
Critz (1)	EBRT + I-125	239	15%	NA
Blasko (46)	EBRT + Pd-103/I-125	NA	7%	Grade 3
Stone (6)	EBRT + Pd-103	40	18%	Grade 2

NA = not available

the actuarial preservation of potency at 3 years with 9 months of hormone therapy and CMT was 43% [22].

CONCLUSION

CMT has emerged as a viable treatment option for localized prostate cancer. Biochemical control rates are comparable to other treatment modalities. In comparison to seed implant alone, there does not appear to be any clear benefits to the use of CMT in low-risk prostate cancer. Although available data is mostly retrospective, there appears to be an increased incidence of treatment-related side effects with CMT compared to implant alone. This increased risk is probably justified in intermediate- and high-risk prostate cancer, where CMT appears to offer improved biochemical control rates over seed implant alone [7].

REFERENCES

1. Critz FA, Tarlton RS, Holladay DA. Prostate specific antigen-monitored combination radiotherapy for patients with prostate cancer: I-125 implant followed by external-beam radiation. Cancer 1995; 75:2383–2391.
2. Partin AW, Kattan MW, Subong EN, Walsh PC, Wojno KJ, Oesterling JE, Scardino PT, Pearson JD. Combination of prostate-specific antigen, clinical stage, and Gleason score to predict pathological stage of localized prostate cancer: A multi-institutional update. JAMA 1997 May 14; 277(18):1445–1451.
3. Blasko J, Ragde H, Cavanagh W, Sylvester J, Grimm P. Long-term outcomes of external beam irradiation and I-125/Pd-103 brachytherapy boost for prostate cancer. Int J Radiat Oncol Biol Phys 1996; 36(Suppl 1):198.
4. Dattoli M, Wallner K, Sorace R, Koval J, Cash J, Acosta R, Brown C, Etheridge J, Binder M, Brunelle R, Kirwan N, Sanchez S, Stein D, Wasserman S. 103Pd brachytherapy and external beam irradiation for clinically localized, high-risk prostatic carcinoma. Int J Radiat Oncol Biol Phys 1996 Jul 15; 35(5):875–879.
5. Zeitlin SI, Sherman J, Raboy A, Lederman G, Albert P. High dose combination radiotherapy for the treatment of localized prostate cancer. J Urol 1998 Jul; 160(1): 91–95.
6. Stone NN, Stock RG. Prostate brachytherapy: Treatment strategies. J Urol 1999 Aug; 162:421–426.
7. Stock RG, Stone NN. The effect of prognostic factors on therapeutic outcome following transperineal prostate brachytherapy. Sem Surg Oncol 1997; 13:454–460.
8. D'Amico AV, Whittington R, Malkowicz SB, Schultz D, Blank K, Broderick GA, Tomaszewski JE, Renshaw AA, Kaplan I, Beard CJ, Wein A. Biochemical outcome after radical prostatectomy, external beam radiation therapy, or interstitial radiation therapy for clinically localized prostate cancer. JAMA 1998 Sep 16;; 280(11): 969–974.
9. Davis BJ, Pisansky TM, Wilson TM, Rothenberg HJ, Pacelli A, Hillman DW, Sargent DJ, Bostwick DG. The radial distance of extraprostatic extension of prostate carci-

noma: implications for prostate brachytherapy. Cancer 1999 Jun 15;; 85(12): 2630–2637.

10. Potters L, Cha C, Ashley R, Freeman K, Waldbaum R, Wang X, Leibel S. The role of external beam irradiation in patients undergoing prostate brachytherapy. Urol Oncol 2000 Apr 1; 5(3):112–117.

11. Holm HH, Juul N, Pedersen JF, Hansen H, Stroyer I. Transperineal 125iodine seed implantation in prostatic cancer guided by transrectal ultrasonography. J Urol 1983 Aug; 130(2):283–286.

12. Blasko JC, Radge H, Schumacher D. Transperineal percutaneous iodine 125 implantation for prostatic carcinoma using transrectal ultrasound and template guidance. Endocurie Hypertherm Oncol 1987; 3:131–139.

13. Stock RG, Stone NN, Wesson MF, DeWyngaert JK. A modified technique allowing interactive ultrasound-guided three-dimensional transperineal prostate implantation. Int J Radiat Oncol Biol Phys 1995 Apr 30; 32(1):219–225.

14. Stock RG, Stone NN, Lo YC, Malhado N, Kao J, DeWyngaert JK. Post-implant dosimetry for I-125 prostate implants: Definitions and factors affecting outcome. Int J Radiat Oncol Biol Phys 2000 Oct 1; 48(3):899–906.

15. Stock RG, Stone NN, Lo YC. Intraoperative dosimetric representation of the real-time ultrasound-guided prostate implant. Tech Urol 2000 Jun; 6(2):95–98.

16. Stone NN, Stock RG, DeWyngaert JK, Tabert A. Prostate brachytherapy: Improvements in prostate volume measurements and dose distribution using interactive ultrasound-guided implantation and three-dimensional dosimetry. Radiat Oncol Investig 1995; 3:185–195.

17. Lo YC, Stock RG, Hong S, Howard V, Stone N. Prospective comparison of intraoperative real-time to post-implant dosimetry in patients receiving prostate brachytherapy. Int J Radiat Oncol Biol Phys 2000; 48(Supp):170.

18. Nag S, Ciezki JP, Cormack R, Dogget S, DeWyngaert K, Edmunson GK, Stock RG, Stone NN, Yu Y, Zelefsky M. Intraoperative planning and evaluation of permanent prostate brachytherapy. Int J Radiat Oncol Biol Phys 2001; 51:1422–1430.

19. Stock RG, Ferrari AC, Stone NN. Does pelvic irradiation play a role in the management of prostate cancer? Oncology 1998 Oct; 12(10):1467–1472.

20. Lawton CA, Winter K, Byhardt R, Sause WT, Hanks GE, Russell AH, Rotman M, Porter A, McGowan DG, DelRowe JD, Pilepich MV. Androgen suppression plus radiation versus radiation alone for patients with D1 (pN+) adenocarcinoma of the prostate (results based on a national prospective randomized trial, RTOG 85–31). Radiation Therapy Oncology Group. Int J Radiat Oncol Biol Phys 1997 Jul 15; 38(5):931–939.

21. Messing EM, Manola J, Sarosdy M, Wilding G, Crawford ED, Trump D. Immediate hormonal therapy compared with observation after radical prostatectomy and pelvic lymphadenectomy in men with node-positive prostate cancer. N Engl J Med 1999 Dec 9; 341(24):1781–1788.

22. Stock RG, Stone NN. Preliminary toxicity and PSA response of a phase I/II trial of neoadjuvant hormonal therapy, Pd-103 brachytherapy, and 3 D conformal external beam irradiation in the treatment of locally advanced prostate cancer. J Brachytherapy: In press.

23. Zelefsky MJ, Fuks Z, Hunt M, Lee HJ, Lombardi D, Ling CC, Reuter VE, Venkatraman ES, Leibel SA. High dose radiation delivered by intensity modulated conformal radiotherapy improves the outcome of localized prostate cancer. J Urol 2001 Sep; 166(3):876–881.

24. Cha CM, Potters L, Ashley R, Freeman K, Wang XH, Waldbaum R, Leibel S. Isotope selection for patients undergoing prostate brachytherapy. Int J Radiat Oncol Biol Phys 1999 Sep 1; 45(2):391–395.

25. Lederman GS, Cavanagh W, Albert PS, Israeli R, Lessing J, Savino M, Volpicella F. Retrospective stratification of a consecutive cohort of prostate cancer patients treated with a combined regimen of external-beam radiotherapy and brachytherapy. Int J Radiat Oncol Biol Phys 2001 Apr 1; 49(5):1297–1303.

26. Beyer D, Nath R, Butler W, Merrick G, Blasko J, Nag S, Orton C. American Brachytherapy Society recommendations for clinical implementation of NIST-1999 standards for 103palladium brachytherapy. The clinical research committee of the American Brachytherapy Society. Int J Radiat Oncol Biol Phys 2000 May 1; 47(2): 273–275.

27. Labrie F, Dupont A, Cusan L, Gomez J, Diamond P, Koutsilieris M, Suburu R, Fradet Y, Lemay M, Tetu B. Downstaging of localized prostate cancer by neoadjuvant therapy with flutamide and lupron: The first controlled and randomized trial. Clin Invest Med 1993 Dec; 16(6):499–509.

28. Soloway MS, Sharifi R, Wajsman Z, McLeod D, Wood DP, Puras-Baez A. Randomized prospective study comparing radical prostatectomy alone versus radical prostatectomy preceded by androgen blockade in clinical stage B2 (T2bNxM0) prostate cancer. The Lupron Depot Neoadjuvant Prostate Cancer Study Group. J Urol 1995 Aug; 154(2 Pt 1):424–428.

29. Bolla M, Gonzalez D, Warde P, Dubois JB, Mirimanoff RO, Storme G, Bernier J, Kuten A, Sternberg C, Gil T, Collette L, Pierart M. Improved survival in patients with locally advanced prostate cancer treated with radiotherapy and goserelin. N Engl J Med 1997 Jul 31; 337(5):295–300.

30. Laverdiere J, Gomez JL, Cusan L, Suburu ER, Diamond P, Lemay M, Candas B, Fortin A, Labrie F. Beneficial effect of combination hormonal therapy administered prior and following external beam radiation therapy in localized prostate cancer. Int J Radiat Oncol Biol Phys 1997 Jan 15; 37(2):247–252.

31. Pilepich MV, Krall JM, Sarraf M, John MJ, Doggett RL, Sause WT, Lawton CA, Abrams RA, Rotman M, Rubin P, Shaky WV, Grignon D, Caplan R, Cox JD. Androgen deprivation with radiation therapy compared with radiation therapy alone for locally advanced prostatic carcinoma: a randomized comparative trial of the Radiation Therapy Oncology Group. Urology 1995 Apr; 45(4):616–623.

32. Shearer RJ, Davies JH, Gelister JS, Dearnaley DP. Hormonal cytoreduction and radiotherapy for carcinoma of the prostate. Br J Urol 1992 May; 69(5):521–524.

33. Zietman AL, Nakfoor BM, Prince EA, Gerweck LE. The effect of androgen deprivation and radiation therapy on an androgen-sensitive murine tumor: an in vitro and in vivo study. Cancer J Sci Am 1997 Jan-Feb; 3(1):31–36.

34. Stock RG, Stone NN, Yeghiayan P. Neoadjuvant androgen suppression and permanent radioactive seed implantation in the treatment of stage T1–T2 prostate cancer. Molecular Urology 1998; 2:121–126.

35. Terk MD, Stock RG, Stone NN. Identification of patients at increased risk for prolonged urinary retention following radioactive seed implantation of the prostate. J Urol 1998; 160:1379–1382.

36. Lee L, Stock RG, Stone NN. The role of hormone therapy in the management of intermediate to high risk prostate cancer treated with permanent radioactive seed implantation. Int J Radiat Oncol Biol Phys:In press.

37. Critz FA, Williams WH, Levinson AK, Benton JB, Holladay CT, Schnell FJ. Simultaneous irradiation for prostate cancer: intermediate results with modern techniques. J Urol 2000 Sep; 164(3 Pt 1):738–741.

38. Dattoli M, Wallner K, True L, Sorace R, Koval J, Cash J, Acosta R, Biswas M, Binder M, Sullivan B, Lastarria E, Kirwan N, Stein D. Prognostic role of serum prostatic acid phosphatase for 103Pd-based radiation for prostatic carcinoma. Int J Radiat Oncol Biol Phys 1999 Nov 1; 45(4):853–856.

39. Ragde H, Elgamal AA, Snow PB, Brandt J, Bartolucci AA, Nadir BS, Korb LJ. Ten-year disease free survival after transperineal sonography-guided iodine-125 brachytherapy with or without 45-Gray external beam irradiation in the treatment of patients with clinically localized, low to high Gleason grade prostate carcinoma. Cancer 1998 Sep 1; 83(5):989–1001.

40. Stock RG, Cahlon O, Cesaretti JA, Kollmeier MA, Stone NN. Combined modality treatment in the management of high-risk prostate cancer. Int J Radiat Oncol Biol Phys 2004; 59:1352–1359.

41. Kaye KW, Olson DJ, Payne JT. Detailed preliminary analysis of 125iodine implantation for localized prostate cancer using percutaneous approach. J Urol 1995 Mar; 153(3 Pt 2):1020–1025.

42. Beyer DC, Priestley JB. Biochemical disease-free survival following 125I prostate implantation. Int J Radiat Oncol Biol Phys 1997; 37:559–563.

43. Wallner K, Roy J, Harrison L. Tumor control and morbidity following transperineal iodine 125 implantation for stage T1/T2 prostatic carcinoma. J Clin Oncol 1996; 14:449–453.

44. Snyder KM, Stock RG, Hong SM, Lo YC, Stone NN. Defining the risk of developing Grade 2 proctitis following 125I prostate brachytherapy using a rectal dose-volume histogram analysis. Int J Radiat Oncol Biol Phys 2001 Jun 1; 50(2):335–41.

45. Gelblum DY, Potters L. Rectal complications associated with transperineal interstitial brachytherapy for prostate cancer. Int J Radiat Oncol Biol Phys 2000; 48:119–124.

46. Merrick GS, Butler WM, Dorsey AT, Galbreath RW, Blatt H, Lief JH. Rectal function following prostate brachytherapy. Int J Radiat Oncol Biol Phys 2000; 48:667–674.

47. Blasko JC, Ragde H, Luse RW, Sylvester JE, Cavanagh W, Grimm PD. Should brachytherapy be considered a therapeutic option in localized prostate cancer?. Urol Clin North Am 1996 Nov; 23(4):633–650.

48. Stock RG, Kao J, Stone NN. Penile erectile function after permanent radioactive seed implantation for treatment of prostate cancer. J Urol 2001; 165:436–439.

49. Potters L, Torre T, Fearn PA, Leibel SA, Kattan MW. Potency after permanent prostate brachytherapy for localized prostate cancer. Int J Radiat Oncol Biol Phys 2001 Aug 1; 50(5):1235–1242.

50. Merrick GS, Butler WM, Galbreath RW. Erectile function after permanent prostate brachytherapy. Int J Radiat Oncol Biol Phys:In press.

EDITORIAL COMMENTARY

Michael J. Droller
Katherine and Clifford Goldsmith Professor of Urology, The Mount Sinai Medical Center, New York, NY, USA

If we accept the premise that radiation therapy is effective in eradicating all cancer cells from the prostate, brachytherapy can be considered highly attractive for several reasons: (a) high doses of radiation are achievable; (b) rapid fall-off of radiation reduces potential radiation toxicity to adjacent structures; (c) dosimetry can be standardized and variability in its delivery minimized; and (d) the method of administration is generally well tolerated.

If we continue with this premise, adjunctive external beam radiation for disease that is *not* organ-confined may conceivably eradicate cells that have escaped but have remained in the immediate proximity of the prostate (either in surrounding soft tissue or regional pelvic lymph nodes).

The application of brachytherapy as described by Stock and Stone in this chapter, with preimplant dosimetry planning, real-time transrectal ultrasound imaging and real-time implant dosimetry modification, and postimplant dosimetry assessment has been accomplished exceedingly well through the exploitation of enhanced imaging, computational, and technological delivery systems that have been developed over the past decade. The efficacy that appears to have been achieved (albeit with somewhat limited follow-up) in the context of an excellent safety profile have led to an increased acceptance of this treatment to the point where it has arguably become a standard of care that is rapidly overtaking surgery as the treatment of choice in the United States for prostate cancer. However, several issues warrant consideration in interpreting efficacies that have been presented and whether further validation is indicated.

In approaching this analysis, it may be worth reviewing the historical context in which brachytherapy for prostate cancer was begun. Until two decades ago, prostate cancer detection was initiated using an abnormal digital rectal examination. This prompted confirmation of the cancer using transrectal finger-guided biopsy. Since clinical suspicion at that time was based on palpable disease (vs. current diagnosis, which is most commonly based on PSA-driven biopsy in a patient with a normal digital rectal exam), diagnosis of prostate cancer was effectively made much later in the evolution of the cancer than today. Apparently successful results currently observed through earlier PSA-driven diagnosis and treatment have been interpreted as reflecting the value of identifying a cancer at an earlier and, therefore, arguably more curable phase. Equally plausible is that the lead-time bias created by the earlier diagnosis could account for the apparent success of treatment, particularly when outcome analysis is limited by observations of only short-term follow-up.

In further considering historical context, prostate cancer was also sometimes diagnosed "incidentally" in the course of performing simple prostatectomy to treat symptoms associated with benign prostatic hyperplasia. In these instances, further treatment for the cancer was thought to be unnecessary since the natural course of disease was observed not to be aggressive unless it was high grade. These patients generally appeared to have long-term survivals that approached normal life expectancy (at that time, life expectancy was 72 years rather than the more than 80 years it is today). Moreover, treatments then were associated with greater morbidity, and there were increased risks for complications.

Previously, treatment of prostate cancer with brachytherapy was accomplished by the direct placement of iodine-125 seeds on exposure of the prostate (often limited) through a retropubic incision. Pelvic lymphadenectomy, done at the time of seed implant, allowed documentation of pelvic lymph node metastases. Findings of a higher incidence of nodal metastases at that time probably reflected the higher clinical stage of disease that was being detected by digital rectal exam.

Unfortunately, the placement of seeds by this approach was inaccurate, dosimetry was compromised by inadequate imaging, and both local and distant treatment failure was frequently experienced in the context of substantial morbidity from both the radiation itself and the inadequacy of the implant technique.

Several events subsequently led to dramatic changes in the diagnosis and treatment of prostate cancer as we know it today. These included the discovery of the prostate-specific antigen (PSA); an increased rate of PSA-driven biopsies in men whose prostates were digitally normal, albeit often enlarged; the consequent diagnosis of increased numbers of men with "subclinical" prostate cancer whose disease might otherwise not have been diagnosed until after digital rectal examination had become abnormal many years later; the development of a surgical technique that would not only make radical dissection of the prostate more anatomic (reducing potential blood loss and allowing preservation of continence) but that would also allow preservation of the neurovascular bundles responsible for maintenance of erectile function; and development of imaging techniques that would allow visualization of enlarged lymph nodes, assessment of prostate size, and evaluation of possible extension of cancer beyond the prostatic capsule with or without involvement of the seminal vesicles.

These developments prompted a change in attitude among men who now believed that they could undergo radical surgery with an intent to cure that would not compromise their quality of life or the risks that previously had been encountered in radical surgery. At the same time, previously undiscovered "subclinical" prostate cancers that had existed untreated in the general population were now being uncovered because of an elevation in PSA thought to reflect the presence of cancer. Both of these developments led to a dramatic increase in the number of radical prostatectomies performed.

As earlier autopsy series had shown an increasing involvement of the prostate by occult cancer as men aged, many men now being diagnosed because of PSA evaluation were considered elderly. Since their normal life expectancy was thought unlikely to extend beyond the natural course of their cancer, or their medical condition was such that it might compromise their suitability to undergo radical surgery, it was generally held that these men should not undergo radical prostatectomy. Although surveillance was therefore suggested to such men, with potential intervention by hormone ablation therapy in the event that progression was detected, many were uncomfortable with this approach and instead chose radiation therapy.

It was these men who became candidates for brachytherapy, especially as the techniques for this procedure became more refined and the ease of application more acceptable. Further, they did not want to undergo a six-week course of external beam radiation, their prostates could be readily imaged by transrectal ultrasound, and the transperineal placement of radioactive seeds (using either a template or real-time ultrasound imaging) could be performed with greater accuracy of dosimetry than had previously been possible. In addition, the morbidity of this approach was considered to be far less, given the apparently lesser risk of this form of radiation to the rectum. Therefore, brachytherapy was provided to these patients as long as there was no evidence of metastatic disease. With new imaging studies, the use of PSA as an indication of whether or not there might be metastatic disease, and application of laparoscopic lymphadenectomy to diagnose the status of pelvic nodes, patients could now be better selected for regional treatment than had previously been possible. However, this also introduced the possibility that stage migration might influence some of the improved results that were obtained.

In analyzing outcomes in these early patients, a number of issues became apparent regarding risk factors for treatment failure and for morbidity of the procedure. This prompted modifications in assessing patients and in designing their seed implant protocol in order to enhance treatment efficacy and minimize treatment morbidity. For example, Stock and Stone were among the first to use real-time transrectal ultrasound in performing seed implants. They were also at the forefront in intensifying and standardizing radiation dosage while maintaining treatment safety. The various steps they took in reaching their current approach are reviewed in this chapter.

However, absent from their outcomes review and from previous reports on the use of brachytherapy and external beam radiation in treating prostate cancer are several caveats that should be considered. As has been suggested in other editorial comments in this volume, many of these caveats could have been addressed by prospective randomized trials. Unfortunately, most observations of treatment results and evidence upon which recommendations for treatment are based (and on which patients make their choices) are from retrospective reviews in which data reflect varying criteria in outcomes assessment, changing patterns of therapy, and comparison of results in historical cohorts. Therefore, selection of patients for contemporary treatment is often based on unspecified or changing rationales.

Patients with Gleason Scores 6 or less appear to have good outcomes with brachytherapy, external beam radiation therapy, radical surgery, and surveillance. Patients who have Gleason Score 7 or higher often have poorer outcomes with each modality. If we compare all such patients (groups with higher and groups with more moderate Gleason Scores) who now undergo aggressive therapy earlier in their course (because their cancer was detected by PSA-driven biopsy rather than by clinical detection), a substantial lead-time bias may have been introduced that itself may account for the improved 5-year survivals reported. Indeed, increased 5-year survival rates may only reflect earlier diagnosis rather than any change impacting the natural course of disease. Even reporting biochemical disease-free survival in the short term may be insufficient given these lead-time issues and early treatment or other exposure to androgen ablation therapy (which has become virtually standard, particularly in high-grade disease).

We might also ask how biochemical treatment failure translates into actual survival. Several reports have commented on durability of survival for many years following radical surgery even after PSA failure. The same may be true with radiation therapy. Indeed, if radiation is effective in eradicating all prostate cancer cells, brachytherapy should be effective in curing patients with prostate-confined disease, and brachytherapy together with external radiation should be effective against disease that has extended outside the prostate and spread to regional lymph nodes. This has not been well documented, and several reports have shown that patients who fail biochemically have disease in their prostates following brachytherapy and/or external radiation.

The increasingly routine use of hormone ablation therapy, often for prolonged periods (9 months–2 years), in conjunction with various radiation regimens adds to the difficulty in interpreting these results. Suppression of PSA levels could just as likely, if not more so, reflect the effects of hormone therapy than the impact of the radiation itself. Since PSA appears to be the standard (and earliest) means of detecting treatment failure, PSA level increases actually precede radiologic evidence of disease progression, its physiologic response to radiation or hormone ablation and its recovery from the effects of these need to be understood better for interpretation of treatment efficacy to be reliably based on PSA recovery.

The morbidity of treatment is another important issue when patients discuss their treatment options. Most patients presume that part of the ease with which they can undergo brachytherapy and external radiation is occasioned by the minimization of side effects and the virtually negligible potential risks associated with these treatments. Given the increased expertise and enhanced technologies that have been brought to bear in the administration of radiation therapy, these presumptions are reasonably valid. However, these treatments are not without their risks. Irritative and obstructive voiding symptoms may occur not only in those who have symptoms of obstruction before radiation treatment but also in those who deny any symptoms beforehand. Decreasing the size of the prostate by hormonal treatment can facilitate radioactive seed placement and increase radiation density with fewer seeds. It can also decrease the degree of obstruction that may result from the edema and bleeding that may accompany seed placement. However, men may still complain of irritative and obstructive symptoms. Also, the expertise in placement of seeds and application of external radiation at a "Center of Excellence" may not translate to a similar expertise that is uniformly available at all treatment sites.

Several additional unanswered questions emerge. First, does treatment actually confer an advantage in patients with more advanced clinical stage (though still regionalized), or those with higher Gleason scores (8–10)? Second, in those patients who are younger (and who therefore have many years potentially at risk either for recurrence by cancer cells that have escaped the effects of radiation or from cancers that develop de novo from the potential carcinogenic effects of radiation), is it possible to document an advantage conferred by such treatment and to select patients who are likely to benefit? Third, how can we factor in lead-time biases introduced by PSA-driven biopsies and earlier diagnosis in the course of the natural history of the disease in considering treatment efficacy in terms of survival? Fourth, in considering length biases as they may relate to outcomes, is it possible that acceleration of disease progression may occur (and whether these patients would have been better off not to have been diagnosed as early, and then only to have been treated when non-PSA driven clinical diagnosis was made)?

Answers to these questions beg for prospective randomized studies in which contemporary nontreated control groups are used in assessing the value of each of our current approaches. Although the concept of low intrinsic biologic potential should be considered in the context of currently increased longevity, aggressive therapy actually may not be needed at all in such patients. Conversely, treatment currently available may not be effective in patients who have disease of particularly high malignant potential.

Dr. Willet Whitmore, considered the father of urologic oncology, encapsulated these concepts when he questioned whether available treatments were effective in those in whom it was necessary or unnecessary for cure when they were likely to be effective but the cancer being treated was of low malignant potential.

"Appropriate treatment implies that therapy be applied neither to those patients for whom it is unnecessary nor to those for whom it will prove ineffective. Furthermore, the therapy should be that which will most assuredly permit the individual a qualitatively and quantitatively normal life. It need not necessarily involve an effort at cancer cure! Human nature in physicians, be they surgeons, radiotherapists, or medical oncologists, is apt to attribute good results following treatment to such treatment and bad results to the cancer, ignoring what is sometimes the equally plausible possibility that the good results are as much a consequence of the natural history of the tumor as are the bad results.''

He understood the value of studying these issues in a prospective manner, and he encouraged the performance of such studies to obtain sufficient information to provide evidence-based advice so that patients and their physicians could make truly well-informed decisions regarding their care. We urgently need to consider these precepts if we are to be able to provide sound advice to our patients in treating their individual disease.

EDITORIAL OVERVIEW

Kenneth B. Cummings

Stock and Stone outline the evolution and logic of combined modality therapy (CMT). They appropriately identify the high-risk patient (Gleason Sum > 7, and PSA > 10.0 ng/mL). They employ a real-time ultrasound guide to needle and seed placement [1] and use an intraoperative dosimetry system [2,3].

The authors review the rationale for sequencing external beam radiation therapy (EBRT) [4–6]. They further review the merits of each isotope, I-125 and Pd-103, and conclude that, to date, no clinical superiority has favored one over the other [7]. Their preference is, first, to implant Pd-103, then, after a two-month break to allow Pd-103 to deliver its radiation, to perform postimplant dosimetry followed by tailored EBRT [8].

Stock found that 9 months of combined androgen blockade and 59.4 Gy of EBRT and Pd-103 brachytherapy resulted in a 4-year freedom-from-PSA-failure rate of 74% in 40 very high-risk prostate cancer patients (Median PSA 16 ng/mL, Gleason > 7 in 77%, and positive seminal vesicle biopsies in 49%) [6].

The authors further conclude that there is an increased risk of treatment-related side effects with CMT compared to implant alone, which is justified to achieve biochemical control in high-risk prostate cancer patients [9].

Droller provides a scholarly review of the contemporary management of localized prostate cancer. His philosophic overview of the past thirty years illuminates many of our current dilemmas.

''Lead-Time'' and ''Length-Time'' bias occasioned by the PSA-driven earlier diagnosis and treatment make short-term reporting of outcomes of treatment unreliable. Disease-specific survival or fifteen-year outcomes are difficult to achieve for competing treatments. He further draws attention to the absence of randomized, controlled clinical trials to answer most of the seminal questions that would permit patients to receive "evidence-based" advice regarding individualization of therapeutic options.

REFERENCES

1. Stock RG, Stone NN, Wesson MF, DeWyngaert JK. A modified technique allowing interactive ultrasound-guided three-dimensional transperineal prostate implantation. Int J Radiat Oncol Biol Phys 1995; 32(1):219–225.
2. Stock RG, Stone NN, Lo YC. Intraoperative dosimetric representation of the real-time ultrasound-guided prostate implant. Tech Urol 2000; 6(2):95–98.
3. Nag S, Ciezki JP, Cormack R, Dogget S, DeWyngaert K, Edmunson GK, Stock RG, Stone NN, Yu Y, Zelefsky M. Intraoperative planning and evaluation of permanent prostate brachytherapy. Int J Radiat Oncol Biol Phys: 2001 Dec. 1:51(5):1422–1430.
4. Critz FA, Tarlton RS, Holladay DA. Prostate-specific antigen-monitored combination radiotherapy for patients with prostate cancer: I-125 implant followed by external-beam radiation. Cancer 1995; 75:2383–2391.
5. Dattoli M, Wallner K, Sorace R, Koval J, Cash J, Acosta R, Brown C, Etheridge J, Binder M, Brunelle R, Kirwan N, Sanchez S, Stein D, Wasserman S. Pd-103 brachytherapy and external beam irradiation for clinically localized, high-risk prostatic carcinoma. Int J Radiat Oncol Biol Phys 1996; 35(5):875–879.
6. Stock RG, Stone NN. Preliminary toxicity and PSA response of a phase I/II trial of neoadjuvant hormonal therapy, Pd-103 brachytherapy, and 3-D conformal external beam irradiation in the treatment of locally advanced prostate cancer. J Brachytherapy: 2002: 1(1):2–10 Review.
7. Cha CM, Potters L, Ashley R, Freeman K, Wang XH, Waldbaum R, Leibel S. Isotope selection for patients undergoing prostate brachytherapy. Int J Radiat Oncol Biol Phys 1999; 45(2):391–395.
8. Stone NN, Stock RG. Prostate brachytherapy: Treatment strategies. J Urol 1999; 162: 421–426.
9. Stock RG, Stone NN. The effect of prognostic factors on therapeutic outcome following transperineal prostate brachytherapy. Sem Surg Oncol 1997; 13:454–460.

8

Cryosurgical Ablation of the Prostate for Prostate Cancer: Background, Technique, and Results

Allan J. Pantuck, Amnon Zisman, and Arie S. Belldegrun
University of California School of Medicine, Los Angeles, California, USA

BACKGROUND AND HISTORICAL PERSPECTIVES

A number of efforts are underway to expand the armamentarium available for the treatment of cancer beyond the traditional three pillars of surgery, chemotherapy, and radiation. One area of active investigation involves an old idea, namely the destruction of tumor tissue using the cytotoxic effects of extreme cold. The therapeutic use of the application of extreme cold for the treatment of disease may be generally termed cryotherapy. Cryosurgery is a form of cryotherapy that focuses on the destructive response to cold and is based on using freezing temperatures to elicit necrosis in tissues exposed to a severe cryogenic injury. Cryodestruction is thought to occur on two levels, causing cellular injury as well as vascular injury and large-scale injury. Mechanisms of immediate, direct cell injury caused by freezing include protein and lipid stress; failure of cell metabolism; shifts in osmolality; formation of crystal ice, which disrupts organelles and membranes; cell shrinkage and expansion; thermomechanical shear stress; and recrystallization during thawing and membrane rupture. On the macroscopic level, delayed injuries occur secondary to vascular damage, microthrombi and tissue ischemia, and increased capillary permeability, which become apparent in tissue 4 to 10 days postsurgery.

The development of cryosurgery as a therapeutic technique, whose roots can be traced back to the 19th century [1], was significantly advanced in 1961 by Cooper and Lee by their introduction of an automated cryosurgical apparatus cooled by liquid nitrogen [2]. Their apparatus, which had controls that regulated the temperature of the freezing surface of its probe, was used to develop a vacuum-insulated, liquid nitrogen-cooled probe for brain surgery for the treatment of parkinsonism and other neuromuscular disorders involving the destruction of the basal ganglia [3].

Three distinct generations of prostate cryoablation may be outlined. Although some experimental work in renal cryosurgery was performed in the 1940s [4], the first real urologic applications of cryosurgery began in earnest in the 1960s, when Gonder et al. developed probes suitable for transurethral freezing of prostatic tissue for the relief of bladder outlet obstruction caused by benign prostatic hypertrophy and prostate cancer [5,6]. Using a vacuum-insulated probe shaped like a urethral sound, the prostate was frozen by direct contact through the prostatic urethra, with the surgeon's finger in the rectum as a rudimentary method of monitoring the freezing process and protecting the patient against rectal freezing. Transurethral cryosurgery was performed without the use of general or regional anesthesia, and appeared to be suitable for elderly and other high-risk patients. Early investigations emphasized possible delayed immunologic mechanisms, such as the development of antiprostate antibodies and postulated an associated clinical benefit, placing cryosurgery as an early foray into prostate immunotherapy [7]. The initial enthusiasm and experimentation with prostate cryosurgery was extended further by extensive use during the 1960s and 1970s with an open, transperineal [8,9] approach employed in order to eradicate prostate cancer. By 1975, a review describing the outcome of 154 prostate cancer patients treated by cryosurgery via the open perineal route between 1969 and 1974 was published [9] and later expanded to a series containing 229 cases [10]. The patients were staged clinically; most of these patients had bulky, locally extensive primary tumors, and one-half had disseminated disease. The authors treated these high-risk patients with a liquid nitrogen cryogenic unit using either a pointed or flat-ended probe. In some instances, tumors had to be cut through to expose the prostate, leaving tumors on the anterior rectal wall. Preliminary analysis suggested comparable survival rates for cryotherapy compared to other treatment modalities available at that time for localized prostate cancer. However, a 20-year follow-up for 51 patients, of whom 40 had Stage C disease, was recently presented by Porter et al., showing a 78% recurrence rate, median overall progression-free survival of only 34 months, and median overall survival of only 75 months [11].

Despite being viewed as a promising new method for killing cancer cells, the technical limitations of the equipment available at that time limited the ability to guide and control the freezing process, which often resulted in either inadequate cancer control or destruction of too much adjacent normal tissue. The experience with the first generation equipment and surgical techniques was ultimately judged to be a devastating failure, mostly due to the unacceptably high rate of local complications [6,11,12]. The high incidence of complications, which included urethral sloughing as well as a 14% rate of urethrorectal and urethrocutaneous fistulas, which often required diverting colostomy [9], delayed further developments in the field for three decades.

Second-Generation Prostate Cryoablation in the 1990s

Second-generation cryoablation was initiated in the United States during the early 1990s [13,14]. The improvement in the technology of cryogen delivery combined with the advances in medical imaging using transrectal ultrasound (TRUS) guidance, which assured accurate real-time control over the placement of cryoprobes and monitoring of ice ball formation [15,16]; percutaneous access capabilities; the use of urethral warming devices capable of adequate protection against urethral sloughing [17]; and the introduction and refinement in the use of prostate-specific antigen (PSA) since the late 1980s, which has led to a stage migration to earlier cancers as well as improved preoperative staging and patient selection, have paved the way for modern cryosurgical ablation of the prostate (CSAP). Using intraoperative ultrasound (US) to monitor the process of tissue freezing was first described by Onik et al. for cryosurgery of the liver and prostate [18]. The ultrasound image guided probe placement and provided a means to perform real-time monitoring of the freezing process.

The improved technique, improved efficacy, and decreased complication rates ultimately led to CSAP being accepted by both the American Urological Association (AUA) and the Health Care Financing Administration (HCFA) as an acceptable option for the management of localized prostate cancer. In 1993, the AUA published a position statement calling CSAP ''investigational,'' making it nearly impossible for providers and manufacturers to receive third-party payment. By 1996, the AUA had removed the experimental label from cryosurgery. However, the Technology Advisory Committee of HCFA ruled that the CSAP literature was lacking in standardized technique, randomized trials, studies with adequate controls groups, and short follow-up, and that the CSAP failed to provide direct comparison to other available treatments. Therefore, in 1996, HCFA adopted a policy of national noncoverage, which went into effect April, 1997 [19].

In 1999, HCFA performed a review of newer data, including pooled data from 5 institutions involving 975 patients treated between 1993 and 1998 [19,20]. This data suggested that for patients in low-, medium-, and high-risk groups, the five-year, biochemical-free survival (BFS) and negative biopsy rates after CSAP were comparable to matched outcomes reported after radiotherapy. The more recent data presented showed 5-year BFS exceeding 70% in some patient groups, and an overall negative biopsy rate of 82% [19,20]. Furthermore, the morbidity data actually showed lower rectal injury rates for CSAP than for radiotherapy, and very low urethral complication rates for patients treated with approved urethral warming catheters. Based on its review of this data, HCFA revised its coverage policy, calling CSAP a "safe and effective as well as medically appropriate" procedure for certain patient populations [19], making CSAP an alternative option to Medicare beneficiaries undergoing this procedure as primary therapy for clinically localized prostate cancer. Effective July 1, 2001, HCFA expanded the national coverage policy for CSAP to include salvage CSAP after radiation, stating that "salvage cryosurgery of the prostate is medically necessary and appropriate only for those patients with localized disease who have failed a trial of radiation therapy as their primary treatment, and meet one of the following conditions: stage T2b and below, Gleason less than 9, or PSA less than 8 ng/mL." Cryosurgery is currently not covered for salvage after failure of any other therapies.

State of the ART CSAP

Third generation prostate cryoablation using gas-driven probes was reported in 2000 [21,22]. Third generation cryosurgery marks the transition from systems circulating liquid nitrogen to gas-driven probes utilizing the Joule-Thompson effect in which pressurized gas is permitted to depressurize through a narrow nozzle located at the tip of the probe (Figure 1). In accordance with the gas coefficient and the dimension of the nozzle, different gaseous elements generate

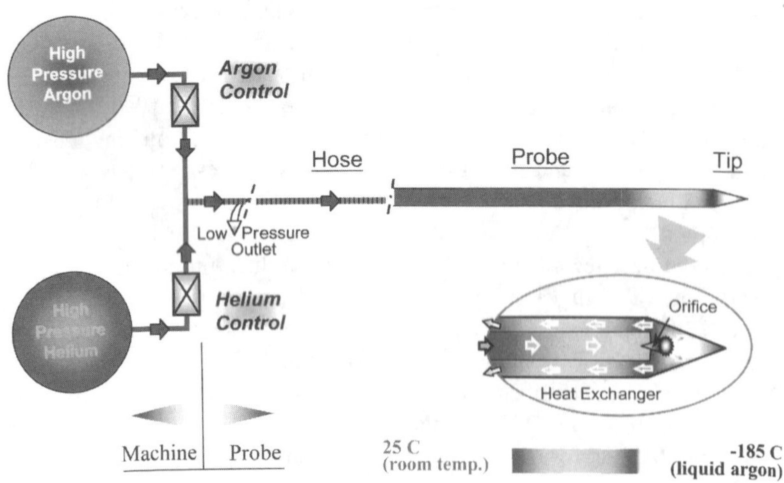

FIGURE 1   Probe design based on the Joule-Thompson effect. High pressurized gas exiting through an orifice in the probe tip undergoes a change in pressure, which results in a change in temperature dictated by its gas coefficient.

different thermal exchange in the area close to the nozzle. The properties of argon make it useful for cooling to $-187°C$, whereas the properties of helium allow it to serve for heating/thawing (defrosting at $+67°C$). Probe designs that permit the operator to select what gas flows through the probe tip at a given time from a selection of different gases with different gas coefficients, adds defrosting capability to the third generation systems, as well as the capability to abruptly transition between cooling and defrosting. Besides allowing this versatility, its main contribution was to permit a dramatic reduction in the diameter of cryoprobes. Use of third-generation, miniaturized equipment was first reported in March 2000 [22]. Ultra-thin probes with sharp tips became feasible, allowing direct transperineal penetration and placement without the necessity of an insertion kit. The small diameter probes enable a change in the technique in which cryoprobes are inserted. The free-hand and operator-dependent probe placement technique using cumbersome insertion kits employed in second-generation procedures, as well as procedures using large diameter third-generation equipment, gave way to a standardized procedure in which the probes can be inserted through a conventional brachytherapy template.

CSAP: MORBIDITY AND COMPLICATIONS

The risks of cryosurgery include the risks of 1–2 hour general anesthesia and the risks associated with cryosurgery itself. Most risks associated with cryosurgery are local and usually are not associated with systemic toxicity. Cryosurgery complications have to be discussed and understood within the same context as the historical perspective that was provided in the introduction. Like the development in cryosurgical technologies, cryosurgical complications can also be assessed as a reflection of the era in which the procedures were performed. Cryosurgery without imaging control in the pre-PSA era, when patient selection was lacking in the 1960s and 1970s, resulted in a very high complication rate. Although good tissue destruction was achieved, this procedure was abandoned for two decades.

In the early 1990s, the use of this procedure was revived mainly because TRUS monitoring was feasible. The era of "modern" prostate cryosurgery is divided into two periods, at least as far as complications are concerned. The first series of modern cryosurgery were performed without an urethral warmer. Although this did not result in the devastating complications as those seen in the early 1960s, a wide array of quite prevalent complications were still noted (i.e., 38% tissue sloughing without a urethral warmer versus 10% tissue sloughing with the use of a urethral warmer) [23]. After the FDA approval of urethral warmers, complications have become rarer and milder, leading to high patient satisfaction: 96% of the patients report that they will choose cryosurgery as treatment option again [24], and 83% of the patients reported no complications at all [25]. The decreasing trend in complication rates as a function of time is illustrated in Table 1, which lists major complications reported by CSAP studies from 1993

TABLE 1 Comparison of the reported complications of CSAP arranged chronologically. Results given in percentages

Reference	Onik, (13)	Miller, (28)	Wieder, (45)	Bahn, (46)	Cox, (47)	Shinohara, (48)	Sosa, (23)	Long, (25)	Badalament, (24)	Zisman, (44)
Year	1993	1994	1995	1995	1995	1996	1996	1998	1999	2001
# of pts.	55	62	79	210	63	65	1467	127	290	69
Fistula	4	0	0	2	3	2	1.4	0	0.4	0
Tissue sloughing	5	1	4		19		10	6	10	1.4
Incontinence		3	3	9	27	2	11	2	4.3	4.4 (SUI)
Pelvic pain				2	11		9.4		12	1.4
Urinary retention		2	10	3	29	17	6.8	12		1.4 (transient obstruction)
Impotence	64			41		86	100		85	67
UTI/sepsis					−/3	20/−	9.1/2.3	2.3/0.8		−/0

to 2001. The extent and severity of complications with CSAP has become clearer: 4.3% mild incontinence, 85% erectile dysfunction in previously potent patients, 0.4% urethrorectal fistulae, and 10% bladder outlet obstruction leading to secondary intervention. Complication rates are comparable with those reported for radical retropubic prostatectomy and radiotherapy [24]. The concern raised by the systemic complication which has been termed the cryoshock syndrome was recently addressed by Seifert et al., who reported only 2 cases out of 5432 subjects (0.04%) who had undergone CSAP in 62 centers [26]. A low rate of other, various complications have also been reported, including bladder neck contracture, 0.8%; urethral stricture, 0.8%; epididymitis, 1.6%; penile numbness, 1.6%; and perirectal abscess, 0.8% [25]. An increased complication rate is reported for salvage cryosurgery done in patients failing radiotherapy [25]: incontinence, 73% (no control, 21%; dribbling, 52%; but only 30% use more then 3 pads per day), obstructive symptoms, 67%; and impotence, 72% [27].

PATIENT SELECTION

Candidates for cryotherapy include patients with histologically confirmed adenocarcinoma of the prostate, clinical stage T1-2, a prostate volume $\leq$40mL, serum PSA $\leq$15ng/mL, and who accept the possibility of postoperative erectile dysfunction. Patients with a PSA >15 ng/mL, but with a negative pelvic lymph node dissection and negative metastatic work-up are also considered candidates. Traditionally, cryoablation has been advocated as being able to eradicate locally advanced disease (small T3) by extending freezing laterally [28]. However, as for any treatment involving locally advanced disease, there is a higher risk of both local and distant failure. Candidates for salvage cryotherapy are similar to those who are eligible for salvage prostatectomy [29,30], and include those with biopsy-proven local recurrence 18m or more postradiation and whose imaging studies and PSA velocity profile are compatible with local failure [31] in the absence of evidence of distant metastasis. Patients who are at high-risk for complications or failure include those who underwent a previous transurethral resection of the prostate (TURP), as this is a group that has been reported to have an increased rate of stress urinary incontinence [32] following cryotherapy. We believe that previous TURP should not be an absolute contraindication for cryosurgery, but we advocate that performers would approach these patients cautiously until they are confident and experienced with the procedure. Radiation failures who have undergone prior TURP should not be considered candidates for cryotherapy unless they are willing to accept the significant risk of total urinary incontinence. Patients with extensive local or systemic disease, those with a diagnosis of transitional cell carcinoma (TCC), incontinence, positive urine culture, permanent urethral catheter, prior fistula formation due to inflammatory bowel disease, previous pelvic surgery or trauma, or uncorrectable clotting defects are usually not considered candidates.

RESULTS OF PRIMARY CSAP

During the past 5 years, a number of reports have been published detailing the results of TRUS guided CSAP as primary treatment for men with prostate cancer. As noted by HCFA, many of these studies have not been randomized—patient selection criteria vary as do the definitions of treatment outcome and, therefore, cure rates. Despite these limitations, it is worthwhile to review the results of a number of these studies to gain some insight into the efficacy and morbidity of modern CSAP.

Investigators at the University of California, San Francisco, published the results of 207 cryosurgical procedures on 176 patients treated between 1993 and 1998, the majority of whom were followed-up for two or more years [33]. Over 60% of these patients had clinically advanced stages, the mean preoperative PSA was over 18 ng/mL and 20% had Gleason scores of 8 or greater. Cryosurgery treatment success was defined as a PSA nadir of less than 0.5 ng/mL, which did not increase by more than 0.2 ng/mL on two consecutive occasions. Using these definitions, 70% of patients reached the defined PSA nadir, of which 43% failed to have an increase. Patients with T1/T2 disease, PSA less than or equal to 10 preoperatively, and Gleason Score less than or equal to 7, and those achieving an undetectable PSA after CSAP had improved outcomes. The majority of patients underwent post-CSAP prostate biopsy, which were positive in 36% of patients. In this series of generally high-risk patients, only 12% were defined as low-risk (PSA less than 10, clinically localized, and Gleason 6 or less). Low-risk patients achieved a 69% rate of BFS at 3 years following CSAP.

Long et al [34] presented the results of 145 consecutive patients with clinical stages of T1a to T3c with a mean and minimum follow-up of 36 and 12 months treated after January 1993. Overall actuarial rate of maintaining a PSA less than 0.3 ng/mL was 59%. The overall actuarial progression free rate at 60 months was 56%. 160 biopsies were performed post-CSAP, of which only 16% showed residual cancer. No significant morbidity was encountered in 85% of patients who had not received radiation prior to CSAP.

The most satisfying data is that which was also published by Long et al [20], which presents the pooled analysis that was presented to HCFA resulting in the current national coverage policy for CSAP as primary therapy for prostate cancer. The strength of this analysis stems from its numbers, intermediate length follow-up, and analysis, which stratified patient-selection criteria and used uniform definitions of cancer-related outcomes. The authors used these standardized definitions to compare the results of CSAP to the results of radiotherapy in similarly risk-stratified patients. A total of 975 patients were analyzed who had undergone CSAP as primary therapy from 1993 to 1998 at five institutions (New England Medical Center, University of California at San Francisco, Urologic Institute of New Orleans, Crittenton Hospital, and Alhambra Hospital). Patients with clinical stage T1 to T4, any PSA level, and any Gleason score were included. Patients with metastatic disease at the time of treatment and those who had received previous radiotherapy were excluded. Patients receiving androgen deprivation therapy preoperatively were considered separately, and median follow-up for the entire group was 24 months.

5-year BFS rates for low-risk patients undergoing CSAP were 76% and 60% using a PSA cut off of less than 1 ng/mL and 0.5 ng/mL, respectively. These results were compared to 5-year BFS rates for low-risk patients undergoing brachytherapy and conformal radiotherapy, which ranged from 67% to 87%. For patients in medium and high-risk categories, 5-year BFS rates ranged from 71% to 36% after CSAP, compared to 58% to 0% following brachytherapy, and 65% to 15% following conformal radiotherapy. Posttreatment positive biopsy rates ranged from 12% to 24% following cryotherapy, from 22% to 26% following brachytherapy, and from 43% to 62% following conformal radiotherapy. A comparison between reported morbidities after radiotherapy and cryoablation, including incontinence, impotence, fistula formation and necessity for postprocedure TURP, demonstrated lower rates of rectal problems after CSAP but higher rates of potency after radiotherapy. Significantly, the use of nonapproved urethral warming devices during CSAP was associated with much higher rates of urethral sloughing, incontinence, and rectal fistulas.

RESULTS OF SALVAGE CSAP

Effective July 1, 2001, HCFA expanded the national coverage policy for CSAP to include salvage CSAP after radiation. The radiation oncology literature suggests that local-recurrence rates as high as 56% may be expected 15 years following radiotherapy [35]. An increasing PSA value after radiation therapy has become the most commonly seen evidence of inadequate local control [36], and at least three quarters of these men will have clinical relapse within 5 years after an increasing PSA is noted [37]. Treatment options for men failing radiation therapy are limited, but include hormonal ablation, salvage radical prostatectomy, salvage cryotherapy, and experimental therapies. Long-term hormone deprivation has a number of associated morbidities, including decreased muscle mass and osteoporosis, and, as with following radical prostatectomy, no good data exists to show improved survival for early- versus late-androgen deprivation following radiation failure. Salvage prostatectomy is a technically challenging operation that is associated with high rates of complications, including severe incontinence and rectal injuries occurring in as many as 15% of patients [29,30]. These grim statistics have spurred studies investigating the efficacy and morbidity of salvage cryotherapy after radiation.

Salvage cryotherapy has been reported to be more technically challenging than primary cryotherapy. A number of good studies have been published with intermediate follow-up that give us a good general picture of what can be expected following salvage cryotherapy, and what patients may be considered the best candidates. Chin et al. presented the results of 118 patients treated with CSAP after biopsy-proven local recurrence [38]. Of 118 patients with a median follow-up of 19 months, 114 had serum PSA nadir less than 0.5 ng/mL. There was an 87% rate of freedom from post–cryohistological failure and 34% freedom from biochemical failure using a stringent 0.5 ng/mL cut off. Predictors of worse outcomes included PSA greater than 10 ng/mL prior to CSAP, Gleason score of 8 or greater before radiotherapy, and advance-stage disease. Glands with volumes greater than 40 cc had higher postoperative PSA, suggesting an upper limit to what can be adequately frozen. Serious complications, including rectourethral fistulas, were seen in 3.3%, and severe incontinence in 6.7%. Predictors of complications included high-volume disease and a prior TURP procedure.

One of the largest experiences to date comes from the University of Texas M.D. Anderson Center where 145 patients were treated between 1992 and 1995 [39,40]. Patients with a pre-CSAP PSA less than 10 ng/mL and Gleason score of less than or equal to 8 achieved better results, with 2-year actuarial disease-free survival rates as high as 74%. Post-CSAP biopsies were positive in 21%, where number of probes used and post-CSAP PSA nadir were variables that predicted positive biopsies in a multivariate analysis. The negative biopsy rate using a 3-probe technique was 62%, compared to 89% using a 5-probe technique [40]. Although some have recently pointed out that urethral warmers have a theoretical risk of sparing cancer close to the urethra [41], no difference in biopsy positivity was observed associated with the use of a urethral warmer in this series of patients. De la Taille has published the Columbia University experience for 43 patients and describes a 66% biochemical recurrence-free rate defined as less than 0.1 ng/mL at 12 months [42]. They describe a 9% post-CSAP incontinence rate and a 5% obstruction rate, but no patients developed rectal fistulas.

Taken as a whole, salvage CSAP after radiation failure is a viable option than can impact local tumor control with the expectation of some morbidity. Treatment failure seen in patients with high-grade, locally advanced disease may be secondary to clinical under-staging and the presence of occult metastases [43]. Patients with a 10-year life expectancy, clinically organ-confined disease, and a PSA less than 10 ng/mL appear to be better candidates. The use of multiple probes may improve freedom from treatment failure. Detectable PSA after salvage CSAP is a strong predictor of treatment failure.

UCLA PROSTATE CRYOSURGICAL ABLATION TECHNIQUE

At UCLA, we have had a broad experience with prostate cryotherapy, using both second- and third-generation cryo-machines. Traditionally, CSAP has been performed using an insertion kit that enables the surgeon to use Seldinger's principle in a multistep fashion in order to place the freezing probes, which have a typical diameter of 3 mm (9.4F), into the prostate. Even for the experienced cryosurgeon, use of these large diameter probes poses some difficulties: placement is time consuming and trauma to surrounding tissues, to some extent, is inevitable. In the classical technique, an 18G echogenic needle is inserted transperineally into the chosen location of the prostate. A 0.038-inch encoring hooked guide wire is inserted through the needle and then the needle is withdrawn. Dilation is performed up to 10F and a specially designed sleeve is inserted over the dilator. The guide wire and the dilator are withdrawn and the cryoprobe is introduced through the sleeve. The sleeve is then pulled back by 2–3 cm and the probe is fixed to the tissue by low-intensity freezing. The same sequence is performed repeatedly until all of the probes are fixed in position and ready to be engaged. Inaccurate positioning or malfunction in each of the 6 steps involved in probe placement may occur. We have recently changed to a new, modified technique that is based on using 17G cryoneedles, instead of the larger diameter cryoprobes, which can be directly inserted into the prostate through a matrix template as in brachytherapy without the need for an insertion kit. It has been our experience that the newer equipment and techniques have reduced patient morbidity and side effects. However, as with any surgical procedure, good results may be more frequently obtained when the technique is standardized. Currently, an ongoing multi-institutional study of third-generation cryosurgical ablation of the prostate is underway, which will hopefully contribute to the development of a standardized surgical approach.

EQUIPMENT

At the present time, there are a number of companies manufacturing equipment suitable for prostate cryotherapy. This list includes Endocare, Cryomedical Sciences (CMS), and Oncura Medical. At UCLA, we recently have adopted the Galil system, which utilizes the third-generation, 17-gauge cryoprobes that can be placed transperineally through a brachytherapy template under TRUS guidance. The Seed-Net system allows groups of up to 5 probes to be bound together into 6 different channels, each of which can be operated independently, enabling freezing and active thawing to be performed in different sectors of the prostate at the same time.

Set Up

General or regional anesthesia is used. Patients are placed in the lithotomy position with careful cushioning. The perineum is placed on the edge of the operating table, 90° to the theater floor, in order to permit access to the US probe-holding device and template (Figure 2). The scrotum is fixed superiorly using 2 stay sutures, and a 16F Foley catheter is inserted.

Prostate Alignment with US Image, Aiming Grid and Insertion Template

A multifrequency biplanar US probe is attached into the holding device adapting cradle, commonly used for brachytherapy. The prostate is imaged and its dimen-

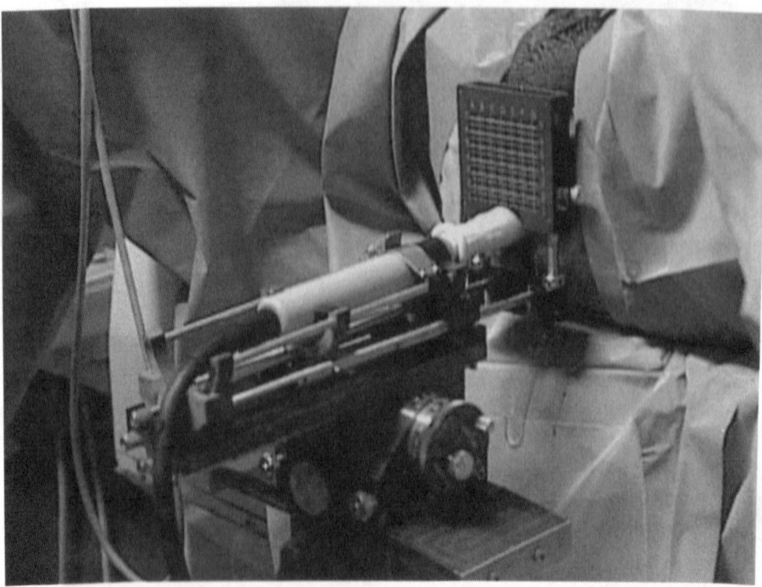

Figure 2 Set-up for CSAP using a brachytherapy stepping device, biplanar transrectal ultrasound probe, and brachytherapy template.

sions measured. The aiming grid software that most modern US machines contain is activated and projected onto the US image of the prostate. The attached probe is lowered posteriorly until slight resistance from the posterior rectal wall is felt or the image of the shiny anterior fibromuscular stroma is lost at 5 MHz. This maneuver opens up the distance between the prostate gland and the rectum, providing a greater safety margin to prevent ischemia of the rectal wall during freezing. A brachytherapy template drilled with a matrix of 85 17-gauge holes is attached to the holding device (Figure 2) and gently fixed against the perineum. The holes in the template are 5 mm apart and correspond to the aiming grid projected on the US image.

Cryoprobe Placement and Insertion

Probe planning and placement is based on the cryobiology of the 17-gauge probe, which produces an ice ball geometry in which a 9 mm radius is achieved at 5 minutes of continuous freezing, and a 13 mm radius at 10 minutes of continuous freezing. The lethal $-20°C$ isotherm is located at a corresponding radius of 7 mm and 10 mm respectively. The 1.5 mm 17-gauge probe creates an ice ball with a length of 27 mm, which begins 5 mm distal to the tip of the probe. The leading edge of the ice ball that is seen on ultrasound, which achieves a freezing temperature of only 0°C, is only 2–3 mm beyond the −20°C zone, making a small difference between the leading edge on ultrasound and the lethal zone. The placement of each probe and the necessity of performing a "pull back" maneuver are estimated based on these characteristics, and spacing the probes at 10 mm intervals generates one large ice ball created by the confluence of each individual, overlapping ice ball. Probes are inserted into desired the loci identified by coordinates on the aiming grid projected on the prostate US image. The actual probes are then inserted through the corresponding holes in the template bearing the same coordinates.

Number of Probes

Up to 30 simultaneously active probes in 6 distinct groups may be employed. Dependent on the prostate size, 84% of the glands may be covered with 10–15 probes (most commonly 12–13), 5% with ≤10 and 11% with 16–17 probes. Cryoprobes are inserted in 3 (prostate height ≤3.5 cm) or 4 (h≥3.5 cm) horizontal rows, 1 cm apart. Each row groups 2–5 probes according to prostate width. Typical configurations employ 2–4 probes in the most anterior row, 4–5 in the posterior row, and almost always 4 probes in the middle rows (Figure 3). Since

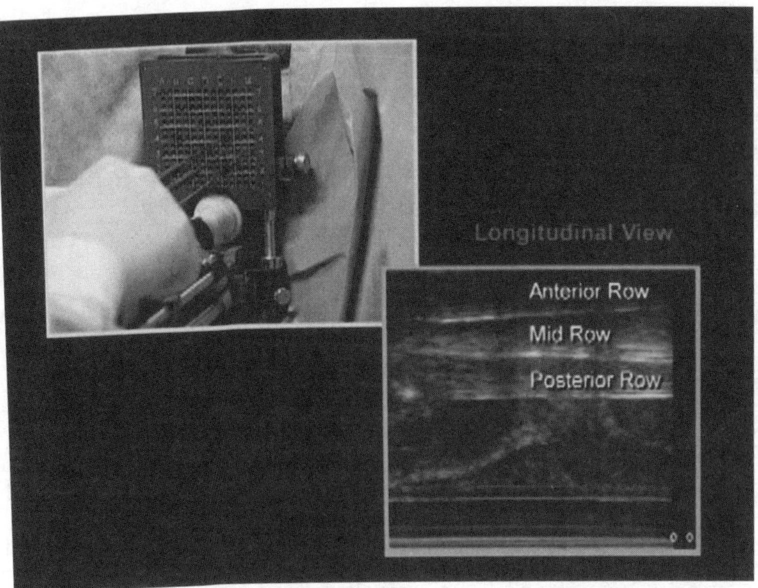

FIGURE 3 Probes are grouped and inserted in a varying number of rows necessary to cover the entire prostate. Lower right inset: probes can be monitored in the sagittal view to position probes up to the base of the prostate.

the ice balls progress longitudinally 5 mm past the probe tip, the probes are advanced into the prostate base and positioned 5–6 mm caudal to the bladder neck. The most posterior row is ideally located 7–8 mm anterior to the prostate capsule (Figure 3). Given the propensity of prostate cancer to invade laterally through the lymphatic spaces and neurovascular branches, we advocate lateral probe placement permitting extraprostatic freezing as well as facilitating killing by early shut down of the arterial supply to the gland. Identification of the entire urethra both in the longitudinal and transverse views is crucial, and may be facilitated by placement of a guidewire or Foley catheter. Each cryoprobe should be placed 8–9 mm away from the urethra. The only probe permitted in the same sagittal plane as the urethra is the middle probe of the posterior row when an odd number of probes is used (usually 3 or 5).

Flexible Cystoscopy, Suprapubic Catheter Placement, and Urethral Warmer Insertion

After all probes are placed, the Foley catheter is gently removed. Any difficulty with catheter removal may indicate that the probes have been wrongly positioned and may traverse the urethral wall. A meticulous 360° examination of the urethra is performed using a flexible cystoscope. In case a misplaced probe is visualized

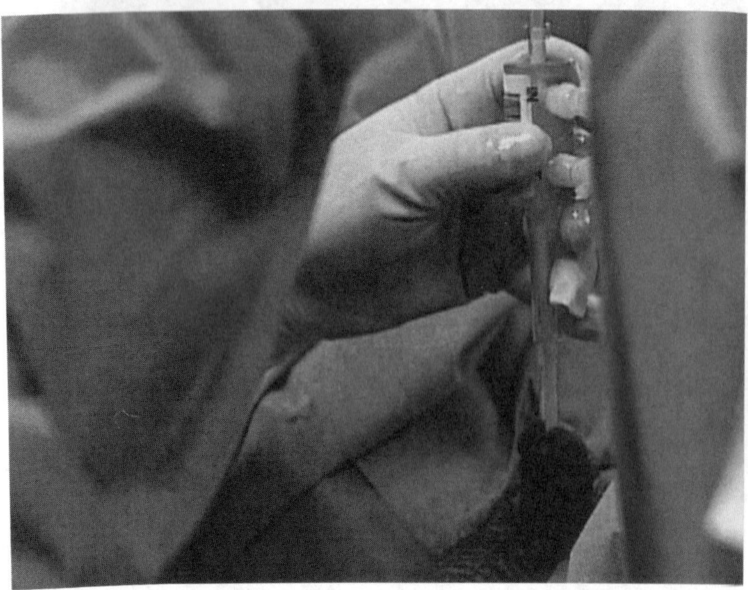

FIGURE 4   The urethral warmer is inserted, having inflow and outflow tracts to rapidly circulate saline warmed to 40 degrees.

in the urethra, it is critical to remove and revise the probe positioning in order to avoid direct urethral freezing or freezing of the circulating urethral warmer fluid. Once the urethra is confirmed to be normal, the bladder is examined and a soft 10–12F suprapubic (SP) catheter may be inserted under vision, closed, and secured to the skin. Some operators do not insert a SP tube, but conclude the procedure with a 16F Foley catheter left indwelling for 24–48 hours. A 0.38 guidewire is inserted through the working channel of the flexible cystoscope, over which the heavily lubricated urethral warming catheter is introduced into the bladder (Figure 4). During the procedure, the bladder is kept near full in order to prevent injury from the rigid tip of the warmer device.

Freezing

The ice ball is anechoic on US, as the sound waves bounce back from, instead of passing through, the ice (Figure 5). Since the US probe is in the rectum, starting to freeze in the posterior row would obliterate visualization of any prostate tissue anterior to the ice ball. In order to maintain US visibility, freezing is instead started with the anterior row of probes and continued posteriorly, preserving good

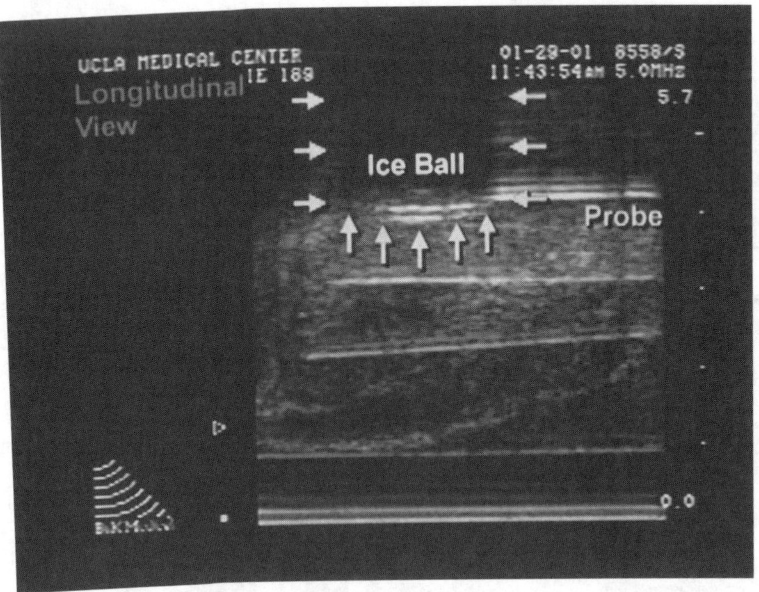

FIGURE 5   The anechoic ice ball is beginning to form as the anterior probes are activated. The leading edge of the ice ball is hyperechoic due to the ice-tissue interface.

US imaging posteriorly where visability is crucial to avoiding rectal injuries. Any uncovered area will be evident at this stage and corrected.

Two cycles of freezing and thawing are advocated. Between cycles, the prostate may be allowed to thaw and regain visibility passively ($\sim$15–20 minutes) or actively ($\sim$7–8 minutes) using helium. In glands longer than the 27 mm long ice-balls, a "pull back" procedure is indicated and employed in order to adequately freeze the zone of apical tissue (Figure 6). Using US, the distance from the apex of the prostate to the distal edge of the ice ball can be measured, and the probes pulled back a corresponding distance. Two additional freeze/thaw cycles are performed at the apex while the base passively thaws. Caution should be paid when freezing the apical tissue, particularly for salvage cryosurgical procedures, since too distal a pullback may damage the external urethral sphincter and compromise continence.

Many surgeons feel that the urethral warming catheter should be left in place until the entire gland is fully thawed. The gland is fully thawed when a full US image of the prostate is regained and no ice balls are seen. In glands up to 40 mL, this image may be reached within 15 minutes of passive thawing. Once the entire prostate has been completely thawed, the warmer catheter is gently removed and the SP tube is opened or, alternatively, the Foley catheter is reinserted over the guidewire and left to gravity drainage.

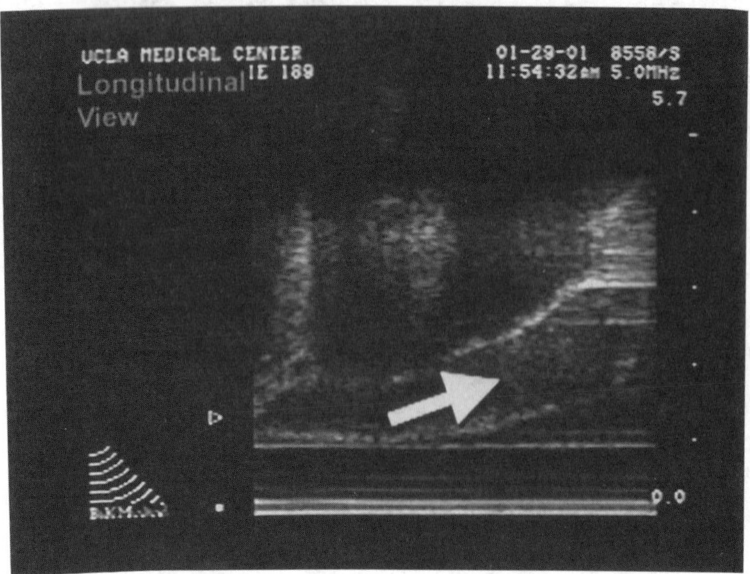

FIGURE 6 a   In glands longer than 27 mm, a rim of apical tissue (arrow) remains unfrozen.

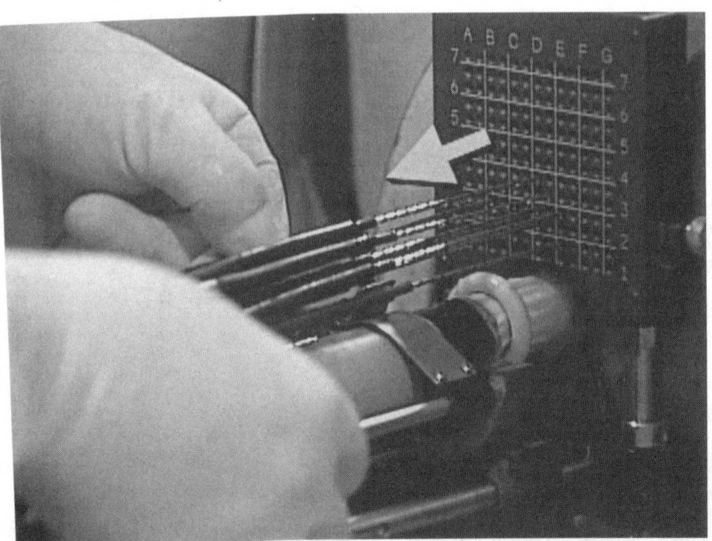

FIGURE 6 b   Using 5 mm graduated marks, the cryoprobes are pulled back to the corresponding distance measured on ultrasound (US) to freeze the apex.

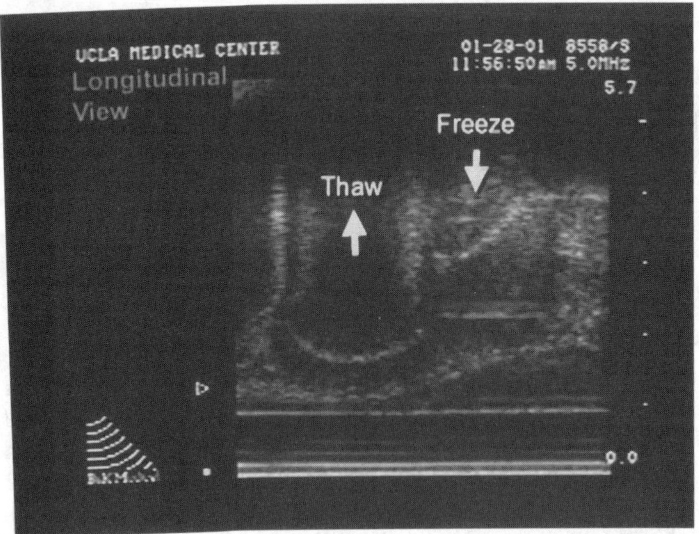

FIGURE 6 c   After pull back, the base ice ball is passively thawing upwards while the apical ice ball is freezing down from anterior to posterior, forming the "double belly" sign.

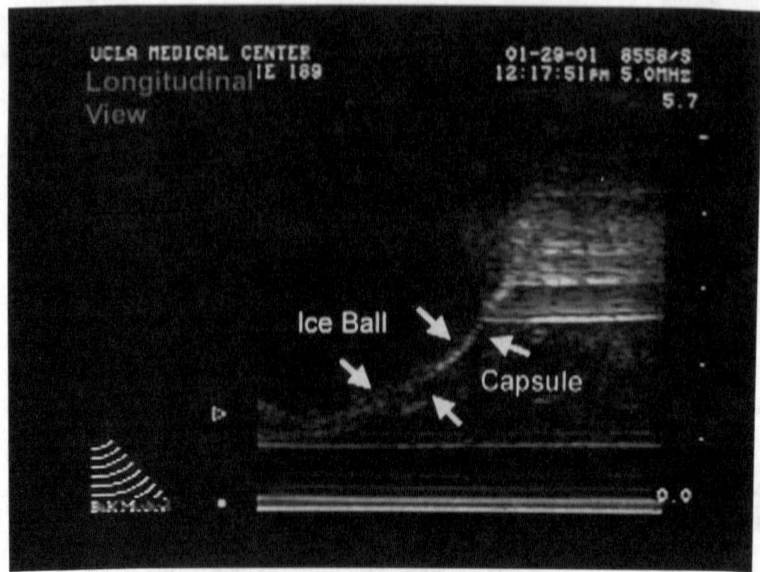

FIGURE 6 d At the conclusion of the apical freeze, no prostate tissue can be seen within the limits of Denonvilliers' fascia, the external sphincter, and the rectourethralis muscle.

Postoperative Care

Patients are discharged home on the same day or on post operation day 1 (POD1). The SP catheter is kept open for 72 hours and then closed for a voiding trial. Patients document urinary and postvoid volumes, and, once normal voiding is regained, the SP catheter is removed.

THIRD GENERATION CSAP: PRELIMINARY RESULTS

Between 1999 and 2000, 69 patients underwent prostate cryoablation using the SeedNet approach in the United States (110 worldwide) [44]. In 43% and 21% of the patients, 3m and 6m follow-up (f/u) PSA is available, respectively. 52% had undetectable PSA and 30% had PSA of less then 0.3 ng/mL. 71% of patients with clinical stage T1c disease had undetectable PSA, and the remaining 2 patients had a PSA less than 0.3 ng/mL. Of 3 patients who had clinical T3 disease, only 1 achieved a 3 m PSA of under 0.3. Thirteen patients had Gleason's score $\geq$7. At 3 m, 7 patients had undetectable PSA and 3 patients had PSA $\leq$0.3. In patients with organ confined disease, no difference in chemical control at 3 m was observed between those with low and high ($\geq$7) Gleason score. No cases of urinary fistula occurred, including 10 cases of salvage cryoablation post-(radiotherapy)XRT. Complications were reported in 6 patients (9%), who were all primary cases who did not undergo XRT, TURP or prior cryoablation: 3 patients had mild stress urinary incontinence (SUI), one had sloughing of the urethra, one had prolonged pelvic pain, and one was noted as having transient obstruction. No secondary intervention was required for any of these patients. Impotence occurred in the majority of patients (67%) who were preoperatively potent.

CONCLUSIONS

Many aspects of the management of prostate cancer remain controversial, and it is difficult to reach a consensus regarding the optimal treatment for clinically localized or locally advanced disease. Prospective, randomized trials comparing different treatment modalities are entirely lacking. Technical improvements in cryotechnology, real-time imaging, urethral warming devices, and preoperative staging have improved efficacy and morbidity results for cryosurgical ablation of the prostate for patients undergoing both primary and salvage therapy. Pre-CSAP patient selection criteria and indicators of post-CSAP outcome success are becoming clearer. The cumulative experience, which is still without sufficient long-term data, supports the notion that CSAP produces favorable results that are similar to risk-matched patients undergoing other forms of therapy for prostate cancer. We have detailed the special features of minimally invasive, third-generation cryogenic equipment based on the Joule-Thompson principal, and the modification in the surgical techniques that are entailed. The preliminary impression is that the new approach generates fewer side effects than those side effects published for second-generation procedures. The final judgement on CSAP is pending. Until then, it remains as one alternative in the management of select patients.

REFERENCES

1. Gage AA. History of cryosurgery. Seminars in Surgical Oncology 1998; 14:99–109.
2. Cooper IS, Lee A. Cryostatic congelation: a system for producing a limited controlled region of cooling or freezing of biologic tissues. J Nerv Ment Dis 1961; 133:259–263.
3. Cooper IS. Cryogenic surgery of the basal ganglia. JAMA 1962; 181:600.
4. Haas GM, Taylor CB. A quantitative hypothermal method for the production of local tissue injury. Arch Pathol 1948; 45:563–580.
5. Gonder MJ, Soanes WA, Smith V. Experimental prostate cryosurgery. Investigative Urology 1964; 1:610–619.
6. Gonder MJ, Soanes WA, Shulman S. Cryosurgical treatment of the prostate. Investigative Urology 1966; 3(4):372–378.
7. Gonder MJ. Cryosurgery in prostate carcinoma: clinical evidence of immunostimulation of host versus tumor. National Cancer Institute Monographs 1978; 49:369.
8. Loening S, Hawtrey C, Bonney W, Narayana A, Culp DA. Cryotherapy of prostate cancer. Prostate 1980; 1(3):279–286.

9. O'Donoghue EP, Milleman LA, Flocks RH, Culp DA, Bonney WW. Cryosurgery for carcioma of prostate. Urology 1975; 05(3):308–316.

10. Bonney W, Fallon B, Gerber W, Hawtrey C, Loening SA, Narayana A, Platz CE, Rose EF, Sail JC, Schmidt JD, Culp DA. Cryosurgery in prostatic cancer: survival. Urology 1982; 19(1):37–42.

11. Porter MP, Ahaghotu CA, Loening SA, See WA. Disease-free and overall survival after cryosurgical monotherapy for clinical stages B and C carcinoma of the prostate: a 20-year followup. Journal of Urology 1997; 158(4):1466–1469.

12. Loening SA, Bonney WW, Fallon B, Gerber WL, Hawtrey CE, Lubaroff DM, Narayana AS, Culp DA. Cryotherapy. Prostate 1984; 5(2):199–204.

13. Onik GM, Cohen JK, Reyes GD, Rubinsky B, Chang Z, Baust J. Transrectal ultrasound-guided percutaneous radical cryosurgical ablation of the prostate. Cancer 1993; 72(4):1291–1299.

14. Lee F, Bahn DK, McHugh TA, Onik GM, Lee FT. US-guided percutaneous cryoablation of prostate cancer. Radiology 1994; 192(3):769–776.

15. Roobottom CA, Jurriaans E, Lanigan D, Dubbins PA, Choa G. Endosonographic monitoring of transurethral cryoprostatectomy. Clinical Radiology 1993; 48(4): 241–243.

16. Littrup PJ, Mody A, Sparschu R, Prchevski P, Montie J, Zingas AP, Grianon D. Prostatic cryotherapy: ultrasonographic and pathologic correlation in the canine model. Urology 1994; 44(2):175–183; discussion 183–184.

17. Cohen JK, Miller RJ. Thermal protection of urethra during cryosurgery of prostate. Cryobiology 1994; 31(3):313–316.

18. Gilbert JC, Onik GM, Hoddick WK, Rubinsky B. Real time ultrasonic monitoring of hepatic cryosurgery. Cryobiology 1985; 22(4):319–330.

19. Whyte JJ, Bagley GP, Kang JL. The Health Care Financing Administration cryosurgery decision: a timely response to new data. Journal of Urology 1999; 162(4): 1386–1387.

20. Long JP, Bahn D, Lee F, Shinohara K, Chinn DO, Macaluso JN. Five-year retrospective, multi-institutional pooled analysis of cancer-related outcomes after cryosurgical ablation of the prostate. Urology 2001; 57(3):518–523.

21. de La Taille A, Benson MC, Bagiella E, Burchardt M, Shabsigh A, Olsson CA, Katz AC. Cryoablation for clinically localized prostate cancer using an argon-based system: complication rates and biochemical recurrence. 2000; 85(3):281–286.

22. Zisman A, Leibovici D, Siegel YI, Lindner A. Prostate cryoablation without an insertion kit using direct transperineal placement of ultrathin freezing probes. Techniques in Urology 2000; 6(1):34–36.

23. Sosa R, Martin T, Lynn K. Cryosurgical treatment of prostate cancer: a multicenter review of complications. Journal of Urology 1996; 155:361–368.

24. Badalament RA, Bahn DK, Kim H, Kumar A, Bahn JM, Lee F. Patient-reported complications after cryoablation therapy for prostate cancer. Urology 1999; 54(2): 295–300.

25. Long JP, Fallick ML, LaRock DR, Rand W. Preliminary outcomes following cryosurgical ablation of the prostate in patients with clinically localized prostate carcinoma. Journal of Urology 1998; 159(2):477–484.

26. Seifert JK, Morris DI. World survey on the complications of hepatic and prostate cryotherapy. World Journal of Surgery 1999; 23(2):109–113; discussion 113–114.

27. Pisters LL, von_Eschenbach AC, Scott SM, Swanson DA, Dinney CP, Pettaway CA, Babaian RJ. The efficacy and complications of salvage cryotherapy of the prostate. Journal of Urology 1997; 157(3):921–925.

28. Miller RJ, Cohen JK, Merlotti LA. Percutaneous transperineal cryosurgical ablation of the prostate for the primary treatment of clinical stage C adenocarcinoma of the prostate. Urology 1994; 44(2):170–174.

29. Lerner SE, Blute ML, Zincke H. Critical evaluation of salvage surgery for radio-recurrent/resistant prostate cancer. Journal of Urology 1995; 154(3):1103–1109.

30. Rogers E, Ohori M, Kassabian VS, Wheeler TM, Scardino PT. Salvage radical prostatectomy: outcome measured by serum prostate specific antigen levels. Journal of Urology 1995; 153(1):104–110.

31. Patel A, Dorey F, Franklin J, de Kernion JB. Recurrence patterns after radical retropubic prostatectomy: clinical usefulness of prostate specific antigen doubling times and log slope prostate specific antigen. Journal of Urology 1997; 158:1441–1445.

32. Saliken JC, Donnelly BJ, Brasher P, Ali Ridha N, Ernst S, Robinson J. Outcome and safety of transrectal US-guided percutaneous cryotherapy for localized prostate cancer. Journal of Vascular and Interventional Radiology 1999; 10(2 Pt 1):199–208.

33. Koppie TM, Shinohara K, Grossfeld GD, Presti JC, Carroll PR. The efficacy of cryosurgical ablation of prostate cancer: the University of California, San Francisco experience. Journal of Urology 1999; 162(2):427–432.

34. Long JP, Fallick ML, Rand W. Increased serum total creatine kinase and creatine kinase isoenzyme MB after cryosurgical ablation of the prostate. Journal of Urology 1997; 157(5):1723–1726.

35. Eastham JA, Kattan MW, Groshen S, Scardino PT, Rogers E, Carlton CE, Lerner SP. Fifteen-year survival and recurrence rates after radiotherapy for localized prostate cancer. Journal of Clinical Oncology 1997; 15(10):3214–3222.

36. Zagars GK, Pollack A, Kavadi VS. Prostate specific antigen and radiation therapy for clinically localized prostate cancer. Int J Radiat Oncol Biol Phys 1995; 32:293–306.

37. Lee FT, Mahvi DM, Chosy SG, Onik GM, Wong WS, Littrup PJ, Scanlon KA. Hepatic cryosurgery with intraoperative US guidance. Radiology 1997; 202(3):624–632.

38. Chin JL, Pautler SE, Mouraviev V, Touma N, Moore K, Downey DB. Results of salvage cryoablation of the prostate after radiation: identifying predictors of treatment failure and complications. Journal of Urology 2001; 165(6 Pt 1):1937–1941; discussion 1941–1942.

39. Pisters LL, Perrotte P, Scott SM, Greene GF, von Eschenbach AC. Patient selection for salvage cryotherapy for locally recurrent prostate cancer after radiation therapy. Journal of Clinical Oncology 1999; 17(8):2514–2520.

40. Izawa JI, Perrotte P, Greene GF, Scott S, Levy L, McGuire E, Madsen L, von Eschenbach AC, Pisiers LL. Local tumor control with salvage cryotherapy for locally recurrent prostate cancer after external beam radiotherapy. Journal of Urology 2001; 165(3):867–870.

41. Leibovich BC, Blute ML, Bostwick DG, Wilson TM, Pisansky TM, Davis BJ, Ramnani DM, Cheng L, Sabo TJ, Zincke H. Proximity of prostate cancer to the urethra: implications for minimally invasive ablative therapies. Urology 2000; 56(5):726–729.

42. de la Taille A, Hayek O, Benson MC, Bagiella E, Olsson CA, Fatal M, Katz AE. Salvage cryotherapy for recurrent prostate cancer after radiation therapy: the Columbia experience. Urology 2000; 55(1):79–84.

43. Catalona WJ. Management of cancer of the prostate. New England Journal of Medicine 1994; 331(15):996–1004.

44. Zisman A, Pantuck AJ, Cohen J, Belldegrun AS. Prostate cryoablation using direct transperineal placement of ultra-thin probes through a 17 gauge brachytherapy template-Technique and preliminary results. Urology 2001:In press.

45. Wieder J, Schmidt JD, Casola G, Sonnenberg E, Stainken BF, Parsons CL. Transrectal ultrasound-guided transperineal cryoablation in the treatment of prostate carcinoma: preliminary results. Journal of Urology 1995; 154(2 Pt 1):435–441.

46. Bahn DK, Lee F, Solomon MH, Gontina H, Klionsky DL, Lee FT. Prostate cancer: US-guided percutaneous cryoablation. Work in progress. Radiology 1995; 194(2): 551–556.

47. Cox RL, Crawford ED. Complications of cryosurgical ablation of the prostate to treat localized adenocarcinoma of the prostate. Urology 1995; 45(6):932–935.

48. Shinohara K, Connolly JA, Presti JC, Carroll PR. Cryosurgical treatment of localized prostate cancer (stages T1 to T4): preliminary results. Journal of Urology 1996; 156(1):115–120; discussion 120–121.

EDITORIAL COMMENTARY

Louis Pisters

Department of Urology, University of Texas MD Anderson Cancer Center, Houston, Texas, USA

As pointed out by Pantuck et al., cryotherapy now is substantially different from what it was in the early to mid-1990s, and is vastly different from its earliest history in the 1960s. New generation cryotherapy machines that are argon-based use small-caliber probes, which, unlike earlier machines, may not require dilation of a tract. The other main technological improvement has been the development of pinpoint size thermocouples that can accurately measure temperatures in critical areas such as around the membranous urethra, along the rectum, and in the neurovascular bundle region. The extensive use of these thermocouples in conjunction with effective urethral warming catheters has dramatically reduced cryotherapy-related treatment complications, particularly in the salvage setting after radiation therapy.

As currently practiced, primary cryotherapy bears striking similarity to prostate brachytherapy. Both procedures are minimally invasive techniques that can be performed in an outpatient setting with spinal or general anesthesia. Both procedures involve transrectal ultrasound-guided transperineal insertion of metal probes into the prostate. In the case of brachytherapy, the metal probes or needles introduce radioactive seeds, whereas in the case of cryotherapy, the probes induce thermal tissue damage. Both brachytherapy and cryotherapy may employ a grid system and computer software to tailor the treatment to the shape and size of the prostate gland. Furthermore, both cryotherapy and brachytherapy lack the 10- to 15-year long-term follow-up that radical prostatectomy and external beam radiation therapy have. The five- to seven-year biochemical results of primary cryotherapy and prostate brachytherapy are quite similar (although there are no randomized prospective studies directly comparing biochemical outcome). The complications of prostate brachytherapy and primary cryotherapy are also similar; both produce transient obstructive symptoms. Both prostate cryotherapy and brachytherapy have a low risk for urinary incontinence and both can adversely affect potency. In the case of prostate cryotherapy, thermocouples can be placed in the area of the neurovascular bundle to help preserve potency in patients with low-risk disease. Thus, primary cryotherapy and brachytherapy have similarities in technique, efficacy, and complications.

In fact, cryotherapy may have several advantages over brachytherapy. Cryotherapy can destroy a biologically heterogeneous population of cancer cells, including cell populations that are resistant to radiation therapy and hormonal therapy (androgen-independent cells). Prostate cryotherapy can be used to treat more extensive prostate cancers than prostate brachytherapy. In particular, the freezing process can be extended beyond the capsule of the prostate to potentially eradicate extracapsular disease in patients with T_3 cancers. Another advantage of cryotherapy is that it can to be repeated, whereas brachytherapy cannot. In general, I believe that a randomized prospective study of primary cryotherapy vs. brachytherapy for patients with low-risk prostate cancer would be an important trial; such a trial would be the only way to prove the superiority of one of these minimally invasive treatments over the other.

In the salvage setting after initial radiation therapy, cryotherapy can be safely performed provided that there is extensive thermocouple monitoring and an effective urethral warming catheter is used. Ghafar et al [1] reported their experience with salvage cryotherapy in 38 patients using the argon-based system. All patients received 3 months of hormonal therapy before salvage cryotherapy. This report demonstrated that when the argon-based system and careful thermocouple monitoring were used, salvage cryotherapy could be performed with a much lower rate of complications than in earlier series [2,3]. In particular, the incidence of incontinence was 8% in their series, which is much lower than the 60–95% rate reported in earlier series [2,3].

The overall effectiveness of salvage cryotherapy deserves close scrutiny. In particular, is salvage cryotherapy really as effective as salvage radical prostatectomy? The available evidence would suggest that it is difficult to ablate or completely eliminate all prostatic epithelium with cryotherapy. In a small study of neoadjuvant cryotherapy before radical prostatectomy, 4 of 7 patients had PT0 disease with no residual tumor in the radical prostatectomy specimen, suggesting that cryotherapy may cure some patients [2]. However, all patients had residual viable benign glands, emphasizing how difficult it is to destroy the entire prostatic epithelium [4].

We compared the biochemical outcome of patients who underwent salvage cryotherapy at M. D. Anderson Cancer Center compared with that of patients who underwent salvage radical prostatectomy at the Mayo Clinic [2]. This study was limited to patients with a presalvage PSA less than or equal to 10 ng/mL, a presalvage therapy Gleason grade of recurrent cancer of 8 or lower, and no hormonal therapy either before or after salvage local therapy. These criteria were designed to minimize bias between the two groups. Fifty-six prostatectomy patients and sixty cryotherapy patients fit the criteria for evaluation. None of the patients received androgen-deprivation therapy until postsalvage biochemical failure. Using the same definition of biochemical failure of two rises in prostate specific antigen above nadir for both groups, the five-year biochemical disease-free survival rate for salvage prostatectomy group was 66% compared to 41% for the salvage cryotherapy group (p = 0.0004). With longer follow-up, these differences became even more pronounced. Although there were not very many patients in either cohort beyond eight years, the seven-year biochemical disease-free survival rate for the salvage radical prostatectomy group remained favorable at 50% compared with only 19% for those who underwent salvage cryotherapy. With current follow-up, there were no differences in cause-specific survival noted between these two groups. In order to make the groups as comparable as possible, a Cox proportional hazards model was performed to adjust for presalvage Gleason score, clinical stage, and presalvage PSA levels. The Cox proportional hazards model confirmed superior biochemical disease-free survival for salvage radical prostatectomy compared with cryotherapy (p = 0.049). The relative risk of biochemical failure was 0.36 for patients undergoing salvage radical prostatectomy compared with salvage cryotherapy [5]. These results strongly suggest that salvage radical prostatectomy was superior to cryotherapy with respect to biochemical disease-free survival for patients with local recurrence after initial radiation therapy.

I believe that salvage prostatectomy and salvage cryotherapy is appropriate for different patient groups. In particular, younger healthy patients should consider salvage prostatectomy for cure. Older patients and those with comorbid conditions may wish to consider salvage cryotherapy. Although many patients who undergo salvage cryotherapy are not cured, it may improve local control and delay the initiation of long-term hormonal therapy and all its attendant side effects. Recent evidence indicates that when newer argon-based systems are used with extensive thermocouple monitoring, salvage cryotherapy can be performed quite safely.

REFERENCES

1. Ghafar MA, Johnson CW, DeLa Taille A, Benson MC, Bagiella E, Fatal M, Olsson CA, Katz AE. Salvage cryotherapy using an argon-based system for locally recurrent prostate cancer after radiation therapy. The Columbia Experience. J Urol 2001; 166: 1333–1338.

2. Pisters LL, von Eshenbach AC, Scott SM, Swanson DA, Dinney CP, Pettaway CA, Babaian RJ. The efficacy and complication of salvage cryotherapy of the prostate. J Urol 1997; 157:921.

3. Bales GT, Williams MJ, Sinner M. Short-term outcomes after cryosurgical ablation of the prostate in men with recurrent prostate carcinoma following radiation therapy. Urology 1995; 46:676.

4. Pisters LL, Dinney CP, Pettaway CA, Scott SM, Babaian RJ, von Eschenbach AC, Troncoso P. A feasibility study of cryotherapy followed by radical prostatectomy for locally advanced prostate cancer. J Urol 1999; 161:509.

5. Leibovich BC, Zinke H, Blute ML, Slezak JM, Izawa J, Madsen L, Scott S, von Eschenbach AC, Pisters LL. Recurrent prostate cancer after radiation therapy: salvage prostatectomy versus salvage cryosurgery. J Urol 2001; 165:389, abstract 1595.

EDITORIAL OVERVIEW

Kenneth B. Cummings

Cryosurgical ablation of the prostate (CSAP) is an evolving technique since its inception in the 1960s and 1970s with an open transperineal approach [1,2]. Pantuck and coworkers provide an excellent background and description of contemporary technique. A distinction needs to be made between primary CSAP and salvage CSAP.

Refinements in the technique of cryoablation with advances in medical imaging using transrectal ultrasound (TRUS) guidance and the assured accurate real-time control over placement of cryo probes and monitoring of the ice ball formation [3,4], percutaneous access capabilities, and the use of urethral warming devices [5] and improved patient selection have advanced the employment of CSAP as primary therapy with curative intent.

Based on a review of current data, Health Care Financing Administration (HCFA) revised its coverage policies calling CSAP "a safe and effective as well as medically appropriate" procedure for certain patients [6], making CSAP an alternative option to Medicare beneficiaries undergoing this procedure as primary therapy for clinically localized prostate cancer.

Effective July 1, 2001, HCFA expanded the national coverage policy of CSAP to include salvage CSAP after radiation, stating that "salvage cryosurgery of the prostate is medically necessary and appropriate only for those patients with localized disease who have failed a trial of radiation therapy as their primary treatment and who meet one of the following conditions: Stage T2b and below, Gleason < 9, or PSA < 8 ng/mL."

Pisters, in his editorial comment, points out that Pantuck's observation of cryotherapy in now is substantially different from what it was in its first and second iterations. As currently practiced, primary cryotherapy bears a striking similarity to prostate brachytherapy. Both procedures are minimally invasive techniques and can be performed in an outpatient setting under spinal or general anesthesia. Technically, both procedures employ transrectal ultrasound-guided perineal insertion of metal probes into the prostate, and, in the case of cryotherapy, the probes induce thermal tissue damage. Both brachytherapy and cryotherapy employ a grid system using computer software to tailor treatment to the shape and size of the prostate gland.

A problem with both procedures is that cryotherapy and brachytherapy lack the 10-year/15-year long-term follow-up that radical prostatectomy or external beam therapy have, and, as such, the results should be considered preliminary. Pisters believes that prostate cryotherapy can be used to treat more extensive prostate cancers than prostate brachytherapy is able to encompass. In particular, the freezing process can be extended beyond the capsule of the prostate to potentially eradicate extracapsular disease in patients with T3 disease.

It will be necessary for a randomized perspective trial comparing primary cryotherapy of the current generation vs. brachytherapy in patients who are at low risk to determine superiority of one of these minimally invasive treatments. Pisters further points out that, in the salvage setting, while initial results with cryoablation were accompanied by significant complications with urethral warming and appropriate patient selection, it can likely be safely performed in current generation [7].

REFERENCES

1. O'Donoghue EP, Milleman LA, Flocks RH, Culp DA, Bonney WW. Cryosurgery for carcinoma of prostate. Urology 1975; 05(3):308–316.

2. Bonney W, Fallon B, Gerber W, Hawtrey C, Loening S, Narayana A, Platz CE, Rose EF, Sail JC, Schmidt JD, Culp DA. Cryosurgery in prostatic cancer: survival. Urology 1982; 19(1):37–42.

3. Roobottom CA, Jurriaans E, Lanigan D, Dubbins PA, Choa G. Endosonographic monitoring of transurethral cryoprostatectomy. Clinical Radiology 1993; 48(4): 241–243.

4. Littrup PJ, Mody A, Sparschu R, Prchevski P, Montie J, Zingas AP, et al. Prostatic cryotherapy: ultrasonographic and pathologic correlation in the canine model. Urology 1994; 44(2):175–183; discussion 183–184.

5. Cohen JK, Miller RJ. Thermal protection of urethra during cryosurgery of prostate. Cryobiology 1994; 31(3):313–316.

6. Whyte JJ, Bagley GP, Kang JL. The health care financing administration cryosurgery decision: a timely response to new data. J Urol 1999; 162(4):1386–1387.

7. Ghafar MA, Johnson CW, DeLa Taille A, Benson MC, Bagiella E, Fatal M, Olsson CA, Katz AE. Salvage Cryotherapy using an argon-based system for locally recurrent prostate cancer after radiation therapy: the Columbia experience. J Urol 2001; 1666: 1333–1338.

9

Postprostatectomy Radiotherapy

Hari Siva Gurunadha Rao Tunuguntla, Suzanne Generao, and Ralph W. de Vere White
Department of Urology, University of California Davis, Sacramento, California, USA

INTRODUCTION

Prostate cancer is the most common cancer in American men, with 180,400 new cases and 31,400 deaths in the year 2001. Histological cancer is noted in the prostates of approximately 42% of men over 50 years of age who die of other causes.

Although prostate cancer is fatal in some patients, most men die *with* rather than *of* their cancer. While the lifetime risk that an American man will be diagnosed with prostate cancer is estimated to be about 11%, the risk of dying from the disease is only 3.6% [1,2]. Optimal management of this cancer requires assessment of cancer risk and side effects and complications of each treatment.

Approximately two-thirds of patients diagnosed with prostate cancer are treated with surgery or radiation. Recent advances in the technique of radical prostatectomy, along with an increase in diagnosis of clinically localized prostate cancer, have led to a progressive increase in the number of radical prostatectomies performed in the United States (54.6 out of 100,000) [3]. There is also a 3–4-fold increase in the number of radical prostatectomies for men 45 to 59, and 2–3-fold increase for those 60 to 69 years-old. Therefore, equal attention should be paid to the cure/disease-free survival and maintaining good quality of life in these relatively younger patients.

Selection of only T1 and T2 patients for radical prostatectomy (RP) results in a very low incidence of residual disease within the tumor bed and a high probability of cure. However, by current clinical and imaging criteria, it is not possible to exclusively select such patients, who are the best candidates for surgery with intent to cure. 30–60% of men undergoing RP are noted to have tumor penetration of the prostatic capsule or positive surgical margins, some of which are likely to relapse biochemically (50,000 men per year have "PSA-only progression") and/or locally [4–7]. Radiotherapy is the most commonly used form of adjuvant treatment in these patients.

CANCER CONTROL FOLLOWING RADICAL PROSTATECTOMY

Radiotherapy depends on the preoperative prostate-specific antigen (PSA) level, Gleason sum from the specimen, pathologic stage, and surgical margin status. While these are good predictors of the likelihood of failure of primary treatment, they are not known to reliably predict the risk of clinical recurrence or the growth rate/pattern of recurrence.

Residual disease is likely in present in the presence of extracapsular disease, positive margins, seminal vesicle/lymph node involvement, and/or poorly differentiated histology [8]. Failure of PSA to drop to undetectable levels within 6 weeks post-RP indicates micrometastases [9–15]. Overall, 30–40% of patients experience post-RP recurrence, and up to 75% of those with extensive extracapsular disease, positive margins, or seminal vesicle involvement have been reported to relapse within 5 years of surgery [10].

Anscher and Prosnitz attempted to segregate seminal vesicle involvement from the positive surgical margin and noted that seminal vesicle involvement is not an independent predictor for local failure, but it is the strongest predictor for distant metastasis [7].

FAILURE PATTERNS OF PROSTATE CANCER FOLLOWING RADICAL PROSTATECTOMY

Post-RP failure is 1 of 3 types: *local residue* of the primary tumor, *biochemical recurrence* ("PSA only progression"), and *clinical recurrence* (local recurrence or distant metastases). Palpable induration at the site of surgery with an elevated PSA or a positive biopsy of the prostatic fossa in the absence of positive chest radiograph, pelvic CT, and bone scan indicate local recurrence. Distant recurrence is defined as evidence of metastases by bone scan or CT with or without concurrent local disease.

"PSA-only Progression" (Biological Failure/Biochemical Recurrence) of Prostate Cancer

"PSA-only recurrence" is currently broadly defined as any elevation of PSA postoperatively after an initial drop to undetectable level. The incidence of biological failure is 2–3 times greater than clinical failure. An ultrasensitive PSA assay may be able to identify relapse 1 to 2 years earlier than the commonly used assay [4]. The median interval from PSA recurrence to cancer death is between 5 and 12 years, depending on the Gleason score.

Postradical Prostatectomy PSA Kinetics

The half-life of PSA is 2.6 days. Thus, the time taken for elimination of all pre-treatment PSA depends on the initial level.

Incidence & Timing of Biochemical Recurrence

Ten to 15% of patients have been reported to develop biochemical recurrence (follow-up, 3–6 years) (Table 1). Most patients have been noted to fail during the first year, whereas no failures have been reported after 6 years, which suggests that post-RP failure is due to clinical understaging [14]. On the other hand, the actuarial post-RP PSA failure rates include 16%, 26% and 34%, at 5, 10 and 15

TABLE 1 Actuarial (PSA-based) 5- and 10-year Nonprogression Rates in Patients Undergoing Radical Retropubic Prostatectomy for Clinical Stage T1 and T2 Prostate Cancer

	PSA Nonprogression rate (%)		
Group	No. of patients	5 Yr	10 Yr
Partin et al., 1993	894	83	70
Trapasso et al., 1994	601	69	47
Catalona and Smith, 1994	925	78	—
Scardino, 1996	623	81	79
Ohori et al., 1994	500	76	73
Zincke et al., 1994	3170	70	52

Adapted from: Eastham JA, Scardino PT. Radical Prostatectomy for Clinical Stage T1 and T2 Prostate Cancer. In: Vogelzang NJ, Scardino PT, Shipley WU, Coffey DS (eds). Comprehensive Textbook of Genitourinary Oncology. 2000: Lippincott Williams & Wilkins, Philadelphia, PA; 722–738; Lightner DJ, Lange PH, Reddy PK, Moore L. Prostate-Specific Antigen and Local Recurrence After Radical Prostatectomy. J Urol 1990; 144:921; Stein A, deKernion JB, Dorey F. Prostate-Specific Antigen Related to Clinical Status 1 to 14 Years After Radical Retropubic Prostatectomy. Br J Urol 1991; 67:626; Morton RA, Steiner MS, Walsh PC. Cancer Control Following Anatomic Radical Prostatectomy: An Interim Report. J Urol 1991; **145**:1197 (14–16,18)

TABLE 2 Actuarial (PSA-based) 5-Year Nonprogression Rates (%) After Radical Retropubic Prostatectomy for Clinically Localized Prostate Cancer According to Clinical Stage, Gleason score in the Biopsy Specimens, Pathologic Stage, and Preoperative PSA

	No. of patients		
	Partin et al. (n=894)	Catalona and Smith (n=925)	Scardino (n=623)
Clinical Stage			
T1a	100	89	94
T1b	91		
T1c	100	99	98
T2a	87		84
T2b	71	85	76
T2c	69		74
Gleason Score			
2–4	98	91	93
5	92		88
6	85	89	83
7	62		60
8–10	46	74	
Preoperative PSA (ng/mL)			
0–4	92	95	94
4.1–10	83	93	78
10.1–20	56	71	79
>20	45		70
Pathologic Stage			
Organ confined	97	91	95
Capsular penetration			82
Seminal vesicle invasion	47		49
Positive lymph nodes	15		29

Adapted from: Eastham JA, Scardino PT. Radical Prostatectomy for Clinical Stage T1 and T2 Prostate Cancer. In: Vogelzang NJ, Scardino PT, Shipley WU, Coffey DS (eds). Comprehensive Textbook of Genitourinary Oncology. 2000: Lippincott Williams & Wilkins, Philadelphia, PA; 722–738; Lightner DJ, Lange PH, Reddy PK, Moore L. Prostate-Specific Antigen and Local Recurrence After Radical Prostatectomy. J Urol 1990; 144:921; Morton RA, Steiner MS, Walsh PC. Cancer Control Following Anatomic Radical Prostatectomy: An Interim Report. J Urol 1991; 145:1197 (14,15,18)

TABLE 3 Disease-Free Survival of pT3, N0 Patients with Seminal Vesicle Invasion

Institution (follow-up, 3–5 years)	N	Adjuvant radiation	Freedom from PSA failure (%)
Boston University	12	No	0
Johns Hopkins	67	No	15
Duke	58	No	36
UCLA	33	No	24
Washington University	15	Yes	53
Massachusetts General	24	Yes	43

Adapted from: Zietman AL. The Role of Radiation as Adjuvant or Salvage Therapy Following Radical Prostatectomy. In: Vogelzang NJ, Scardino PT, Shipley WU, Coffey DS (eds). Comprehensive Textbook of Genitourinary Oncology. 1996: Williams & Wilkins, Baltimore, MD; 782–790 (30)

years, respectively [16,17]. 35% to 70% of men with positive margins/seminal vesicle invasion, and 55% to 95% of those with a Gleason score ≥ 8 progress to biochemical failure (Table 2 and Table 3).

PSA that increases rapidly post-RP after an initial drop to undetectable levels indicates metastatic disease, whereas men whose PSA remains undetectable for longer periods (1 to 4 years) and then gradually increases have local recurrence in the prostatic bed [16]. In addition, *PSA velocity* (>0.75 versus <0.75 ng/mL/yr) and *doubling time* (<6 months versus >12 months) predict the type of clinical recurrence (distant versus local) [19–21].

PSA recurrence precedes clinical recurrence by 18–24 months. There is a direct correlation between the PSA level at 3–6 months and the disease-free interval [22]. Seventy percent of patients with early positive PSA progress within the first three years following RP. The median interval from PSA recurrence to cancer death is between 5 and 12 years, depending on the Gleason score.

Persistently Detectable PSA Following Radical Prostatectomy

This is a worse prognostic sign, and is due to either a large residue left within the tumor bed or, more likely, the presence of metastatic disease [13,23–27]. Its incidence is higher in the presence of extracapsular disease, positive surgical margins, and seminal vesicle invasion (Table 4).

FACTORS INFLUENCING POSTPROSTATECTOMY CANCER PROGRESSION

Clinical Stage and Pathological Stage

Patients with pathologic localized prostate cancer have excellent ($>90\%$) 5-year freedom from PSA recurrence [28,29], whereas the majority of patients with

TABLE 4 Detectable PSA Following Radical Prostatectomy

	Organ confined	Caps. Inv. positive or (+) margins	S. V.
No. Pts.	93	59	23
Detectable PSA	15%	29%	39%
PSA Median (Range)	0.8 (0.4–42)	0.9 (0.4–41)	1.2 (0.4–38)
F/U (mos.)	32	36	27

Adapted from: Stein A, deKernion JB, Smith RB, Dorey F, Patel H. Prostate-Specific Antigen Levels After Radical Prostatectomy in Patients with Organ-Confined and Locally Extensive Prostate Cancer. J Urol 1992; 1 47 : 942–946 (16)

involvement of either seminal vesicles or lymph nodes have been reported to progress by 5 years. The metastatic failure rates in men with Gleason score ≥ 8, positive seminal vesicles, or positive lymph nodes include 95%, 86% and 100%, respectively [16].

Preoperative Serum PSA and Gleason Score

Direct correlation has been noted between preoperative serum PSA and post-RP progression, especially in those with >10 ng/mL preoperative PSA [15]. In addition, poorly differentiated tumors with higher Gleason sum have been shown to progress faster.

Surgical Margin Status

Positive surgical margins are defined as the presence of cancer cells at the inked margin of resection. Stamey and associates described 2 distinct variants of positive margins, those associated with extracapsular extension of the tumor and those resulting from inadvertent surgical incision through the capsule into the intracapsular cancer [31]. Patients with ≥ 10 ng/mL preoperative PSA, biopsy Gleason score ≥ 7, multiple positive biopsies, or clinical stage T2b, T2c or T3 cancer have a higher risk of positive margins [32].

Partin et al. and Pound et al. have drawn a prognostic distinction between focal and extensive positive margins by *step-sectioning* the prostate specimen [33–35]. The majority of men with positive margins are noted to have focally positive margins. Forty percent of those with focally positive margins progress over 5 years compared to 65% with extensively positive margins. A positive margin at the prostatic base is associated with the highest secondary treatment rate [19]. Positive surgical margins, however, have no prognostic significance in presence of lymph node/seminal vesicle involvement.

Extracapsular Disease Versus Positive Surgical Margin(s)

Stage pT3 cancers fall into 2 categories, those with extracapsular disease and those with positive surgical margins. Schild and associates reported a doubling of the risk of PSA recurrence when extracapsular disease was compared with organ-confined disease. Recurrence rates in those with extracapsular disease, high-grade cancer (Gleason sum ≥ 7), and positive surgical margins equal the recurrence rates in men with seminal vesicle invasion [16]. Frazier et al. reported that 68% of those with specimen-confined extracapsular disease are disease free at 4 years compared with only 34% of those with positive margins [36].

PATHOLOGY OF RADICAL PROSTATECTOMY SPECIMEN

Whole mount sections have the advantage of maintaining architectural orientation in addition to producing fewer sections (about 6) for the pathologist to evaluate, and are useful for studying tumor distribution in the prostate and for determining tumor volume by quantitative image analysis. Compared to standard sectioning, step-sectioning of the totally embedded prostatectomy specimen (as practiced in some centers), has not been shown to provide additional histopathologic information in terms of detection of positive margins or extraprostatic extension of the tumor [37]. However, no study correlating the type of sectioning with PSA recurrence and clinical outcome is available to date.

PREDICTION OF PSA-ONLY PROGRESSION, LOCAL FAILURE, AND DISTANT FAILURE

In addition to the previously discussed factors, certain cellular and molecular markers that recently have been found to be associated with post-RP PSA recurrence include DNA ploidy, angiogenesis, p53, p27, bcl-2 and Ki-67 status [38–41]. Partin and associates developed a biostatistical model equation that divides post-RP patients into 3 groups of low-, intermediate-, and high-risk for biochemical failure. A sigmoidal transformation of PSA, prostatectomy Gleason sum, and specimen confinement (margin status) are incorporated into the following equation that calculates the relative risk of recurrence, R_w, as:

$$R_w = (0.061 \times PSA_{ST}) + (0.54 \times \text{postop. Gleason sum}) + (1.87 \times \text{specimen confined})$$

The initial challenge is to determine whether the PSA originates from local recurrence or from distant metastases (or both) (Table 5). Better criteria aimed at differentiating local from distant failure enable enrollment of only those with local failure for effective pelvic radiotherapy, and spare patients with metastatic disease unnecessary radiation.

TABLE 5 Role of Gleason Score, Pathologic Stage, and Timing of PSA
Recurrence in Prediction of Postradical Prostatectomy Recurrence Pattern

Variable	Local recurrence	Distant metastases with or without local recurrence
Number	41 (34%)	88 (66%)
Gleason score		
2–4	0%	0%
5–6	55%	45%
7	39%	61%
8–10	11%	89%
Pathologic stage		
Organ confined	40%	60%
Capsular penetration with negative surgical margins	54%	46%
Capsular penetration With positive surgical Margins	48%	52%
Seminal vesical Invasion	16%	84%
Micrometastases to Pelvic lymph nodes	7%	93%
Timing of PSA recurrence		
In year 1	7%	93%
Within years 1–2	10%	90%
After year2	61%	39%
After year 3	74%	26%

Adapted from: Pound CR, Partin AW, Epstein JI, Walsh P. Prostate-Specific Antigen After
Anatomic Radical Retropubic Prostatectomy. Urol Clin North Am 1997; 24(2):395–406 (12)

DIAGNOSIS OF POSTRADICAL PROSTATECTOMY CANCER PROGRESSION

Post-RP recurrences almost always manifest initially as a rise in the PSA. It is
extremely rare to have a clinical recurrence in the absence of a detectable PSA.

Digital Rectal Examination (DRE) and Biopsy of the Prostatic Bed

DRE is unreliable for the detection of local failure. Prostatic bed biopsy may be
helpful in presence of an abnormal DRE and a rising PSA, is positive in 30% of

patients with a rising PSA and normal DRE [44], and is invariably negative in those with an abnormal DRE but an undetectable PSA [45,46].

Bone Scan, Abdominopelvic CT Scan and MRI

Imaging studies to detect metastatic disease generally have a low yield in the majority of patients with post-RP biochemical recurrence [47–50]. They are neither sensitive nor specific to identify and localize recurrent disease unless PSA is high or the rate of PSA increase is >20 ng/mL/year.

Early post-RP failure is rarely associated with a positive bone scan, which has a low yield for detection of recurrence at <8 ng/mL [48]. Without systemic/bony symptoms, the probability of a positive bone scan is <5% until the total PSA level has increased to 40–45 ng/mL [49].

Prostascint Scan ([111]Indium Capromab Pendetide Scan)

Prostascint scan uses a radioactive monoclonal antibody (In-111 labeled capromab pendetide) to attack the prostate-specific membrane antigen (PSMA). It was initially hoped that Prostascint scan would improve selection for salvage local treatment.

It has a positive predictive value of 50%, negative predictive value of 70%, sensitivity of 75%, specificity of 86%, and accuracy rate of 81% [51]. In addition, the test is operator dependent and requires special training for reading the scans. Bowel and vascular structures may cause false-positive scans, and no histological confirmation of post-RP recurrences identified with *Prostascint scan* have been reported to date [52]. Overall, the utility of *Prostascint scan* is currently limited due to difficulties associated with interpretation.

Should the Urethrovesical Anastomosis Be Biopsied in Patients with Postradical Prostatectomy Biochemical Recurrence?

As it is a sound practice to histologically document recurrent cancer before further treatment is undertaken, biopsy may seem logical when local recurrence is suspected or when there is a post-RP palpable abnormality. However, biopsy of the vesicourethral anastomosis is mostly imprecise and experience to date suggests that the overall chance of documenting recurrent cancer with one biopsy is <50%.

Foster et al. and Connolly et al. advocate prostate bed/anastomotic biopsy and reported biopsy-confirmed recurrences in 54% of patients, with two-third of patients having recurrence diagnosed on the first biopsy and two-third of recurrences being found at the anastomotic site [53,54]. Ninety percent of recurrences were seen as a hypoechoic lesion and PSA level at biopsy correlated with positive biopsy (28% positive biopsy rate for PSA level <0.5 and 70% for >2 ng/mL).

On the other hand, Fowler et al. reported that transrectal ultrasound-guided (TRUS) biopsy of the anastomosis was positive in 78% of men with a palpable lesion, 40% of patients with an abnormal TRUS, but only 23% with normal DRE and TRUS, and concluded that routine TRUS-guided anastomotic biopsy is not indicated, and use of PSA and PSA doubling time is sufficient for clinical diagnosis of recurrence [55]. In addition, the response to radiation therapy has been shown to be similar among those with negative or positive biopsies.

PSA doubling time of <6 months indicates rapidly progressive disease and histological confirmation of cancer in such a setting is not warranted. Biopsy is also not warranted if the patient is well informed about the nature of further therapy and does not express an interest in pursuing treatment.

TREATMENT OF POSTRADICAL PROSTATECTOMY DISEASE PROGRESSION

Treatment of PSA-only Progression

Currently, treatment of post-RP biochemical recurrence is controversial. This controversy arises from the fact that, to date, no adjuvant therapy has been proven to prolong survival. Options include observation, conventional external beam radiotherapy (CRT) to the prostatic bed, and conformal 3-D external beam radiation with dose escalation and hormonal therapy. Only radiation therapy is discussed in this chapter.

Prior to the use of PSA as a biochemical indicator of recurrence, relapse post-RP was noted with a change in DRE or evidence of metastatic disease. *Delaying radiation until patients were found to have a positive DRE is clearly very different from radiotherapy given when the PSA begins to rise.* The use of PSA has caused stage migration. 10% compared to 30% of patients present with metastatic disease. 2% versus 22% are found to have positive nodes at surgery. 15% versus 30% have positive margins. This trend has rendered the current patient population quite different from the preceding populations studied. Historical data comparing immediate versus delayed post-RP radiotherapy is no longer relevant given that patients are presenting much earlier. Failure after local therapy (RP or radiotherapy) is now the second most common way in which prostate cancer presents. The issue of adjuvant versus delayed radiotherapy is, therefore, a relevant clinical problem.

Radiation Dose and Morbidity

The optimal dose of radiation therapy is the one that maximizes tumor control with minimum morbidity, and this will vary (45 to 64 Gy) according to the estimate of the residual disease burden. Valicenti et al. reported that radiation doses of ≥64.8 Gy are superior to prevent future biochemical failures of pT3N0 prostate cancers [56].

Radiation doses can be tailored with 45 to 54 Gy being given to those with undetectable PSA and specimen-confined pT3 disease, 55 to 64 Gy to those with positive margins, and 64 to 68 Gy as salvage therapy for a delayed rise in PSA. Doses >64 Gy were found to be more effective than lower doses, with little morbidity over a median follow-up of 2 years [57], although the long term morbidity is a concern.

Radical prostatectomy is associated with the risks of incontinence and urethral stricture, among others. One concern regarding post-RP radiotherapy is that it will interfere with healing and may exacerbate incontinence and stricture following surgery. However, studies have shown that doses that yield excellent local control have an acceptably low risk (5–15%) of these complications [58–62].

Genital/lower limb edema has been reported to occur in 0–21% of patients (median, 9%) [58–62]. With the extent of pelvic lymph-node dissection now routinely done in patients with prostate cancer, lower limb edema is rarely seen following adjuvant radiation. Severe (grade 3 to 4) gastrointestinal complications are rare (0–12%, median, 4%), and urethral strictures occur in 5–10% of patients.

Eighty-two percent of patients treated with nerve sparing prostatectomy and radiotherapy have been reported to lose potency, compared to 54% of nonirradiated patients.

Timing of Radiation Therapy for Postradical Prostatectomy PSA-only Progression (Adjuvant Versus Delayed Salvage Radiation)

Even if one is going to use postoperative radiation, there is no consensus regarding the ideal timing of intervention. No randomized study has been reported to prove or disprove that adjuvant radiotherapy (given for positive resection margins or pT3 disease with undetectable PSA) gives a survival advantage over delayed salvage radiotherapy (given to those with a rising PSA following an initial drop to undetectable level or post-RP palpable recurrence), and results of nonrandomized case series have been conflicting (Table 6). The results of Southwest Oncology Group (SWOG) *intergroup* study 8794, which randomized pathologic stage C cases to radiation versus observation will at the earliest only be available in the year 2005.

Proponents of adjuvant radiation contend that the currently utilized PSA assays will not detect a recurrence smaller than 10^7 to 10^8 cells, nor does PSA identify the site of recurrence. On the other hand, pathologic findings at the time of surgery can predict stage progression and can be reliably used to distinguish patients at risk for local recurrence from those likely to fail distantly. Post-RP

TABLE 6 Comparison of Postradical Prostatectomy Adjuvant versus Delayed Radiotherapy

Author	No. of patients (Adjuvant/Salvage)	Follow-up (mos.)	Adjuvant RT			Salvage RT		
			Overall survival	Disease-free survival	Local control	Overall survival	Disease-Free survival	Local control
McCar thy	27/37	33	–	67%	–	–	54%	–
Morris	40/48	31	–	81%	–	–	48%	–
Nudell	36/35	35	–	80%	–	–	55%	–
Vicini	38/19	48	83%	67%	–	100%	24%	–
Valicenti	52/27	36/46	–	93%	–	–	44%	–

Adapted from: Anscher MS. Adjuvant Radiotherapy Following Radical Prostatectomy Is More Effective and Less Toxic than Salvage Radiotherapy for a Rising Prostate Specific Antigen. Int J Cancer (Int Radiat Oncol Invest) 2001; 96:91–93 (61)

adjuvant pelvic radiotherapy, when given to those at high risk for local recurrence (but at low risk for distant metastases), results in a higher biochemical relapse-free rate (bRFR) and fewer side effects (due to the lower dose of radiation) than when delayed until the PSA begins to rise [63,64]. The reported outcomes (5-year bRFR) over a follow-up period of 3.7 years include 81% for adjuvant radiotherapy, 19% for delayed salvage radiotherapy, and 0% for those with palpable disease. Salvage RT is most successful in those with a preradiotherapy PSA <2 ng/mL or Gleason score <7 [65]. However, all available data supporting adjuvant radiotherapy is retrospective, in a small number of patients (12 or less), most had positive surgical margins.

Although immediate adjuvant radiation can significantly reduce the risk of relapse, survival data from randomized trials are not available [66]. On the other hand, two-thirds of patients with post-RP rising PSA can be salvaged with delayed radiotherapy, if administered before the PSA rises to >1.1 ng/mL.

The difficulty in radiating patients with positive margins is that approximately 30% may not have failed local therapy and will be subjected to the morbidity associated with immediate radiotherapy. Approximately 10% of margin positive patients will have metastatic disease and derive no benefit from radiotherapy. The remaining 60% will have better survival from immediate radiation. However, if radiotherapy is delayed until PSA recurrence, the doubling time may be used to differentiate local versus metastatic disease before proceeding. The American Society for Therapeutic Radiology and Oncology (ASTRO) consensus report recommends salvage radiotherapy (6,400 cGy to the prostatic bed) before PSA rises to >1.5 ng/mL [67], at which level, adjuvant radiotherapy and delayed salvage radiation have similar outcome.

Delayed radiotherapy may result in poorer urinary control in 5–10% of patients, which is due to the higher doses of radiation required [68].

Future studies should examine the issue of adjuvant versus delayed salvage radiation in a randomized, prospective fashion.

Three-Dimensional Conformal External Beam Radiotherapy as Salvage Treatment for a Rising Postprostatectomy PSA

Koper et al., Sandler et al., and Wilder et al. reported that 3-D conformal external beam radiotherapy (CRT) (in 1.8 to 2.0 Gy daily fractions to a total dose of 60.6 to 74.2 Gy) delivered to the prostatic fossa results in less toxicity [69–71]. In those with a preradiotherapy PSA of ≤1.0 ng/mL, 3-D CRT has been reported to yield a 2-year biochemical disease-free survival rate of 67%, compared to 20% for those with a PSA of ≥1.0 ng/mL. A positive microscopic margin has no impact on the outcome and 25% of those with poorly differentiated cancer have been reported to be disease free. Genitourinary and gastrointestinal complications occurred in 29% and 21% of patients, respectively. All patients who are potent at the start of treatment remain potent. Salvage 3-D CRT appears to be well tolerated and less expensive than prolonged hormonal therapy in such patients.

Postradical Prostatectomy Radiotherapy Outcome

Response to radiotherapy is associated with preradiotherapy PSA and postrecurrence PSA doubling time [72], the former being the most important prognostic factor [73]. Patients who are in need of and stand to gain (in terms of progression-free survival) from adjuvant therapy such as radiation include those with Gleason scores ≥8, positive seminal vesicles/lymph nodes, or a PSA recurrence within the first year post-RP. On the other hand, these are also the very patients in whom adjuvant radiation is less effective.

Radiation is considered successful if serum PSA remains undetectable (<0.2 ng/mL) for at least 2 years after the last radiation treatment, and unsuccessful if a detectable PSA is identified during follow-up [28]. Cadeddu et al. reported that 21% of men had an undetectable PSA (<0.2 ng/mL) for ≥2 years following radiotherapy. Late (>5 years post-RP) recurrences have a response rate of 44% [28]. Schild et al. reported 90% 5-year bRFR following adjuvant radiotherapy

TABLE 7 External Beam Radiotherapy Outcome for "PSA only progression" After Radical Prostatectomy

Reference	No. of patients	Tumor stage	Mean PSA at start of radiation	PSA Response (ng/mL)	Follow-up (mean, months)
Schild et al.	46	B	0.9	<0.3	36–50
		C			
Morris et al.	48	T3	1.7	Undetectable	31
Cadeddu et al.	57	T2	2.2	Undetectable	31
		T3			24
Garg et al.	78	T2	2.8		25
		T3			
		T4			
		N1			
Egawa et al.	32	T2	2.2		25.6
		T3			
		N1			

Adapted from: Cadeddu JA, Partin AW, DeWeese TL, Walsh PC. Long-term Results of Radiation Therapy for Prostate Cancer Recurrence Following Radical Prostatectomy. J Urol 1998; 159:173–178; Schild SC, Buskirk SJ, Wong WW, et al. The Use of Radiotherapy for Patients with Isolated Elevation of Serum Prostate Specific Antigen Following Radical Prostatectomy. J Urol 1996; 156:1725; Morris MM, Dallow KC, Zeitman AL, et al. Adjuvant and Salvage Irradiation Following Radical Prostatectomy for Prostate Cancer. Int J Radiat Oncol Biol Phys 1997; 38:731; Garg MK, Tekyi-Mensah S, Bolton S, et al. Impact of Postprostatectomy ProstateSspecific Antigen Nadir on Outcomes Following Salvage Radiotherapy. Urology 1998; 51:998; Egawa S, Matsumoto K, Suyama K, et al. Limited Suppression of Prostate-Specific Antigen After Salvage Radiotherapy for Its Isolated Elevation After Radical Prostatectomy. Urology 1999; 53:48 (28, 73–76) compared to 40% for RP alone (Table 7) [74]. Adjuvant radiation results in 5-, 10- and 15-year actuarial bRFR were 84%, 74% and 66%, respectively [17].

ANDROGEN BLOCKADE AND RADIOTHERAPY

Addition of hormone therapy to radiotherapy for post-RP biochemical recurrence appears to be effective only for a low-volume disease. In addition, long-term hormone therapy is more expensive and may result in loss of libido, impotence, decreased bone density with risk of a fracture, and reduced quality of life. The addition of a short course of androgen deprivation in patients receiving 3-D CRT does not improve PSA relapse-free survival in any of the risk groups (79).

The Radiotherapy Oncology Group (RTOG) is currently conducting a prospective, randomized study (Protocol 96–01) comparing 64.8 Gy post-RP radiotherapy plus a placebo for 2 years versus 64.8 Gy post-RP radiotherapy plus the antiandrogen, bicalutamide for 2 years in those with normal activity, with a life expectancy of >10 years, and without evidence of metastases.

SUMMARY AND CONCLUSIONS

Postradical prostatectomy "PSA-only progression" is a common problem facing the contemporary urologist. Sixty percent of such patients may have local disease, 15–20% have distant disease, and 20–25% may have both. Treatment options include observation, immediate adjuvant radiotherapy, delayed salvage radiotherapy, and hormone therapy. Two-thirds of patients with postprostatectomy-rising PSA can be salvaged with radiotherapy. The three settings for potentially curative postradical prostatectomy radiotherapy include an adjuvant therapy following prostatectomy, a salvage following PSA rise indicative of recurrence, and a salvage for those with a clinically evident local recurrence (palpable, biopsy-proven, or both).

Radiotherapy is provides durable benefits (with mild and self-limited long-term morbidity) to men with low PSA ($\leq$1.5 ng/mL) at recurrence; longer (>12 months) postrecurrence PSA doubling time, and delayed (2–3 years following prostatectomy) PSA recurrence in the absence of adverse pathological features, such as Gleason scores $\geq$8 and positive seminal vesicles or lymph nodes. Early, short-term hormone therapy is not beneficial for PSA-only recurrence.

Adjuvant radiotherapy may improve biochemical and local relapse in men with multiple positive-surgical margins or extensive extracapsular disease. Data regarding its survival advantage are forthcoming. When administered before the PSA rises to >1.1 ng/mL in those without palpable recurrence, delayed salvage radiotherapy is safe, effective, and protective, exposing fewer patients to unnecessary/nonbeneficial therapy.

REFERENCES

1. Landis SH, Murray T, Bolden S, Wingo PA. Cancer statistics, 1999. Ca Cancer J Clin 1999; 49:831.
2. Stanford JL, Stephenson RA, Coyle LM, et al. Prostate Cancer trends 1973–1995, NIH Pub. No. 99–4543 Bethesda MD, Ed. SEER Program: National Cancer Institute, 1999.
3. Stephenson RA. Population-based prostate cancer trends in the PSA era: data from the Surveillance, Epidemiology, and End Results (SEER) Program. 1998. Monogr Urol 1998; 19:3.
4. Moul JW. Prostate specific antigen only progression of prostate cancer. J Urol 2000; 163:1632–1642.
5. Wingo WJ, Tong T, Bolden S. Cancer statistics, 1995. CA 1995; 45:8–30.
6. Partin AW, Kattan MW, Subong ENP, et al. Combination of prostate-specific antigen, clinical stage, and Gleason score to predict pathological stage of localized prostate cancer. J Am Med Assoc 1997; 277:1445–1451.
7. Anscher MS, Prosnitz LP. Multivariate analysis of factors predicting local relapse after radical prostatectomy-possible indications for postoperative radiotherapy. Int J Radiat Oncol Biol Phys 1991; 21:941–947.
8. Paulson DF, Moul JW, Robertson JE, et al. Postoperative radiotherapy of the prostate for patients undergoing radical prostatectomy with positive margins, seminal vesicle involvement and/or penetration through the capsule. J Urol 1990; 143:1178–1182.
9. Patel A, Dorey F, Franklin J, et al. Recurrence patterns after radical retropubic prostatectomy:Clinical usefulness of prostate specific antigen doubling times and log slope prostate specific antigen. J Urol 1997; 158:1441–1445.
10. Paulson DF, Robertson CN. Positive margins: is adjunctive radiation therapy indicated?. Acta Oncol 1991; 30:263–265.
11. Nasseri KK, Austeinfeld MS. PSA recurrence after definitive treatment of clinically localized prostate cancer. AUA Update Series 1997; 16:32–37.
12. Pound C, Partin AW, Epstein J, Walsh P. PSA after anatomic radical prostatectomy: Patterns of recurrence and cancer control. Urol Clin North Am 1997; 24(2):395–406.
13. van den Ouden D, Hop WCJ, Kranse R, Schroder FH. Tumor control according to pathological variables in patients treated by radical prostatectomy for clinically localized carcinoma of the prostate. Br J Urol 1997; 79:203–211.
14. Eastham JA, Scardino PT. Radical Prostatectomy for Clinical Stage T1 and T2 Prostate Cancer. In Vogelzang NJ , Scardino PT , Shipley WU , Coffey DS(), Eds. Comprehensive Textbook of Genitourinary Oncology. Philadelphia. PA: Lippincott Williams & Wilkins, 2000:722–738.
15. Lightner DJ, Lange PH, Reddy PK, Moore L. Prostate-specific antigen and local recurrence after radical prostatectomy. J Urol 1990; 144:921–926.
16. Stein A, deKernion JB, Smith RB, Dorey F, Patel H. Prostate-specific antigen levels after radical prostatectomy inpatients with organ-confined and locally extensive prostate cancer. J Urol 1992; 147:942–946.
17. Han M, Partin AW, Pound CR, et al. Long-Term Biochemical Disease-Free and Cancer-specific Survival Following Anatomic Radical Retropubic Prostatectomy. Urol Clin North Am 2001; 28:555–565.

18. Morton RA, Steiner MS, Walsh PC. Cancer control following anatomic radical prostatectomy: an interim report. J Urol 1991; 145:1197.

19. Grossfeld GD, Chang JJ, Broering JM, et al. Impact of positive surgical margins on prostate cancer recurrence and the use of secondary cancer treatment: Data from the CaPSURE Database. J Urol 2000; 163:1171–1177.

20. Danella J, Steckel J, Dorey F, Smith RB, deKernion JB. Detectable prostate-specific antigen levels following radical prostatectomy: relationship of doubling time to clinical outcome [abstract]. J Urol 1993; 149:447A.

21. Pound CR, Partin AW, Eisenberger MA, Chan DW, Pearson JD, Walsh PC. The natural history of progression of prostate cancer after PSA recurrence following radical prostatectomy. JAMA 1999 May 5; 281(17):1591–1597.

22. Hudson MA, Robertson JE, Humphrey PA, et al. Clinical use of prostate specific antigen in patients with prostate cancer. J Urol 1989; 142:1011–1017.

23. Pruthi RS, Johnstone I, Tu IP, Stamey TA. Prostate specific antigen doubling times in patients who have failed radical prostatectomy:correlation with histologic characteristics of the primary cancer. Urology 1997; 49:737–742.

24. Lange PH. Prostate-specific antigen for staging prior to surgery and for early detection of recurrence after surgery. Urol Clin North Am 1990; 17:813–817.

25. Lange PH, Lightner DJ, Medini E, Reddy PK, Vessella R. The effect of radiation therapy after radical prostatectomy in patients with elevated prostate-specific antigen levels. J Urol 1990; 144:927–932.

26. McCarthy JF, Catalona WJ, Hudson MA. Effect of radiation therapy on detctable serumprostate-specific antigen levels following radical prostatectomy: early versus delayed treatment. J Urol 1994; 151:1575–1578.

27. Link P, Freiha FS, Stamey TA. Adjuvant radiation therapy in patients with detectable prostate-specific antigen following radical prostatectomy. J Urol 1991; 145:532–534.

28. Cadeddu JA, Partin AW, DeWeese TL, et al. Long-term results of radiation therapy for prostate cancer recurrence following radical prostatectomy. J Urol 1998; 159: 173–178.

29. Frazier HA, Robertson JE, Humphrey PA, Paulson DF. Is prostate-specific antigen of clinical importance in evaluating outcome after radical prostatectomy? J Urol 1993; 148:516–518.

30. Zietman AL. The role of radiation as adjuvant or salvage therapy following radical prostatectomy. In Vogelzang NJ , Scardino PT , Shipley WU , Coffey DS(), Eds. Comprehensive Textbook of Genitourinary Oncology. Baltimore. MD: Williams & Wilkins, 1996:782–790.

31. Stamey TA, Villers AA, McNeal JE, Link PC, Freiha FS. Positive surgical margins at radical prostatectomy: importance of the apical dissection. J Urol 1990; 143: 1166–1172.

32. Wieder JA, Soloway MS. Incidence, etiology, location, prevention and treatment of positive surgical margins after radical prostatectomy for prostate cancer. J Urol 1998; 160:299–315.

33. Partin AW, Pound CP, Clemens JQ, Epstein JI, Walsh PC. Serum PSA after anatomic radical prostatectomy. Urol Clin North Am 1993; 20:713–725.

34. McNeal JE, Villars AA, Redwine EA, Freiha FF, Stamey TA. Capsular penetration in prostate cancer. Significance for natural history and treatment. Am J Surg Pathol 1990; 14:240–247.

35. Partin AW, Borland RN, Epstein JI, Brendler CB. Influence of wide excision of the neurovascular bundle(s) on the prognosis in men with clinically localized prostate cancer with established capsular penetration. J Urol 1993; 150:142–148.

36. Frazier HA, Robertson JE, Humphrey PA, Paulson DF. Is prostate-specific antigen of clinical importance in evaluating outcome after radical prostatectomy? J Urol 1993; 149:516–518.

37. Sakr WA, Grignon DJ. Practice parameters, pathologic staging, and handling radical prostatectomy specimens. Urol Clin North Am 1999; 26(3):453–463.

38. Partin AW, Piantadosi S, Marshall FF. Selection of men at high risk for disease recurrence for experimental adjuvant therapy following radical prostatectomy. Urology 1995; 45:831–838.

39. Isaacs JT. Molecular markers for prostate cancer metastasis. Developing diagnostic methods for predicting the aggressiveness of prostate cancer. Am J Pathol 1997; 150:1511–1521.

40. Kattan MW, Eastham JA, Stapleton AM, et al. A preoperative nomogram for disease recurrence following radical prostatectomy for prostate cancer. J Natl Cancer Inst 1998; 90:766–771.

41. D'Amico AV, Whittington R, Malkowicz SB, et al. Pretreatment nomogram for prostate-specific antigen recurrence after radicalprostatectomy or external-beam radiation therapy for clinically localized prostate cancer. J Clin Oncol 1999; 17: 168–172.

42. Saleem MD, Sanders H, El Nasser MA, El-Galley R. Factors predicting cancer detection in biopsy of the prostatic fossa after radical prostatectomy. Urology 1997; 51:283–286.

43. Takayama KT, Lange PH. Radiation therapy for local recurrence of prostate cancer after radical prostatectomy. Urol Clin North Am 1994; 21:687–699.

44. Richie JP. Management of patients with positive surgical margins following radical prostatectomy. Urol Clin North Am 1994; 21:717–723.

45. Epstein JI, Pizov G, Walsh PC. Correlation of pathologic findings with progression after radical retropubic prostatectomy. Cancer 1993; 71:3582–3593.

46. Malkowitz SB. Serum PSA elevation in the post-radical prostatectomy patients. Urol Clin North Am 1996; 23:665–675.

47. Cher ML, Bianco FJ, Lam JS, et al. Limited role of radionuclide bone scintigraphy in patients with prostate specific antigen elevations after radicalprostatectomy. J Urol 1998; 160:1387–1391.

48. Manzone TA, Malkowitz SB, Schnall MD, Langlotz CP. Use of endorectal MR imaging to predict prostate carcinoma recurrence after radical prostatectomy. Radiology 1998; 209:537–542.

49. Hinkle GH, Burgers JK, Neal CE, et al. Multicenter radioimmunoscintigraphic evaluation of patients with prostate carcinoma using indium-111 capromab pendetide. Cancer 1998; 83:739–747.

50. Kahn D, Libertino JA. 111 Indium-capromab pendetide in the evaluation of patients with residual or recurrent prostate cancer after radical prostatectomy. J Urol 1998; 159:2041–2047.

51. Foster LS, Jajodia P, Fournier G, et al. The value of prostate specific antigen and transrectal ultrasound guided biopsy indetecting prostatic fossa recurrences following radical prostatectomy. J Urol 1993; 149:1024–1028.

52. Connolly JA, Shinohara K, Presti JC, et al. Local recurrence after radical prostatectomy: characteristics in size, location, and relationship to prostate-specific antigen and surgical margins. Urology 1996; 47:225–231.

53. Fowler JE, Brooks J, Pandey P, et al. Variable histology of anastomotic biopsies with detectable prostate specific antigen after radical prostatectomy. J Urol 1995; 153:1011–1014.

54. Valicenti RK, Gomella LG, Ismail M, et al. Durable efficacy of early postoperative radiation therapy for high pT3N0 prostate cancer: the importance of radiation dose. Urology 1998; 52(6):1034–1040.

55. Pisansky TM, Kozelsky TF, Myers RP, Hillman DW, Blute ML, Buskirik SJ, et al. Radiotherapy for isolated serum prostate specific antigen elevation after prostatectomy for prostate cancer. J Urol 2000; 163(3):845–850.

56. Jacobson GM, Smith JA, Stewart JR. Post-operative irradiation for pathologic stage C prostate cancer. Int J Radiat Oncol Biol Phys 1987; 13:1021–1024.

57. Ray GR, Bagshaw MA, Freiha F. External beam radiation salvage for residual or recurrent local tumor following radical prostatectomy. J Urol 1984; 132:926–930.

58. Pilepich MV, Walz BJ, Baglan RJ. Postoperative irradiation in carcinoma of the prostate. Int J Radiat Oncol Biol Phys 1984; 10:1869–1873.

59. Petrovich Z, Lieskovsky G, Langholz B, Luxton G, Jozsef G, Skinner DG. Radiotherapy following radical prostatectomy in patients with adenocarcinoma of the prostate. Int J Radiat Oncol Biol Phys 1991; 21:949–954.

60. Hanks GE, Dawson AK. The role of external beam radiation therapy after prostatectomy for prostate cancer. Cancer 1986; 58:2406–2410.

61. Anscher MS. Adjuvant radiotherapy following radical prostatectomy is more effective and less toxic than salvage radiotherapy for a rising prostate specific antigen. Int J Cancer 2001; 96(2):91–93.

62. Van Cangh P, Richard F, Lorge F, et al. Adjuvant radiation therapy does not cause urinary incontinence after radical prostatectomy: results of a prospective randomized study. J Urol 1998; 159:164–166.

63. Catton C, Gospodarowicz M, Warde P, et al. Adjuvant and salvage radiation therapy after radical prostatectomy for adenocarcinoma of the prostate. Radiother Oncol 2001; 59(1):51–60.

64. Schild SE. Radiation therapy (RP) after prostatectomy: the case for salvage therapy as opposed to adjuvant therapy. Int J Cancer 2001; 96(2):94–98.

65. Cox JD, Gallagher MJ, Hammond EH, et al. Consensus statements on radiation therapy of prostate cancer: guidelines for prostate re-biopsy after radiation and for radiation therapy with rising prostate-specific antigen levels after radical prostatectomy. American Society for Therapeutic Radiology and Oncology Consensus Panel. J Clin Oncol 1999; 17:1155.

66. Anscher M. Salvage radiotherapy after radical prostatectomy. In Greco C, Zelefsky M(), Eds. Radiotherapy of prostate cancer. Amsterdam: Harwood Academic Publishers, 2000:335–341.

67. Koper PCM, Stroom JC, Putten WLJV, et al. Acute morbidity reduction using 3DCRT for prostate carcinoma: a randomized study. Int J Radiat Oncol Biol Phys 1999; 43:727–734.

68. Sandler HM, McLaughlin PW, Haken RK, Addison H, Forman J, Lichter A. Three dimensional conformal radiotherapy for the treatment of prostate ancer: low risk of chronic rectal morbidity observed in a large series of patients. Int J Radiat Oncol Biol Phys 1995; 33:797–801.

69. Wilder RB, Hsiang JY, Ji M, Earle JD, de Vere White R. Preliminary Results of Three-Dimensional Conformal-Radiotherapy as Salvage Treatment for a Rising Prostate-Specific Antigen Level Postporstatectomy. Am J Clin Oncol 2000; 23(2): 176–180.

70. Leventis AK, Shariat SF, Kattan MW, et al. Prediction of response to salvage radiation therapy in patients with prostate cancer recurrence after radical prostatectomy. J Clin Oncol 2001; 19(4):1030–1039.

71. Crane CH, Rich TA, Read PW, Sanfilippo NJ, Gillenwater JY, Kelly MD. Preirradiation PSA predicts biochemical disease-free survival in patients treated with postprostatectomy external beam irradiation. Int J Radiat Oncol Biol Phys 1997; 39:681–686.

72. Schild SE, Pisansky TM. The Role of Radiotherapy After Radical Prostatectomy. Urol Clin North Am 2001; 28:629–637.

73. Schild SC, Buskirk SJ, Wong WW, et al. The use of radiotherapy for patients with isolated elevation of serum prostate specific antigen following radical prostatectomy. J Urol 1996; 156:1725–1729.

74. Morris MM, Dallow KC, Zeitman AL, et al. Adjuvant and salvage irradiation following radical prostatectomy for prostate cancer. Int J Radiat Oncol Biol Phys 1997; 38:731–736.

75. Garg MK, Tekyi-Mensah S, Bolton S, et al. Impact of post-prostatectomy prostate-specific antigen nadir on outcomes following salvage radiotherapy. Urology 1998; 51:998–1002.

76. Egawa S, Matsumoto K, Suyama K, et al. Limited suppression of prostate-specific antigen after salvage radiotherapy for its isolated elevation after radical prostatectomy. Urology 1999; 53:148–154.

77. Zelefsky MJ, Leibel SA, Gaudin PB, et al. Dose escalation with three-dimensional conformal radiation therapy affects the outcome in prostate cancer [see comments]. Int J Radiat Oncol Biol Phys 1998; 41:491–500.

EDITORIAL COMMENTARY

H. Ballentine Carter

Professor of Urology and Oncology, The James Buchanan Brady Urological Institute, The Johns Hopkins Medical Institutions, Baltimore, MD, USA

Large institutional series now report that 25–50% of men experience PSA progression of disease after radical prostatectomy [1]. Many of these men would be considered candidates for postprostatectomy radiotherapy on the basis of adverse pathologic features after surgery (adjuvant radiotherapy), or on the basis of a rising PSA in the absence of radiographic evidence of distant disease (salvage radiotherapy). However, eradication of residual disease postprostatectomy with radiotherapy is only possible for those men who have residual disease confined to the prostatic bed (pelvis) because distant disease will not be affected by any localized therapy. Currently, it is not possible to identify those men who will benefit from radiotherapy prior to recurrence because the presence of residual disease localized to the pelvis (without distant disease) cannot be accurately predicted by pathologic criteria, serum markers, or radiographic imaging. In addition, there are no convincing data that demonstrate that men who receive postprostatectomy radiotherapy have improved survival when compared to those men who receive no therapy. The available information from uncontrolled comparisons of those men who did and did not receive postprostatectomy radiotherapy are difficult to interpret due to selection bias and short follow-up for a disease with a long natural history in the absence of treatment. Thus, there is no consensus on the administration of radiotherapy postprostatectomy either as adjuvant or salvage therapy. The authors have reviewed this difficult subject and have made recommendations based on available information.

In the **adjuvant** setting, radiotherapy given postprostatectomy (based on adverse pathologic findings) to reduce the risk of local recurrence exposes a substantial proportion of men to unnecessary treatment—either because they would have done well without radiotherapy or because of the presence of unrecognized distant disease. For example, Han et al.[2], demonstrated that those men with capsular penetration and a positive surgical margin who have a Gleason Score of 7 disease or above almost never benefit from radiotherapy because of the presence of distant metastatic disease, and those men with seminal vesicle invasion and lymph node metastases have distant disease for which radiotherapy will not be effective. The high-risk group for which postprostatectomy adjuvant radiotherapy may have benefit are those men with capsular penetration and a positive surgical margin who have a Gleason score less than 7, but have a 15-year biochemical recurrence-free survival of 58% [1]. Thus, postprostatectomy adjuvant radiotherapy for these men would have been unnecessary in the majority of cases. Furthermore, there is no strong evidence that adjuvant radiotherapy will lead to improved outcomes when compared to salvage radiotherapy at the time of PSA recurrence for suspected isolated localized disease. My bias is to selectively use radiotherapy in those men postprostatectomy for **salvage** of residual disease that is suspected to be localized based on pathologic information from the radical prostatectomy specimen and the pattern of PSA failure.

After radical prostatectomy, approximately 30% of men who are carefully selected for the presence of localized disease will have a biochemical recurrence within 10 years [1]. It has been estimated that approximately 25% of isolated PSA failures have a local recurrence as the source of the PSA. When PSA failures occur, which men are most likely to have local recurrence only and therefore, [??] most likely to benefit from salvage postprostatectomy radiotherapy? The temporal relationship between the detectable PSA and surgery and the pathologic features of the radical prostatectomy specimen provide helpful information. Those men with a Gleason Score 8 disease (or above), seminal vesicle invasion or lymph node metastases, or a PSA recurrence within the first year after surgery rarely—if ever—have a durable response to radiotherapy [3]. Those men with Gleason Scores of 7 or less who have no seminal vesicle invasion or lymph nodal disease and have a PSA recurrence beyond 1 year after surgery are more likely to have a durable response to radiotherapy [3]. Short-term data suggest that a durable response to salvage radiotherapy is more likely if radiotherapy is delivered when the PSA is less than 2 ng/mL, and if at least 6400cGy is delivered to the prostatic bed [4].

REFERENCES

1. Han M, Partin AW, Pound CR, Epstein JI, Walsh PC. Long-term biochemical desease-free and cancer-specific survival following anatomic radical retropubic prostatectomy. The 15-year Johns Hopkins experience. Urol Clin North Am 2001; 28:555–565.
2. Han M, Pound CR, Potter SR, Partin AW, Epstein JI, Walsh PC. Isolated local recurrence is rare after radical prostatectomy in men with Gleason 7 prostate cancer and positive surgical margins: therapeutic implications. J Urol 2001; 165:864–866.
3. Cadeddu JA, Partin AW, DeWeese TL, Walsh PC. Long-term results of radiation therapy for prostate cancer recurrence following radical prostatectomy. J Urol 1998; 159:173–177.
4. Cox JD, Gallagher MJ, Hammond EH, Kaplan RS, Schellhammer PF. Consensus statements on radiation therapy of prostate cancer: guidelines for prostate re biopsy after radiation and for radiation therapy with rising prostate-specific antigen levels after radical prostatectomy. American Society for Therapeutic Radiology and Oncology Consensus Panel. J Clin Oncol 1999; 17:1155.

EDITORIAL OVERVIEW

Kenneth B. Cummings

It is axiomatic that only those patients with residual disease in the pelvis following radical prostatectomy will benefit from radiation therapy. The authors provide an excellent assessment of cancer control following radical prostatectomy. Additionally, they focus, with appropriate references, on the patterns of failure and the relationship to pathologic stage, Gleason sum, and timing and slope of PSA progression.

PSA that increases rapidly post–radical prostatectomy after becoming immeasurable most likely indicates metastatic disease; this contrasts with men in whom PSA remains undetectable for longer periods (1–4 years), and then gradually increases with or without the presence of palpable disease in the prostatic fossa [1]. In addition, PSA velocity (> .75 vs. < .75 ng/mL per year) and doubling times (< 6 months vs. > 12 months) predict the type of clinical recurrence, local vs. distant [2–4].

Large institutional series report PSA progression of 25–50% following radical prostatectomy, which estimate that 25% of all PSA failures are a consequent of local disease, the problem is defining that 25% [5]. The authors address the timing of post–radical prostatectomy radiation therapy as (a) adjuvant, based on pathological findings after surgery, vs. (b) salvage, for those with rising PSA thought due to local disease. They appropriately address criteria for patient selection and the appropriate therapeutic recommendation is three-dimensional (3D) conformal radiation therapy (3DCRT) to a dose of 64 Gy [6].

The selection for postprostatectomy radiation remains the greatest challenge. Ballantine allows that the authors have achieved a careful review of a difficult subject. In his commentary, he states that, currently, it is not possible to identify those men who will benefit from radiotherapy prior to recurrence because of the presence of residual disease localized in the pelvis (without distant disease) and that is it impossible to accurately predict from pathologic criteria, serum markers, or radiographic imaging, who these patients are. He additionally states that there is no convincing data to demonstrate that men who receive postprostatectomy radiotherapy have an overall improved disease-free survival compared to those men to receive no radiation therapy.

Because most of the current information is from uncontrolled series and due to selection bias and short follow-up time, it is impossible to draw conclusions. Having said this, he would allow that there is no consensus regarding the administration of radiotherapy postprostatectomy either as adjuvant or salvage therapy. His review of the Hopkins series would define a group at high risk for postprostatectomy local failure who might benefit from adjuvant radiation therapy as those patients who have capsular for penetration and a positive surgical margin with a Gleason Score less than 7.

However, the 15-year biochemical recurrence-free survival is 58% for this group. It would, therefore, be necessary to treat nearly two-thirds of these patients to be able to benefit the presumed third who need this treatment. He does make a clear case for those patients who will not benefit from radiation postprostatectomy (Gleason Score 8 disease or above, seminal vesicle invasion or lymph node metastasis, or PSA recurrence within the first year after surgery) [7]. He further allows that those men with Gleason scores less than 7 who have no seminal vesicle invasion or lymph node disease and whose PSA recurrence is beyond 1 year are more likely to have a durable response to radiotherapy [7]. The consensus of both authors is that a durable response is more likely to be achieved if radiation is initiated when the PSA is less than 2 ng/mL.

REFERENCES

1. Stein A, deKernion JB, Smith RB, Dorey F, Patel H. Prostate-specific antigen levels after radical prostatecotmy in patients with organ-confined and locally extensive prostate cancer. J Urol 1992; 147:942–946.

2. Grossfeld GD, Chang JJ, Broering JM, Miller DP, Yu J, Flanders SC, Henning JM, Stier DM, Carroll PR. Impact of positive surgical margins on prostate cancer recurrence and the use of secondary cancer treatment: data from the CaPSURE database. J Urol 2000; 163:1171–1177.

3. Danella J, Steckel J, Dorey F, Smith RB, deKernion JB. Detectable prostate-specific antigen levels following radical prostatectomy: relationship of doubling ime to clinical outcome [abstract]. J Urol 1993; 149:447A.

4. Pound CR, Partin AW, Eisenberger MA, Chan DW, Pearson JD, Walsh PC. The natural history of progression of prostate cancer after PSA recurrence following radical prostatectomy. JAMA 1999; 281(17):1591–1597.

5. Han M, Partin AW, Pound CR, Epstein JI, Walsh PC. Long-term biochemical disease-free and cancer-specific survival following anatomic radical retropubic prostatectomy: the 15-year Johns Hopkins experience. Urol Clin North Am 2001; 28:555–565.

6. Cox JD, Gallagher MJ, Hammond EH, Kaplan RS, Schellhammer PF. Consensus statements on radiation therapy of prostate cancer: guidelines for prostate re-biopsy after radiation and for radiation therapy with rising prostate-specific antigen levels after radical prostatectomy. American Society for Therapeutic Radiology and Oncology Consensus Panel. J Clin Oncol 1999; 17:1155.

7. Cadeddu JA, Partin AW, DeWeese TL, Walsh PC. Long-term results of radiation therapy for prostate cancer recurrence following radical prostatectomy. J Urol 1998; 159:173–177.

10

Androgen Deprivation for Men with PSA-Only Failure Following Radical Prostatectomy: When?

Donald L. Trump

Professor of Medicine, Senior Vice President for Clinical Research and Chairman of Medicine, Roswell Park Cancer Institute Buffalo, New York, USA

There are many contentious issues in the clinical management of prostate—many of which result from our inability or unwillingness to subject important clinical questions to the cold steel of well-designed, adequately powered, randomized and controlled clinical trials. Among the issues, about which uncertainty remains, are the comparative efficacy of prostatectomy and definitive irradiation for localized prostate cancer; the comparative or additive benefits of brachytherapy and techniques of external beam irradiation; and the role of androgen deprivation—neoadjuvant or adjuvant following prostatectomy. There is even debate regarding the role of androgen deprivation (AD) in patients with metastatic, but asymptomatic disease. The uncertainty regarding this latter question is particularly surprising given that AD was demonstrated to have a major clinical benefit in men with advanced prostate cancer more than 60 years ago. This is not to imply that asking and answering any of these questions would be easy; in fact, some questions may be impossible to ask in the setting of a controlled clinical trial (e.g., prostatectomy versus irradiation). Nonetheless, there is considerable room for improvement in the vigor with which randomized clinical trials are applied to the numerous important questions in the care of men with prostate cancer.

With that as a preamble, one might expect that a discussion of the timing of AD following "PSA failure" in patients who have undergone prostatectomy would be very short indeed. There are no randomized clinical trial data which address this issue. Nonetheless, hundreds of men find themselves in this situation each year. There are approximately 180,000 men diagnosed with prostate cancer each year, and 90% (162,000) have localized disease. Sixty percent of these men undergo either prostatectomy or irradiation (n = 97,000). If the posttreatment recurrence rate is 30%—30,000 men each year experience failure after local therapy, and approximately half of these men have had prostatectomy. In the vast majority of such men, failure is signaled first by a detectable or rising PSA. Few of these men have radiographic evidence of disease. The "charge" of this discussion is to outline the use of AD in such patients. Lacking clinical trial data that address this issue directly, one must base decisions on the natural history of "PSA failure" after prostatectomy and draw inferences from studies in related situations. Unfortunately, there are limited data regarding the natural history of PSA failure following prostatectomy. A major challenge in determining the natural history of PSA failure is the substantial delay, which often occurs between "PSA failure" and symptomatic or radiographic evidence of metastatic disease. Notably, the survival of such men following prostatectomy may be a decade or more. Also confounding the determination of natural history is that most investigators who have carried out large numbers of prostatectomies have not rigorously controlled the use of systemic therapy in such men so that the number of patients from whom one might derive a sense of natural history of untreated disease is small. The best described series of patients who experienced PSA failure following prostatectomy is that of Dr. Patrick Walsh at the Brady Urologic Institute, Johns Hopkins University School of Medicine, described eloquently by Pound et al. in the *Journal of the American Medical Association* in 1999 (2). Pound and colleagues described 315 patients who underwent anatomic radical prostatectomy by Dr. Walsh and subsequently developed a detectable PSA—defined as a PSA >0.2ng/mL (Hybritech-Tandem and the TOSOH assays). The Hopkins group has steadfastly pursued a policy of withholding systemic and local therapy in such men. Of the 315 patients who developed PSA failure, only 11 received any therapy until radiographic or symptomatic progression was documented. Hence, a group of 304 men, carefully followed, is available to assess the natural history of this clinical situation. The outcomes in these patients are important to review in detail. Table 1 notes the clinical and pathological features of the tumors in these men.

Factors predictive of early clinically evident metastases following prostatectomy included the interval from surgery to PSA detection (short, <2years), PSA

TABLE 1 Pathological and Clinical Characteristics of 304 Patients Who Developed PSA Recurrence Following Prostatectomy

Pathologic Gleason Score	
5	15 (4.9%)
6	41 (13.5%)
7	151 (49.7%)
8–10	97 (31.9%)
Pathologic Stage	
Organ-confined	31 (10.2%)
Capsular Penetration (Gleason <7)	30 (9.9%)
Capsular Penetration (Gleason ≥7)	108 (35.5%)
Seminal Vesicals Involved	52 (17.1%)
(negative nodes)	
Positive Lymph Nodes	83 (27.3%)
Year of PSA Recurrence	
1–2	136 (44.7%)
3–5	97 (31.9%)
6–9	59 (19.4%)
≥ 10	12 (4%)

After Pound et al. J Amer Med Assoc 1999; 281 : 1591–1597

doubling time (<10 months), and Gleason score (Gleason ≥7). Of, 103 men who developed metastatic disease, 43% have died of prostate cancer; no man who has developed metastatic disease has died of any other cause. Median survival (actuarial) after recognition of metastases was slightly less than five years. The only variable predictive of survival was the interval between surgery and detectable metastatic disease: an interval of 1–3 years was associated with a median survival of slightly less than five years, while for men whose metastases were detected more than eight years following prostatectomy median survival has not been reached.

Few other sets exist that provide additional or complementary information to this carefully acquired and extensive experience. However, there are limitations to these data: follow-up is relatively short—only 36% of these patients have been followed for more than 10 years, and the number of men with metastases is small. Hence any generalizations which can be made from the group are limited.

In the clinical situation of PSA-only failure following prostatectomy, one might take either the ''glass is half full'' (GIHF) or the ''glass is half empty'' (GIHE) approach. On the GIHF side, there are clearly a number of men in whom the natural history of PSA progression after anatomic prostatectomy is prolonged. Overall, there is a median time-to-radiographic-disease progression of 96 months, and the expected median survival is 36–48 months from the point when AD is initiated. This defines a group of men with a 50% chance of living $\geq$ 10 years. It is important to note that the estimated survival for normal men ages 50–59 and 60–69 years of age is 20.4–27.7 years and 13.5–19.6 years, respectively (3). For the GIHE position, on the other hand, the analysis of Pound et al. allows the definition of men with a very poor prognosis—high Gleason grade, short disease-free interval. Unfortunately, without a prospective, ideally randomized clinical trial, one can not necessarily predict whether the poor prognosis group is the group least likely, or most likely, to benefit from "adjunctive" or "early" AD therapy, (AD) Intuitively, one might posit that these poor prognosis patients are destined to develop rapidly progressive disease and should clearly be offered ADT—on the other hand, these rapidly progressive tumors, perhaps with amplified or mutated growth stimulatory signals (e.g., Her2/neu, EGFR, TGFβ, IGFR, AR, VDR) may be less likely to benefit from "simple" AD. Perhaps tumors in this setting are less dependent on androgens for growth and more likely to develop androgen independence quickly due to genomic "instability." Careful molecular studies of these tumors, and prospective randomized trials, are required to answer this question. Until such data are available, whether the "good risk" or the "poor risk" postprostectomy patients should received ADT is a matter of bias, conjecture, and "clinical judgement."

If the groups of patients with "PSA failure" postprostatectomy that should received ADT is unclear, perhaps we should be guided by analyses of the benefits of ADT and toxicity of ADT in other patient populations.

First, how good is ADT? It could be argued that ADT is the **best** therapy that exists for **any** adult epithelial tumor—only curative, cisplatin-based chemotherapy for germ-cell tumors is better. Ninety-five percent of patients who undergo ADT "respond," if you accept a substantial PSA decrease as a "response." Fifty percent of patients with disseminated prostate cancer are still alive at 24 months. This stands in contrast to the median survival of patients with disseminated colorectal cancer of 12–18 months (4,5), advanced lung cancer of 3–4 months (6,7), metastatic breast cancer of 12–24 months (8), and metastatic gastric cancer of 4 months (9,10). Six to ten percent of patients with advanced prostate cancer are alive and well at 10 years following ADT (11–15). Progress since the pioneering work of Huggins and Hodges in 1941 has been painfully slow (16). ADT for prostate cancer *is* very good treatment for advanced cancer. In experimental models, early AD may prevent the emergence of androgen-independent cell populations. Nonumura and colleagues developed clonal cell lines of the Shionogi tumor (an androgen-dependent breast-cancer cell line in mice) (17). The cloned cells when stimulated by testosterone were noted to secrete growth factors with growth stimulatory effects on both androgen-independent and androgen-dependent subclones, suggesting that withdrawal of androgens may limit the production of other factors that may promote the growth of tumor cells but do not regress with androgen deprivation. Other studies show that androgens stimulate the production of angiogenic compounds such as the vascular endothelial growth factor (VEGF) in benign and malignant tissues. This suggests androgen deprivation may inhibit the growth of androgen-independent cells by reducing the production of angiogenic compounds critical for the growth of tumor masses. Isaacs et al. have shown that androgen deprivation prolongs survival of animals with small prostate tumors compared to animals with larger tumors (18,19). By inhibiting tumor cells when the tumor burden is small, recurrence may either be delayed or prevented. These well-designed preclinical studies support the concept that early ADT is effective.

There are randomized clinical trials that address this issue. The earliest studies were conducted in 1967 by the Veterans Affairs Cooperative Urological Research Group (VACURG) and assessed more than 1750 patients with clinical stages A B C, and prostate cancer (20). The patients were randomized to no therapy until disease progression (placebo), surgical castration, 5 mg of diethylstilbestrol (DES), and surgical castration with 5 mg of DES. No survival benefit was seen in any group. Therapy with DES was associated with increased cardiovascular morbidity and mortality. Although the results from the initial VACURG study were negative in terms of overall survival, a reanalysis suggests that the 5 mg dose of DES may slow disease progression and decrease death from prostate cancer compared to those patients in whom therapy was delayed until disease progression (placebo) (21). A further study compared the results of three doses of DES:—0.2, 1.0, and 5 mg—versus placebo (22). The 5 mg dose was terminated early because of toxicity, for and the 0.2 mg dose was considered ineffective for inducing castration. Delayed time to disease progression was noted in men treated with the less toxic dose of 1 mg of DES compared to placebo; subsequent reanalysis suggested that a survival benefit was present, but limited to patients with stage D disease and high-grade tumors (22). The results of the VACURG studies form the basis of the argument that early ADT does not improve survival.

The positive inferences drawn in the preceding discussion could derive from the hazardous process of retrospective, unplanned subgroup analysis. Among the factors that make it difficult to extrapolate the results of the VACURG studies to the care of patients now are: (1) staging differences—the staging in VACURG consisted of acid phosphatase, bone radiographs, and physical examination; (2) patients have access to better medical care and are generally seen earlier in the course of disease due to PSA testing; and (3) ADT therapies are better tolerated today, hence compliance with ADT may be considerably improved. Walsh and colleagues have reassessed the VACURG studies, focusing on the comparisons of orchiectomy and placebo patients, arguing that these are the only groups whose analysis is not confounded by the use of DES, which was associated with increased mortality and, likely, diminished compliance (23). In restricting analysis to these groups, one finds no indication of improved survival in the patients undergoing orchiectomy. This supports the argument that earlier ADT is not useful, but is confounded by the fact that this analysis relies on subgroup analysis resulting in rather small group sizes.

There are three contemporary studies which address, in a randomized and controlled fashion, the role of early versus delayed ADT in prostate cancer. The Medical Research Council (MRC) in Great Britain compared the outcome of immediate ADT, consisting of surgical or medical castration started at diagnosis, to ADT deferred until disease progressed in patients with symptomatic locally advanced or metastatic disease (T2-4, MO-1) (24). In this study, 938 men were randomized to immediate ADT (n = 469) or deferred treatment until evidence of symptoms (n = 465). The patients were followed for a median period of 6 years. Overall, there was reduced mortality from prostate cancer in the early treatment group (203 deaths versus 257 deaths, p value = 0.001). Subgroup analysis did not show a significant overall survival difference in the M_o group, where 81 of 256 patients (32%) who received early ADT died compared to 119 patients of 244 patients (49%) who received delayed ADT. This trial also showed differences in the distant metastasis rate in M_0 patients and rates of local progression and development of pain. There were fewer complications (spinal cord compression, urethral obstruction and pathologic fracture) in the early ADT group (11%) compared to the deferred group (21%). A criticism of this study is that 29 patients in the delayed group did not receive treatment. However, the design of the study was a randomized trial with intent to treat analysis, and the 29 patients died before treatment was initiated. Another criticism of this trial is that the follow-up schedule for patients receiving delayed ADT was not clearly defined. Therefore, it is argued that delayed patients did not get appropriate care and initiation therapy at the right time—or indeed for some—ever. While this is a valid study design, it also **emphasizes** the hazards of delayed therapy. An updated analysis of this trial published only in abstract form reports no overall survival advantage in either arm for patients with locally advanced disease, though disease-specific survival in the immediate treatment arm remains significantly improved statistically (25).

EORTC study 22863 showed that the combination of adjuvant (early) ADT and external beam radiation therapy (EBRT) improves survival in patients with high-risk, locally advanced disease (T3–4 N_0, M_0 or T1–2 N_1, M_O WHO histologic grade 3) – compared to EBRT alone (26). Patients were randomized to radiation therapy alone (n = 208) or radiation therapy with ADT LHRH agonist, goserelin) for 3 years and oral cyproterone acetate for one month (n = 207). Bolla and colleagues reported the results after a median follow-up of 4 years. Local control, disease, free survival, and overall survival were superior in patients treated with ADT. One of the criticisms of this study is that it did not compare early ADT, versus deferred ADT, but rather early ADT versus no ADT with radiation therapy. It seems unlikely, however, that the patients who progressed never received ADT. Critics also note that the outcome of the radiation-only group was noted to be "poorer than expected," suggesting these patients in some way were selected. But the power of a randomized study is that such biases are expected to be equally distributed in both arms. Randomized clinical trials are the answer to "expectations" of physicians—especially when those "expectations'' are based on anecdote or selected patient series. This study clearly shows that adjunctive (early) ADT can improve survival.

The Radiation Therapy Oncology Group (RTOG 85–31) studied patients with locally advanced disease, as well as patients who were treated with prostatectomy, and found to have positive margins or seminal vesical involvement (T1–2, N_1, M_0 or T3–4, N_{0-1} M_0) (27,28). Patients were randomized to radiation therapy alone (n = 468) or radiation therapy with indefinite medical or surgical ADT (n = 477). Patients assigned to radiation therapy crossed over to ADT after disease progression. After a median follow up of 5 years, patients who received adjunctive (early) ADT had superior disease-free survival, rate of distant metastases, and delayed local failure (p<0.0001). A survival benefit was seen in the subgroup of patients with – Gleason score of 8–10. Although the study does not show an overall survival difference, follow-up is relatively short. An earlier RTOG (86–10) study looked at the impact of a short duration of ADT given prior to and during radiation compared to irradiation only in men with localized prostate cancer. This study revealed benefits of 'early' ADT (28). RTOG 86–10 randomized 456 patients with T2–T4 N_0, M_0 prostate cancer to radiation therapy alone or ADT with goserelin acetate and flutamide two months before and during radiation therapy. With six years of follow-up, patients who received ADT showed no overall survival benefit, but a significant improvement in local failure, distant metastases, biochemical disease-free survival, and disease-free survival (p <0.001) (29,30). An ongoing RTOG trial (94–08) will address the effect of ADT given to patients two months prior to and during radiation therapy in more favorable prognosis patients with early stage (T1b, T2b, N_0, M_0 and PSA <20). Notably studies of hypothetically "better risk" patients (RTOG 85–31 and 86–10) demonstrated encouraging early markers of successful therapy (improved disease-free survival), and it is not illogical to suggest that longer follow-up may be required in these "better risk" patients.

A prospective randomized Eastern Cooperative Oncology Group (ECOG) trial assessed prostate cancer patients found to have positive lymph nodes following radical prostatectomy and lymphadenectomy (T1–2, N_1, M_0) (31). The study randomized 46 patents to early ADT with surgical or medical castration and 52 patients to delayed therapy at the time of disease progression. The study participants were followed for a median of seven years. A significant survival advantage was seen in men on the early ADT arm. The trial has been criticized because of the inability to accrue the planned number of patients, the small number of patients studied, and the lack of central pathology review for consistent Gleason grading. On the other hand, the power calculations used to determine sample size were set to detect a specified difference, and, because of the large difference that was found between the two groups, the smaller sample size still supports the conclusion that early ADT is superior. The study has also been criticized because patients in the delayed arm had lower survival rates than other contemporary studies, that is, the control arm patients did worse "than expected" (32,33). The patients in the ECOG trial reflected a varied prostate cancer population consisting of older men from multiple institutions, including VA and county hospitals. In contrast, men from other studies were younger, probably wealthier, and drawn from the tertiary centers. Patients in each arm of the ECOG trial were comparable in terms of clinical and pathological features, including Gleason scores. However, since pathological specimens were not centrally reviewed, concern has been expressed that an imbalance in prognostic factors may have occurred.

There are few data which allow one to estimate current patterns of care or the standard of practice with regard to the use of adjunctive ADT or ADT in patients with PSA failure. Concern has been expressed that the studies of adjuvant ADT following surgery or irradiation will persuade more and more physicians to administer ADT. Whether these studies have influenced practice patterns is uncertain. Prior to the publication of the 2 randomized trials of ADT following local therapy, Wasson and colleagues surveyed urologists and found that 66% recommend ADT for "PSA-only failure" following prostatectomy—even though most did not believe ADT would increase survival (34). More recently, Potosky and colleagues questioned a sample of men diagnosed within 1 year after a diagnosis of invasive localized prostate cancer (35); 37% of these 661 men had received ADT therapy within one year of diagnosis of localized prostate cancer for whom no local therapy was undertaken. These studies do indicate the widespread use of ADT for men with prostate cancer which is localized or for men who have PSA-only failure.

Since there are no definitive data regarding the use of ADT in men with PSA-only progression following prostatectomy, one must consider the risk of ADT therapy. While ADT does not induce life-threatening side effects if orchiectomy or LHRHa ($+/-$ antiandrogen) are used, ADT is associated with toxicity—diminished potency, loss of libido, weight gain, loss of muscle strength, breast tenderness, and swelling, hot flashes, and osteoporosis are the primary toxicities of ADT. The magnitude and importance of these side effects is uncertain. These side effects are difficult to measure and have not been well quantitated. Potosky and colleagues recently described a relevant study, though in a different population of patients. Using SEER data, this investigative group (the Prostate Cancer Outcomes Study [PCOS]) evaluated 661 men who were diagnosed to have localized prostate cancer and had not undergone local therapy. One year after diagnosis, 37% (245) had received ADT 63% and (416) had received no additional therapy. Compared to baseline status, the men receiving ADT reported loss of libido, impotence, and reduced activity substantially more often than men on no therapy. Interestingly, men who were treated with ADT had tumors with higher Gleason scores (>6), their PSAs were higher (>20 ng/mL) and they were more often clinical stage T2 than men who were not treated. Satisfaction with their treatment was higher among men on ADT as was the likelihood of feeling that they were free of cancer. Thus, while ADT caused symptoms, as a generalization, men who chose ADT were pleased with the status of their therapy. Osteoporosis is a complication of ADT that is poorly characterized. More than 50% of men on ADT develop osteoporosis. If the complication rate of osteoporosis in this setting is similar to the complications that occur in postmenopausal women, hip fracture, vertebral fracture, and mortality are substantially more likely in these men. This potential, combined with the expected long duration of ADT in men with a long natural history, such as those undergoing ADT for PSA-only recurrence, suggests that the morbidity of ADT and osteoporosis may be realized only in the future. Bisphosphonates, however, clearly prevent loss of bone mineral in men receiving ADT (36).

In the absence of data, what is a clinician to do? First and foremost, there should be a national, randomized trial of this question. Men are receiving ADT—but they are not being studied to understand whether ADT for PSA-only failure is rational. My own practice while I await the conduct of this much-desired study is the following:

For men with PSA recurrence following prostatectomy:

1. Prostascint, bone and, CT scan of chest, abdomen, and pelvis.
2. If Prostascint is negative or suggests local (prostatic fossa) recurrence, I utilize irradiation.
3. If scans are negative, I would repeat scans at 12–18 month intervals.
4. I would enter patients on clinical trials of new approaches for prostate cancer (e.g., novel agents, immunologic or bone-targeted therapies). We are currently evaluating high-dose calcitriol in this setting.
5. I would withhold ADT, if the patient is comfortable withholding therapy, until the PSA is 15–20ng/mL, assuming radiographs, physical examination, and clinical assessment are normal.

Unfortunately, there are no data to guide my decision; I have arbitrarily chosen 15–20 ng/mL as the "cut off" past which I begin to lean toward ADT. There are no data of which I am aware to justify this cutoff. My rationale is as follows:

- PSA values in men with overt metastases who are entered on trials of ADT are often in the 75–100 ng/mL range (37).
- There are data suggesting that PSA values >50 ng/mL are often associated with the discovery of radiographic evidence of skeletal metastases (38).
- I do believe that early androgen deprivation will be found to reduce mortality, based on the randomized studies cited, the limitations of the arguments against early ADT, and the general "truism" in cancer therapy—effective systemic therapy applied in situations of high risk very often lead to improved survival. This is the paradigm that has lead to improved survival rates in breast, gastric, bladder, and colorectal cancer. Systemic therapies in these diseases are often only modestly effective in the setting of clearly evident metastatic disease.

- I believe early ADT in men with prostate cancer should ideally begin before any evidence of progressive disease based on radiographic or physical examination.

I fully understand that these arguments are largely philosophical and may be proven wrong when the proper randomized trials are completed. However, these are the biases that I carry, and I try to explain them fully to my patients as I discuss the use of ADT in situations where the only evidence of disease is a detectable PSA.

REFERENCES

1. SEER web page:http://seer.cancer.gov Data on treatment obtained using SEER-Stat 3.0 software and data from public use CD-ROM, 1973–1997, January 2001.

2. Pound CR, Partin AW, Eisenberger MA, Chan DW, Pearson JD, Walsh PC. Natural history of progression after elevation following prostatectomy. J Amer Med Assoc 1999; 281(17):1591–1597.

3. National Vital Statistics Report, 2002.

4. Bruckner HW, Motwani BT. Chemotherapy of advanced cancer of the colon and rectum. Semin Oncol 1991; 18:443–455.

5. Rougier P, Paillot B, LaPlanche A, Morvan F, Seitz JF, Rekacewicz C, Laplaige P, Jacob J, Grandjouan S, Tigaud JM, Fabri MC, Luboinski M, Ducreux M. 5-Fluorouracil (5-FU) continuous intravenous infusion compared with bolus administration. Final results of a randomised trial in metastatic colorectal cancer. Eur J Cancer 1997 Oct; 33(11):1789–1793.

6. Bonomi PD, Finklestein DM, Ruckdeschel JC, et al. Combination chemotherapy versus single agents followed by combination chemotherapy in stage IV non-small cell lung cancer: a study of the Eastern Cooperative Oncology Group. J Clin Oncol 1989; 7:1602–1609.

7. Le Chevalier T, Brisgand D, Douillard J, et al. Randomized study of vinorelbine and cisplatin versus vinorelbine alone in advanced non-small cell lung cancer: results of a European multicenter trial including 612 patients. J Clin Oncol 1994; 12: 360–364.

8. Ross MB, Buzdar AU, Smith TL, Eckles N, Hortobagyi GN, Blumenschein GR, Freireich EN, Gehan EA. Improved survival of patients with metastatic breast cancer receiving chemotherapy. Comparison of consecutive series of patients in the 1950s, 1960s and 1970s. Cancer 1985; 55:341–346.

9. Bruckner HW, Chesser MR, Wong H, Mandeli J. A folate biochemical modulation regimen for gastric cancer therapy. J Clin Gastroenterol 1991; 134:384–391.

10. Webb A, Cunningham D, Scarffe JH, Harper P, Norman A, Joffe JK, Hughes M, Mansi J, Findlay M, Hill A, Oates J, Nicolson M, Hickish T, O'Brien M, Iveson T, Watson M, Underhill C, Wardley A, Meehan M. Randomized trial comparing epirubicin, cisplatin, and fluorouracil versus fluorouracil, doxorubicin, and methotrexate in advanced esophagogastric cancer. J Clin Oncol 1997 Jan; 15(1):261–267.

11. Eisenberger MA, Blumenstein BA, Crawford ED, Miller G, McLeod DG, Loehrer PJ, Wilding G, Sears K, Culkin DJ, Thompson IM, Bueschen AJ, Lowe BA. Bilateral orchiectomy with or without flutamide for metastatic prostate cancer. N Engl J Med 1998 Oct 8; 339(15):1036–1042.

12. Schellhammer P, Sharifi R, Block N, Soloway M, Venner P, Patterson AL, Sarosdy M, Vogelzang N, Jones J, Kolvenbag G. A controlled trial of bicalutamide versus flutamide, each in combination with luteinizing hormone-releasing hormone analogue therapy, in patients with advanced prostate cancer. Casodex Combination Study Group Urology 1995; 45:745–752.

13. Crawford ED, Eisenberger MA, McLeod DG, Spaulding JT, Benson R, Dorr FA, Blumenstein BA, Davis MA, Goodman PJ. A controlled trial of leuprolide with and without flutamide in prostatic carcinoma. N Engl J Med 1989 Aug 17; 321(7): 419–424.

14. Wechsel HW, Zerbib M, Pagano F, Coptcoat MJ. Randomized open labeled comparative study of the efficacy, safety and tolerability of leuprorelin acetate 1M and 3M depot in patients with advanced prostatic cancer. Eur Urol 1996; 30(Suppl 1):7–14; discussion 19–21.

15. Maximum androgen blockade in advanced prostate cancer: an overview of the randomised trials. Prostate Cancer Trialists' Collaborative Group. Lancet 2000 Apr 29; 355(9214):1491–1498.

16. Huggins C, Hodges CV. Studies on prostate cancer: effect of castration, of estrogen and of androgen injection on serum phosphatases in metastatic carcinoma of the prostate. Cancer Res 1941; 1:293–297.

17. Nonomura N, Nakamura N, Uchida N, Noguchi S, Sato B, Sonoda T, Matsumoto K. Growth-stimulatory effect of androgen-induced autocrine growth factor(s) secreted from Shionogi carcinoma 115 cells on androgen-unresponsive cancer cells in a paracrine mechanism. Cancer Res 1988 Sep 1; 48(17):4904–4908.

18. Isaacs JT. The timing of androgen ablation therapy and/or chemotherapy in the treatment of prostatic cancer. Prostate 1984; 5(1):1–17.

19. Henry JM, Isaacs JT. Relationship between tumor size and the curability of metastatic prostatic cancer by surgery alone or in combination with adjuvant chemotherapy. J Urol 1988 May; 139(5):1119–1123.

20. Treatment and survival of patients with cancer of the prostate. The Veterans Administration Cooperative Urological Research. Group Surg Gynecol Obstet 1967 May; 124(5):1011–1017.

21. Byar DP, Corle DK. Hormone therapy for prostate cancer: results of the Veterans Administration Cooperative Urological Research Group studies. NCI Monogr 1988(7):165–170.

22. Byar DP. Proceedings: The Veterans Administration Cooperative Urological Research Group's studies of cancer of the prostate. Cancer 1973 Nov; 32(5):1126–1130.

23. Walsh PC, Deweese TL, Eisenberger M. A structured debate: Immediate versus deferred androgen suppression in prostate cancer—Evidence for deferred treatment. J Urol 2001; 166:508–516.

24. Immediate versus deferred treatment for advanced prostatic cancer: initial results of the Medical Research Council Trial. The Medical Research Council Prostate Cancer Working Party Investigators Group. Br J Urol 1997 Feb; 79(2):235–246.

25. Kirk D. Immediate vs deferred hormone treatment for prostate cancer. How safe is androgen deprivation? Medical Research Council—Prostate Working Party Investigators Group. Br J Urol 2000; 86:220, (suppl) (abstr).

26. Bolla M, Gonzalez D, Warde P, Dubois JB, Mirimanoff RO, Storme G, Bernier J, Kuten A, Sternberg C, Gil T, Collette L, Pierart M. Improved survival in patients with locally advanced prostate cancer treated with radiotherapy and goserelin. N Engl J Med 1997 Jul 31; 337(5):295–300.

27. Pilepich MV, Caplan R, Byhardt RW, Lawton CA, Gallagher MJ, Mesic JB, Hanks GE, Coughlin CT, Porter A, Shipley WU, Grignon D. Phase III trial of androgen suppression using goserelin in unfavorable-prognosis carcinoma of the prostate treated with definitive radiotherapy: report of Radiation Therapy Oncology Group Protocol 85–31. J Clin Oncol 1997 Mar; 15(3):1013–1021.

28. Lawton CA, Winter K, Murray K, Machtay M, Mesic JB, Hanks GE, Coughlin CT, Pilepich MV. Updated results of the phase III Radiation Therapy Oncology Group (RTOG) trial 85–31 evaluating the potential benefit of androgen suppression following standard radiation therapy for unfavorable prognosis carcinoma of the prostate. Int J Radiat Oncol Biol Phys 2001 Mar 15; 49(4):937–946.

29. Pilepich MV, Krall JM, al-Sarraf M, John MJ, Doggett RL, Sause WT, Lawton CA, Abrams RA, Rotman M, Rubin P, et al. Androgen deprivation with radiation therapy compared with radiation therapy alone for locally advanced prostatic carcinoma: a randomized comparative trial of the Radiation Therapy Oncology Group. Urology 1995 Apr; 45(4):616–623.

30. Pilepich MV, Winter K, Roach, et al. M. Phase III RTOG Trial 86–10 of androgen deprivation before and during radiotherapy in locally advanced carcinoma of the prostate. Proc ASCO 1998; 17:308a.

31. Messing EM, Manola J, Sarosdy M, Wilding G, Crawford ED, Trump D. Immediate hormonal therapy compared with observation after radical prostatectomy and pelvic lymphadenectomy in men with node-positive prostate cancer. N Engl J Med 1999; 341(24):1781–1788.

32. Seay TM, Blute ML, Zincke H. Long-term outcome in patients with pTxN + adenocarcinoma of prostate treated with radical prostatectomy and early androgen ablation. J Urol 1998 Feb; 159(2):357–364.

33. Cadeddu JA, Partin AW, Epstein JI, Walsh PC. Stage D1 (T1–3, N1–3, M0) prostate cancer: a case-controlled comparison of conservative treatment versus radical prostatectomy. Urology 1997 Aug; 50(2):251–255.

34. Wasson JH, Fowler FJ, Barry MJ. Androgen deprivation therapy for asymptomatic advanced prostate cancer in the prostate specific antigen era: a national survey of urologist beliefs and practices. J Urol 1998; 159:693–696.

35. Potosky AL, Reeve BB, Clegg LX, Hoffman RM, Stephenson RA, Albertsen PC, Gilliland FD, Stanford JL. Quality of life following localized prostate cancer treated initially with androgen deprivation therapy or no therapy. J Natl Cancer Instit 2002; 94:430–437.

36. Smith MR, McGovern FJ, Zeitman AL, Fallon MA, Hayden DL, Schonfeld DA, Kantoff PW, Finklestein JS. Pamidronate to prevent bone loss during androgen-deprivation therapy for prostate cancer. New Engl J Med 2001; 345:948–955.

37. Eisenberger MA, Blumenstein BA, Crawford ED, Miller G, McLeod DG, Loehrer PJ, Wilding G, Sears K, Culkin DJ, Thompson IM, Bueschen AJ, Lowe BA. Bilateral orchiectomy with or without flutamide for metastatic prostate cancer. N Engl J Med 1998; 339:1036–1042.

38. Pantelides ML, Bowman SP, George NJ. Levels of prostate specific antigen that predict skeletal spread in prostate cancer. Br J Urol 1992; 70:299–303.

EDITORIAL COMMENTARY

Mario A. Eisenberger

R. Dale Hughes Professor of Oncology and Urology, The Johns Hopkins University, Baltimore, MD, USA

ANDROGEN DEPRIVATION FOR MEN WITH PSA-ONLY FAILURE FOLLOWING RADICAL PROSTATECTOMY: WHEN?

The optimal time for initiation of androgen deprivation treatment (ADT) in patients with prostate cancer represents one of the many unresolved controversies associated with this modality of treatment in this disease. Most of the data derives from studies conducted primarily during the last 4 decades of the 20th century, and the observations on these studies have traditionally served as the basis for discussions involving this challenging issue.

As discussed in Dr.Trump's chapter, there is no definitive evidence that immediate androgen deprivation offers a survival advantage over deferred treatment in patients with metastatic disease (M+)+ [1–4]. The main advantage of early treatment in these patients is reflected by a delay in disease progression and, consequently, a significant reduction in the incidence of prostate cancer–associated serious morbidities such as pain, urinary obstruction, transfusion requirements, and spinal cord compression. It is frequently argued that, in these studies, implementation of deferred treatment was not uniformly applied because it was left primarily at the discretion of treating physicians, which could potentially limit the conclusions. In all studies involving patients with M+ disease, initiation of deferred treatment was based on the clinical development of new evidence of disease and/or symptoms and was not driven primarily by changes in PSA levels. At this point the recommendation is to immediately treat all patients with radiological or other clinical evidence of distant metastasis.

There is a large body of data on clinical trials designed to study the role of combined radiation therapy and ADT as the initial treatment for patients with clinically localized prostate cancer [5]. The primary goal of the combined ADT + radiation approach is to enhance the benefits of both modalities at the primary disease level based on their biological interaction; however, in view of the systemic effects of ADT, it may be entertained that treatment is designed to enhance local and distant disease. Clinical trials testing the role of adjuvant/neoadjuvant ADT with primary external beam radiation (EBRT) to the prostate suggest a survival benefit for some patients with palpable primary tumors (T2 +). As expected and shown in early trials, ADT resulted in prolongation of time to disease progression. Radiation Therapy Oncology Group (RTOG) studies with combined hormonal therapy and radiation in patients have formed the foundation for the combined approach in North America. The data in various studies suggest a survival benefit for the combined approach **only in subsets** of patients based on their Gleason Scores and PSA levels. Preliminary subset analyses of 2 different studies (RTOG 8610 and 9202) and more mature information in another study (RTOG 8531) suggest that good-risk patients (Gleason 6 or less) may benefit from a relatively short course of neoadjuvant plus concomitant ADT and EBRT (4 months), whereas patients with Gleason of 8 or higher will most likely benefit from a longer course of ADT of two years only RTOG 853 demonstrated an improvement in overall survival with permanent hormonal therapy and radiation. EORTC study 22863, which included poor risk patients (based on clinical stage and Gleason scores) is the only study that demonstrated an **overall** survival advantage for the combined approach employing 3 years on ADT plus EBRT vs. EBRT alone. Ongoing trials in the United States designed to address the effects of combined ADT and EBRT in the different groups of patients should provide a better definition of the benefits of ADT in patients receiving primary EBRT. None of these studies was designed to address the question of immediate vs. deferred treatment since strict criteria for implementation of deferred treatment was not predefined. Again, these studies did not utilize the PSA test as the criteria for initiation of deferred treatment.

The data on the surgical adjuvant ADT is more limited. There are very few well-conducted clinical trials, and none of the studies provides a definitive conclusion. The surgical adjuvant study reported by ECOG investigators in patients with surgically treated, pathologically staged, stage D1 (N + , M0) patients, despite its shortcomings [6,7], provides the best contemporary data on the subject. The results of this study were succinctly reported and discussed by Dr. Trump. As with the data reported in patients with M + disease and in the radiation series, the ECOG study was designed to implement ADT at the time of objective disease progression (evidence of new sites of disease on physical exam and/or x-rays or scans) and not based on evidence of PSA relapse.

In another large, international, multi-institutional, prospectively randomized, placebo-controlled study of 8,000 patients with clinically localized disease treated with a variety of local treatments (surgery or a form of radiation) or no local treatment were randomized to immediate (''adjuvant'') treatment with bicalutamide (150 mg/day) or an identical placebo. This large prospective randomized study (which actually represents 3 different studies analysed under one umbrella) is also known as the early prostate cancer study. The benefits regarding disease progression observed are certainly not unexpected since they represent a known effect of early endocrine treatment. In view of its premature disclosure, it is doubtful that the results of this study will ever provide any reliable definitive information on survival. However with a median follow-up of 5.4 years in the watchful waiting group there were 25% of deaths on the bicaluta-Arm compared to 20% on placebo (HR-1.2, 95% C.I., 1.0–1.5)

Can one extrapolate from the existing data that the use of ADT should be routinely considered in all patients where the only evidence of disease activity is a rise in serum PSA levels? My answer is a categorical *no*! Prior to discussing the potential merits of ADT in these patients, it becomes imperative to evaluate our current knowledge about their natural history. The best information regarding the outcome of these patients is the data derived from our own institution involving patients who underwent a radical retropubic prostatectomy and received no ADT until evidence of distant metastasis. The Johns Hopkins experience initially reported by Pound et al. [9] clearly indicates a spectrum of outcomes ranging from a large proportion of patients who, in view of their long natural history, are unlikely to develop clinical evidence of metastatic disease during their lifetime to those that presented with evidence of bone metastasis with a median time to progression (from the first evidence of PSA relapse until bone scan progression) of about 4 years. Important predictors of outcome in that report included time of PSA relapse following radical prostatectomy (before or after 2 years), gleason score of the prostatectomy specimen (7 or less vs. 8–10) and PSA doubling time (>10.8 months or ≤10.8 months). At this time our current data suggest that the PSADT is the most important prediction for development of distant metastasis and prostate cancer specific survival [10,11]. While the Johns Hopkins experience continues to be updated, physicians, at this point, have information from existing data to identify the group of patients at high risk for early development of metastasis in whom early interventions may be a reasonable consideration. It is important to note, however, that simply identifying the patient's risk is not a sufficient argument for implementing treatment. The role of ADT in these patients should be tested in well-designed, prospectively randomized clinical trials.

Undoubtedly, the most important therapeutic limitation of ADT is hormone independence. Evidence of clonal heterogeneity usually is present at very early stages of the disease and hormone independence is an early biological manifestation of prostate cancer. The apoptotic cascade that follows androgen deprivation kills a significant portion of prostate cancer cells, but is not curative both in laboratory models and humans [12]. In the Dunning R3327 rat adenocarcinoma model of early treatment, when tumors are smaller than 2.0 cm, treatment prolongs survival but is not curative [13]. Additional laboratory experiments clearly indicate that tumor cell proliferation continues even after the maximum effects of apoptosis have been reached and the activation of survival pathways appears to be amplified [12,14]. Long-term benefit of ADT in animals (equivalent to survival in humans) is greatly dependent on tumor burden, and the data suggest that only very small tumors will benefit from this approach. While these data would support the hypothesis for the conduct of adjuvant trials, it is unlikely that such approach (ADT) by itself is sufficiently active to result in a significant survival advantage when tumor burden is most likely above the threshold required for cures or major long-term benefits, such as in patients with recurrent disease. This argument is supported by the clinical data available thus far.

As the controversy involving the issue of "early vs. deferred" hormone therapy perpetuates itself in proportion to the development of the mechanism of immortality of a cancer cell, patients and physicians alike need to deal with the quandary on what to do when prostate cancer relapses biochemically. Once again, our specialty is plagued and punished by our inability to address and adequately answer critical clinical questions that influence standards of care. It seems that urological oncologists always "know the answers" and possess the unique ability to fail when it comes to addressing critical questions. In our own institution, we make vigorous attempts to offer these patients the opportunity to enter into reasonable studies either in our own center or elsewhere. Unfortunately, at this point, most studies are only available in a few select institutions and involve only a handful of the several promising new compounds developed in oncology. Many of these difficulties relate to the fact that methodology for drug development in this population is unclear at the present time. Similarly, there are no large-scale trials conducted by the U.S cooperative groups specifically designed to address standard-of-care issues in this patient population. Some of the critical questions regarding the management of these patients are best answered (perhaps even **only** answered) within the context of well-designed prospective studies. Among these are: study of the natural history, prognostic factors, role of surrogate endpoints, assessment of treatment effects, and a prospective validation of outcome measures, among others. In view of the magnitude of the problem and the extent of unanswered questions. and given the wealth of laboratory and clinical information describing the limitations of ADT, we recommend that treatment be witheld as long as possible in those patients who are not enrolled in clinical trials.

REFERENCES

1. Byar DP, Corle DK. Hormone therapy for prostate cancer: results of the Veterans Administration Cooperative Urological Research Group studies. NCI Monogr 1988; 7:165.
2. Byar DP. Proceedings: the Veterans Administration Co-operative Urological Research Group's studies of cancer of the prostate. Cancer 1973; 32:1126–1130.
3. Immediate versus deferred treatment for advanced prostatic cancer: initial results of the Medical Research Council. Prostate Cancer Working Party Investigators Group. Br J Urol 1997; 79:235–246.
4. Walsh PC, DeWeese TL, Eisenberger MA. A structured debate: immediate versus deferred androgen suppression in prostate cancer-evidence for deferred treatment. J Urol 2001; 166:508–516.

5. D'Amico AV. Radiation and hormonal therapy for locally advanced and clinically localized prostate cancer. Urology 2002; 60(suppl 3A):32–38.

6. Messing E, Manola J, Sarosdy M, Wilding G, Crawford ED, Trump D. Immediate hormonal therapy compared with observation after radical prostatectomy and pelvic lymphadenectomy in men with node-positive prostate cancer. N Engl J Med 1999; 341:1781–1788.

7. Eisenberger MA, Walsh PC. Early androgen deprivation for prostate cancer?. N Engl J Med 1999; 341:1837–1838.

8. See WA, Wirth MP, McLeod DG, et al. Bicalutamide as immediate therapy either alone or as adjuvant to standard care of patients with localized or locally advanced prostate cancer: First analysis of early prostate cancer program. J Urol 2002; 168: 429–435.

9. Pound CR, Partin AW, Eisenberger MA, et al. Natural history of progression after PSA elevation following radical prostatectomy. JAMA 1999; 281:1591–1597.

10. Lassiter LK, Eisenberger MA. The dilemma of patients with a rising PSA level after definitive local therapy for prostate cancer. Seminars in Urological Oncology. 2002; 20:146–154.

11. Laufer M, Pound CR, Carducci M, Eisenberger MA. The management of patients with rising prostate specific antigen after radical prostatectomy. Urology 2000; 55: 395–396.

12. Denmeade SR, Lin XS, Isaacs JT. Role of programmed (apoptotic) cell death during the progression and therapy for prostate cancer. Prostate 1996; 28:251–265.

13. Isaacs JT. The timing of androgen ablation and/or chemotherapy in the treatment of prostatic cancer. Prostate 1984; 5:1–9.

14. Green DR, Evan GI. A matter of life and death. Cancer Cell 2002; 1:19–30.

EDITORIAL COMMENTARY

Edward M. Messing

Professor and Chair, Department of Urology, University of Rochester Medical Center, Rochester, NY, USA

The arguments presented by Dr. Trump and the subsequent guidelines he provides, in the absence of direct clinical trials addressing the question of the timing of androgen deprivation in PSA-only failures following radical prostatectomy, are quite solid, and I am in agreement with almost all of them. This should not come as a great surprise, since we were coinvestigators on the ECOG study referred to in his article[1]. That study, although probably the closest prospective randomized controlled trial available for the circumstance that Dr. Trump was asked to discuss, did not directly address the question of PSA failure after prostatectomy. For example, we do not know if patients in the deferred arm of that study had received androgen ablative therapies upon biochemical failure rather than at the time of positive bone scans (which is when such treatment was administered in the overwhelming majority of observed men) whether the differences in survival (which now, at ten years median follow-up, are immediate treatment:

72.3% and deferred: 49.0% [p = 0.025] for overall survival; and immediate treatment: 87.2% and deferred: 56.9% [p = 0.001] for disease-specific survival) would have occurred. It should be remembered that, despite the patients in the ECOG study having nodal metastases and the majority in each arm having large primary tumors with extraprostatic extent, they had only miniscule quantities of disease when hormone therapy was initiated. Indeed, roughly 80% of patients in both arms had undetectable PSAs after their surgeries at the time of randomization. This is distinctly different from all of the other studies to which Dr. Trump refers, in which patients had much larger quantities of cancer at the time of initiating hormone therapy.

That the quantity of prostate cancer cells might predict both the intensity and longevity of the response to hormone therapy should come as no surprise. First, cancers are known to stimulate their own growth through autocrine, juxtacrine, and paracrine mechanisms, the last two of which are negated when there is a low tumor burden. In addition, the incidence of hormonally independent prostate cancer cells has been estimated in an elegant xenograph tumor model[2] to be between one per 10^5 to one per 10^6 cells. In this model, the original human tumor xenograft was obtained from osseous metastases in a patient whose cancer already had progressed in the face of standard androgen ablative therapy. Thus, it is likely that in the hormonally "naïve" cancer, the incidence of androgen independent cells is far lower. One could ask, in terms of the ECOG study, when PSA was undetectable whether there were so few prostate cancer cells (i.e., below 10^5 to 10^6 cancer cells) remaining that no denovo androgen independent cells existed when androgen ablative therapy was started. That, at 10 years follow-up in that study, fewer than 30% of all patients receiving immediate androgen deprivation have demonstrated any sign of disease recurrence (even biochemical failure), and that less than 13% have succumbed to their disease, indicates that, while patients may not be cured of their malignancy, the quantity of androgen independent cells they had was very few.

However, it is not known how many prostate cancer cells are necessary to produce a detectable and rising PSA level. While this number undoubtedly varies with different tumor and host characteristics, it is quite possible that often far more than 10^6 cancer cells must be present before PSA becomes detectable in serum. Were this the case, numerous androgen independent cancer cells would already exist at the time of initiating androgen ablative therapy, if it was started when PSA became detectable. In such circumstances, while overall tumor growth initially would be suppressed, this may not translate into dramatic improvements in survival[3,4].

Another question that Dr. Trump raises is, even if androgen ablative therapies could retard disease progression and ultimately prolong prostate cancer specific survival, if not overall survival, would all patients who were PSA failures after radical prostatectomy require such therapy? At least part of the answer will await future clinical trials, but, in the absence of specific information, the data reported by Pound, et al.[5] and what is known about the patient's life expectancy (based on current health status, other comorbidities, lifestyle, inheritance, etc.) must be considered. In general, for patients who have a high likelihood of progressing to metastatic disease within 5 years (Gleason 8–10 cancers, PSA doubling times of 10 months or less, or having developed a detectable PSA 2 years or less postprostatectomy), and certainly those who share more than one of these features[5], the likelihood of having systemic disease (even in the face of imaging studies, including a Prostascint scan, that are negative for disease outside the prostatic bed) is quite high. Furthermore, these are exactly the patients who tend to fail most commonly when they have received salvage prostatic-bed radiation following prostatectomy [6]. It would be in this group particularly that I would recommend the use of androgen ablative therapy. Whether such treatment associated with the morbidities that Dr. Trump has outlined are justified for men with more favorable prognostic indicators is more debatable, and, in this group, salvage radiation or even observation until far later in the course of the disease would seem appealing. If radiation was chosen, commencing it before PSA reaches 1 to 1.5 ng/mL appears to be important to maximize its benefit [7]. Again, the guidelines that Dr. Trump provides seem quite reasonable for most of these patients.

Two related questions that warrant discussion are, what exactly defines PSA failure after prostatectomy and what other means of androgen ablation, such as the use of high dose antiandrogens or intermittent hormonal therapy—both of which may lessen some of the morbidities of standard castrative therapy—might be worth investigating?

In terms of the definition of PSA failure, some patients have a detectable, but not rising PSA after prostatectomy. This observation was addressed in a retrospective series by Amling et al., who reported that over 50% of the patients whose maximal PSAs within 3 years after prostatectomy were at .2–.29 ng/mL did not, following 7 more years of observation, experience PSA progression, while only 28% of patients whose PSAs reached .4–.49 ng/mL by 3 years postsurgery did not (and about 25% of those whose PSAs did not subsequently progress received treatment at the .40–.49 ng/mL value—perhaps explaining their failure to progress) [8]. The authors advocated using .4ng/mL as the definition of PSA failure. While in these days of microassays and frequent PSA monitoring (particularly once the PSA becomes detectable on a microassay), most patients (and many urologists) do not feel comfortable withholding treatment until a value of .4 ng/mL is reached, it should be remembered that many patients with a PSA in the .2 ng/mL range or below would not have progressed if left untreated. Which patients in the .2 ng/mL to .4 ng/mL range need treatment, or benefit from it, can best be answered in a prospective clinical trial. However, in studies where additional tissue is removed at the time of prostatectomy, even in very experienced hands, the frequent identification of residual normal prostatic glands and acini may explain the benign outlook in some patients whose PSAs become detectable after surgery [9]. In patients where the PSA becomes undetectable again after either radiation or androgen ablative therapy, the undetectable PSA should not be taken as conclusive evidence that cancer was present at the time these salvage treatments were administered.

In terms of alternative means of androgen ablation that are already available, the two that have been most widely tested are high does antiandrogens or intermittent hormone therapy. The latter, when first advocated by Herr et al., was used primarily to improve quality of life, particularly sexual functioning [10]. Subsequently, this has been suggested by others as well [11]. However, intermittent therapy is more difficult to schedule in someone who has a very low PSA (e.g., under .1 ng/mL or even under .2 ng/mL) than in the patient with metastatic disease who, as Dr. Trump correctly points out, usually has PSAs in the 40 to 50 ng/mL range. For instance, both how long to maintain an undetectable PSA level, which would be quickly achieved in almost all men, and, after cessation of treatment, what PSA level would trigger restarting hormonal therapy are uncertain.

Similarly, while antiandrogens alone appear to have less of an impact on libido, erectile functioning, hematocrit, fatigue, and bone density than castrative therapies[12], specific studies to quantify the effects, particularly in slender Caucasians who tend to have the highest risk for osteoporotic fractures with prolonged castrative therapies[13], have not been well established.

Moreover, if either treatment will be as effective as standard castrative approaches in terms of arresting the tumor is unknown. Additionally, there are significant incremental costs (since high-dose antiandrogens alone are currently neither approved by the FDA nor paid for by most commercial insurance companies, and intermittent therapy usually is administered with total androgen blockade) which must be kept in mind in view of the roughly 30,000+ men each year who, as Dr. Trump correctly indicated, are likely to be PSA failures after prostatectomy. The economic magnitude of such treatment regimens are not trivial, particularly if non traditional hormone approaches are to be administered over very long periods of time. In the absence of specific data confirming the benefits of either of these two approaches in terms of efficacy or morbidity, I usually recommend antiandrogens alone for few postprostatectomy PSA failures, except for those men who have an extremely strong desire to retain libido and potency. For the majority of patients with PSA failure after prostatectomy, I support using the guidelines offered by Dr. Trump.

REFERENCES

1. Messing EM, Manola J, Sarosdy M, Wilding G, Crawford ED, Trump D. Immediate hormonal therapy compared with observation after radical prostatectomy and pelvic lymphadenectomy in men with node-positive prostate cancer. N Engl J Med 1999; 341(24):1781–1788.

2. Craft N, Chhor C, Tran C, et al. Evidence for clonal outgrowth of androgen-independent prostate cancer cells from androgen-dependent tumors through a two step process. Cancer Research 1999; 59:5020–5036.

3. The Medical Research Council Prostate Cancer Working Party Investigators Group. Immediate versus deferred treatment for advanced prostatic cancer: initial results of the Medical Research Council Trial. Br J Urol 1997; 79:235–246.

4. The Veterans Administration Cooperative Urological Research Group. Treatment and survival of patients with cancer of the prostate. Surg Gynecol Obstet 1967; 124:1011–1017.

5. Pound CR, Partin AW, Eisenberger MA, Chan DW, Pearson JD, Walsh PC. Natural history of progression after PSA elevation following prostatectomy. J Amer Med Assoc 1999; 281(17):1591–1597.

6. Slawin KM. Radiation therapy after radical prostatectomy: why patience is a virtue! The case for salvage radiation therapy. Reviews in Urology 2002; 4:90.

7. Kadmon D. Radiation therapy after radical prostatectomy: strike early, strike hard! The case for adjuvant radiation therapy. Reviews in Urol 2002; 4(2):87.

8. Amling CL, Bergstralh EJ, Blute ML, Slezak JM, Zincke H. Defining prostate specific antigen progression after radical prostatectomy: what is the most appropriate cut point?. J Urol 2001; 165(4):1146–1151.

9. Shah O, Melamed J, Lepor H. Analysis of soft tissue margins during radical retropubic prostatectomy. J Urol 2001; 165:1943–1948.

10. Herr H. Intermittent hormone therapy for advance prostate cancer. J Urol 1987; 137:255A (abstract).

11. Akukura K, Bruchovsky N, Goldenberg SL, et al. Effects of intermittent androgen suppression on androgen-dependent tumors: apoptosis and serum prostate-specific antigen. Cancer 1993; 71:2782–2790.

12. Iversen P, Tyrrell C, Karisary A, et al. Casodex (bicalutamide) 150 mg monotherapy compared with castration in patients with previously untreated nonmetastatic prostate cancer: results from two multicenter randomized trials at a median follow-up of 4 years. Urology 1998; 51:389.

13. Oefelein MG, Ricchuiti V, Conrad W, et al. Skeletal fracture associated with androgen suppression induced osteoporosis: the clinical independence and risk factors for patients with prostate cancer. J Urol 2001; 166(5):1724–1728.

EDITORIAL COMMENTARY

E. David Crawford

Professor of Surgery and Radiation Oncology, University of Colorado Health Sciences Center, Denver, Colorado, USA

Hormone therapy or androgen deprivation for prostate cancer has historically been considered a palliative, but not curative, treatment. Its use has been reserved for evidence of progressive, recurrent, or symptomatic disease, i.e., metastatic cancer [1]. Nevertheless, as mentioned by Dr. Trump, this is an effective therapy for a lot of men. Ninety-five percent respond, and, in 10%, this ''response'' lasts 10 years: this may even be labeled a cure. This is certainly better than current therapies for metastatic colon, breast, and lung cancers.

The significant side effects associated with hormone treatment and their impact on quality of life for patients with prostate cancer are reasons clinicians have traditionally delayed its use until advanced-stage disease. Yet, radiotherapy, brachytherapy, and prostatectomy, which are considered potentially curative, have at least as much impact and as many side effects as hormone treatment.

Nearly two-thirds of newly diagnosed patients with prostate cancer are now treated with radiation or surgery. Nonetheless, a significant number of patients with successful initial treatment will experience ''biochemical'' failure: a rise in PSA levels after local therapy has failed. For example, patients with Gleason Scores of 8–10 have a 75% risk of recurrence within 4–5 years [2]. In our revision to the A-B-C-D staging system, this category was designated as D1.5, signifying its intermediate classification [3]. It is in this growing population of patients that hormone therapy is being used more frequently, and more controversially, than previously. As mentioned by Dr. Trump, we do not have a large randomized clinical trial to address the proper therapy in men with biochemical failure.

In discussions of the merits of the earlier use of hormone therapy in patients with prostate cancer, the prevailing notion that such therapy is not curative needs to be reexamined. Although optimal combination treatment with radiation and hormone therapy has been established for patients at high risk for disease recurrence, similar regimens for adjuvant use of hormone therapy in patients who have undergone radical prostatectomy have not been defined. We have compiled data showing 10-year survival rates of 5% to 7% for patients with metastatic disease who were treated with hormone therapy [4]; by some definitions, these patients would be considered cured.

In his article, Trump carefully reviews current evidence in the literature showing that early hormone therapy confers a survival advantage to some patients with prostate cancer.

Several studies conducted in patients representing disease stages sharing similar characteristics to biochemical failure have revealed a survival advantage from earlier treatment. Several of these studies—the Veterans Administration studies [5], the Medical Research Council study [6], studies with hormone therapy plus adjuvant radiation [7,8], and the Eastern Cooperative Oncology Group (ECOG) study [9]—are reviewed. These studies may help guide clinicians in treating patients with biochemical failure. My conclusions are a little different than Dr. Trump, focusing on even earlier therapy. Below is my synopsis:

VETERANS ADMINISTRATION STUDIES (T3)

Three initial studies were undertaken by the Veterans Administration Cooperative Urological Research Group (VACURG) between 1960 and 1975. Patients were randomized to receive therapy with diethylstilbestrol (DES) or orchiectomy in the first study, increasing doses of DES in the second, and DES and placebo in the third. Pooled analyses of all three studies demonstrated a slight advantage in survival in favor of early hormone initiation in patients with T3 tumors [5]. Complicating these analyses were the high rates of death because of cardiovascular disease in patients treated with DES. Nonetheless, patients with more advanced disease did show a clear survival benefit from hormonal treatment initiated immediately following diagnosis.

MEDICAL RESEARCH COUNCIL STUDY

The Medical Research Council study randomized patients with nonmetastatic T3 disease to one of two arms: either early, lifelong hormone therapy in conjunction with orchiectomy or therapy with a luteinizing hormone releasing hormone (LHRH) agonist or delayed therapy begun at the appearance of symptoms [6]. Early treatment was associated with a decreased incidence of comorbid events, including urinary retention, pathologic fractures, and ureteric obstruction. The study showed a significant survival advantage among the patients who received early hormone intervention (Figure 1) [6].

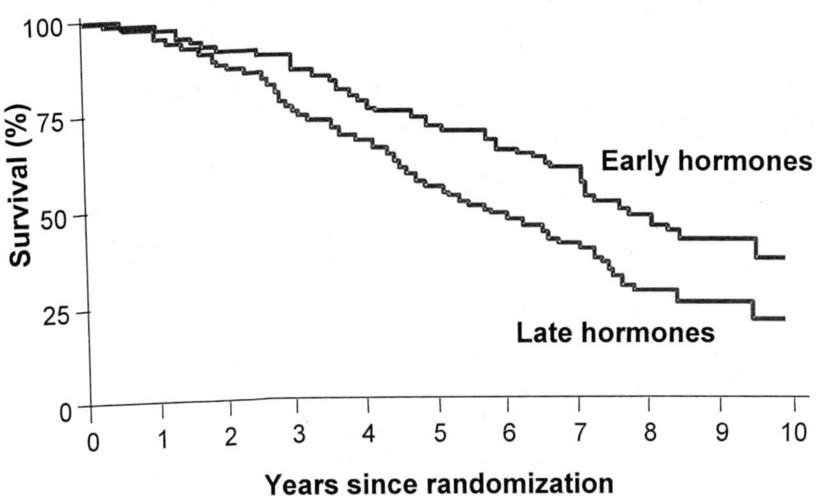

FIGURE 1　Nonmetastatic disease: survival benefit for earlier hormonal therapy. Reprinted with permission from Medical Research Council Prostate Cancer Working Party Investigators Group [6].

HORMONAL THERAPY PLUS RADIATION: THE EUROPEAN ORGANIZATION PLUS RADIATION AND RADIATION THERAPY ONCOLOGY GROUP 8610

The European Organization for Research and Treatment of Cancer (EORTC) documented that 3 years of adjuvant treatment with an LHRH agonist combined with external irradiation significantly improved local control and survival in patients with locally advanced prostate cancer (T3), compared with radiation therapy alone (Figure 2) [8]. Kaplan-Meier estimates of overall survival at 5 years were 79% in patients who received combination therapy and 62% in patients who received radiation alone. Of the patients receiving combined therapy, 85% were disease free at 5 years, compared with only 48% of those treated with radiation monotherapy.

Another trial, testing 4 months of hormone therapy plus radiation vs. radiation along among patients with locally advanced prostate cancer, was conducted by the Radiation Therapy Oncology Group (RTOG 8610) [7]. The results revealed improved local control in the patients receiving combined therapy (84% vs. 71%), as well as lack of biochemical failure (46% vs. 21%). Long-term follow-up studies indicated that combination therapy was associated with highly significant im-

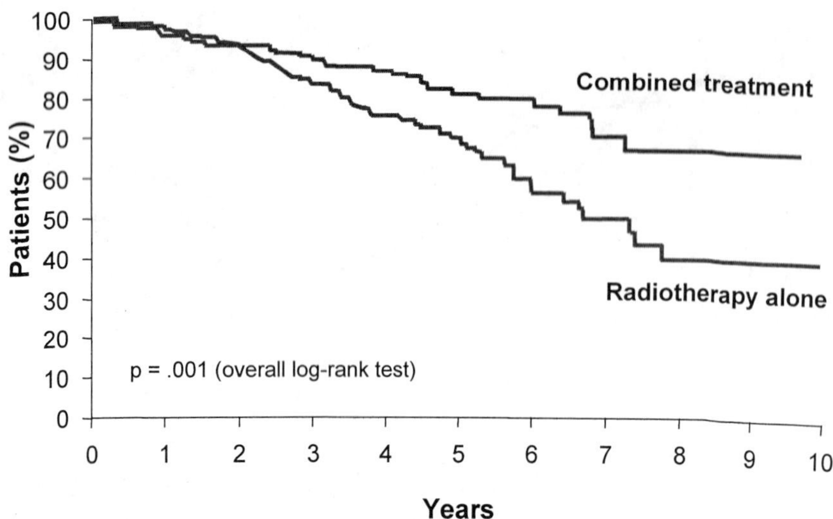

FIGURE 2   Nonmetastatic disease: survival benefit of radiation plus LHRH agonist analogue therapy. The overall survival rate at 5 years was 79% (95% confidence interval (CI), 72%–86%) for combined LHRH therapy and radiation, vs. 62% (95% CI, 52%–72%) for radiation alone. Reprinted from Ref. [7].

provement in local control, reduction in disease progression, and longer overall survival in patients with lower Gleason scores [8].

EASTERN COOPERATIVE ONCOLOGY GROUP (D1)

In a study conducted by the Eastern Cooperative Oncology Group (ECOG), patients who had undergone radical prostatectomy and pelvic lymphadenectomy and who were found to have nodal metastases (D1) were randomly assigned to immediate treatment with initiation of antiandrogen therapy (n = 47) or to observation until disease progression (n = 51) [9]. Median followup was 7.1 years (range, 3 to 10 years). Patients receiving immediate antiandrogen therapy demonstrated improved survival and reduced risk of recurrence, in addition to decreased morbidity (Table 1), as compared with the patients who were merely observed. The median PSA at which treatment was initiated in the observation arm was between 12 and 15 ng/mL. Disease-specific survival rates at 10 years of follow-up were 94.6% for patients receiving early treatment vs. 68.6% for those receiving late hormone therapy. Likewise, progression-free survival rates at 10 years were 75% for those receiving early treatment vs. 18.8% for those in whom treatment was delayed (Figure 3) [10]. Although this was a small study, these differences in overall survival and progression-free survival were significant. Approximately 70% of patients in this study had an undectable PSA when randomized. So, men in this trial actually had less disease, as ascertained by serum PSA, than men with a rising PSA. This is a clinical trial that seems to support very early treatment for biochemical failure.

Identifing factors that predict a poor outcome may help define a subgroup of patients who would derive significant benefit from early hormone treatment. A number of studies have assessed the prognostic value of different measures that correlate with the risk of distant failure. Analyses based on 10-year actuarial estimates of PSA outcomes after radical prostatectomy identified 3 risk groups of

TABLE 1. Early v. Late Hormonae Therapy: Survival and Disease Progression After a Median Follow-up of 7.1 Years

	Immediate Hormonae Therapy (n = 47)	Observation (n = 51)	p Value
Death (prostate cancer)	6.4%	31.4%	< .01
Progression	14.9%	82.4%	< .001

Data from Reft. (9).

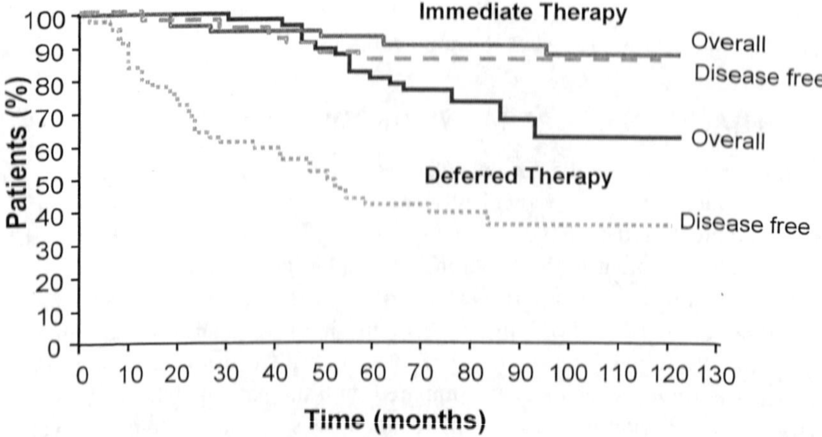

FIGURE 3   ECOG: disease-free and overall survival. Kaplan-Meier estimates of overall survival and disease-free survival in patients receiving immediate versus deferred hormonal therapy. Adapted from Ref. [9].

patients by preoperative PSA levels, biopsy Gleason Score, and clinical category (Table 2) [10]. Other prognostic indicators that correlate with poor outcome and may influence therapy selection include a Gleason sum of 8 or more, positive seminal vesicle (pT3b), tumor invasion of adjacent structures (pT4), nodal metastases (N1), and positive surgical margins [11]. Nomograms that can make accurate predictions of PSA failure have been developed and validated [12]. We have developed several artificial neural network programs to predict outcome. These can be found at www.prostatecalculator.org

TABLE 2.   Survival and Recurrence Rates Among Risk Groups for PSA Failure

Risk Group	Disease Stage	Gleason Score	PSA (ng/mL)	Relative Risk of PSA Failure (Study Cohort)	10-Year PSA Failure-Free Survival
Low	T1c to T2a	≤ 6	≤ 10	1	83%
Intermediate	T2b	7	10-20	3.8 (CI, 2.6-5.7)	46%
High	T2C or higher	≥ 8	> 20	9.6 (CI, 6.6-13.9)	29%

CI = confidence interval
Data from Ref. (10).

The use of chemotherapy in prostate cancer has generally produced poor response rates, and, for this reason, like hormone therapy, it has been relegated to palliative treatment of late-stage, hormone-refractory disease. However, experience in breast and colon cancers suggests that adjuvant chemotherapy, if it is administered at an earlier stage when tumor burden is low, may be more effective than previously thought. In breast and colon cancers, chemotherapy significantly improves survival when used early as an adjuvant therapy [??] but, in the metastatic setting, it provides little benefit [12,13]. When considering the adjuvant use of chemotherapy in patients with prostate cancer, however, the clinician must weigh the risks against the benefits, as the safety profile of cytotoxic therapy may be unacceptable in asymptomatic men whose only qualifying criterion is a rising PSA level.

A important question is, why wait for biochemical failure and then argue about treatment? We can define a group of men who are at risk of failing and then consider the use of adjuvant therapy in these men. The Southwest Oncology Group (SWOG) recently launched an international, randomized trial, SWOG-9921/Cancer and Leukemia Group B (CALGB), to examine the role of adjuvant chemotherapy for patients at high risk (as defined by Gleason Score, tumor size, and margin status) of relapse after radical prostatectomy [15]. The patients are randomly assigned to treatment for 2 years with adjuvant androgen deprivation therapy either alone or combined with mitoxantrone plus oral prednisone following surgery. Radiation therapy may also be administered at the investigator's discretion. The primary study end points are overall survival and disease-free survival among these high-risk patients with localized prostate cancer.

SUMMARY

Biochemical failure is common following a number of local therapies, including radical prostatectomy. There are no large, randomized clinical trials to address the timing and type of therapy. Therefore, decisions need to be made based on data in other stages of prostate cancer. Several trials support a survival advantage with early hormone intervention for prostate cancer. The Medical Research Council trial clearly shows a decrease in comorbid events and a survival advantage in patients with T3 disease. The RTOG study also showed an advantage. Cooperative group studies have demonstrated a significant advantage among patients with microscopic nodal disease. Thus, these studies provide a rationale for investigating the use of early hormone therapy in patients with a rising PSA level after failed local therapy. The same hypothesis, that early treatment can offer a survival advantage, is being evaluated in the SWOG 9221/CALGB trial to determine whether chemotherapy has a place in the treatment of early stage patients at risk for developing metastatic disease. Ongoing studies are evaluating such factors as the length of therapy and the choice of agents and modalities in selected patient groups. Future studies should continue this important work of identifying patients who are at a heightened risk of disease progression and who might prolong their survival with adjuvant therapies. The side effects of these therapies must be weighed against potential benefits. I agree with most of Dr Trump's conclusions: patients should be entered into clinical trials, we should be testing novel new agents and approaches, and the side effects of treatment must be weighed against potential benefits. However, in men with biochemical failure, I treat before the PSA gets "to 15 or 20 ng/mL." This was the same value in the observation arm of the positive node study discussed earlier in which a difference was observed for earlier therapy. So consider treatment when PSA is less than 2 ng/mL. This should give some time to evaluate PSA velocity. The next question is how long do you treat? Should it be lifelong? Should it be for a set period of time, 1, 2, 3, 5 years? Again, we only have some data from the previously discussed trials, which varied from 3 years to lifelong.

REFERENCES

1. Crawford ED, De Antoni EP, Labrie F, Schroder FH and Geller J. Endocrine Therapy of Prostate Cancer: Optimal Form and Appropriate Timing. J Clin Endocrin & Metab 80(4):1062–1078, 1995.

2. Roach M, Lu J, Pilepich MV, et al. Predicting long-term survival, and the need for hormonal therapy: a meta-analysis of RTOG prostate cancer trials. Int J Radiat Oncol Biol Phys 2000; 47:617–627.

3. Crawford ED, Blumenstein BA. Proposed substages for metastatic prostate cancer. Urology 1997; 50:1027–1028.

4. Crawford D, Faulkner J, Thompson I, et al:. Ten-year survival in patients with metastatic (M+) prostate cancer (CAP): analysis of Southwest Oncology Group (SWOG) 8894 [abstract]. Last update: 2002. Available at: http://aua.agora.com/abstractviewer/av_view.asp Accessed July 2, 2002.

5. Byar DP, Corle DK. Hormone therapy for prostate cancer: results of the Veterans Administration Cooperative Urological Research Group Studies. U.S. Department of Health and Human Services, Public Health Service. NIH 1988:165–170.

6. Medical Research Council Prostate Cancer Working Party Investigators Group. Immediate versus deferred treatment for advanced prostatic cancer: initial results of the Medical Research Council Trial. Br J Urol 1997; 79:235–246.

7. Bolla M, Gonzalez D, Warde P, et al. Improved survival in patients with locally advanced prostate cancer treated with radiotherapy and goserelin. N Engl J Med 1997; 337:295–300.

8. Pilepich MV, Krall JM, Al-Sarraf M, et al. Androgen deprivation with radiation therapy compared with radiation therapy alone for locally advanced prostatic carcinoma: a randomized comparative trial of the Radiation Therapy Oncology Group. Urology 1995; 45:616–623.

9. Messing EM, Manola J, Sarosdy M, et al. Immediate hormonal therapy compared with observation after radical prostatectomy and pelvic lymphadenectomy in men with node-positive prostate cancer. N Engl J Med 1999; 341:1781–1788.

10. D'Amico AV, Whittington R, Malkowicz SB, et al. Predicting prostate specific antigen outcome preoperatively in the prostate specific antigen era. J Urol 2001; 166:2185–2188.
11. Graefen M, Karakiewicz PI, Cagiannos I, et al. Validation study of the accuracy of a postoperative nomogram for recurrence after radical prostatectomy for localized prostate cancer. J Clin Oncol 2002; 20:951–956.
12. Ross PL, Gerigk C, Gonen M, et al. Comparisons of nomograms and urologists' predictions in prostate cancer. Semin Urol Oncol 2002; 20:82–88.
13. Duric V, Stockler M. Patients' preferences for adjuvant chemotherapy in early breast cancer: a review of what makes it worthwhile. Lancet Oncol 2001; 2:691–697.
14. Crawford ED. Immediate versus delayed therapy for prostate cancer. Family Urology 2002; VI:18–21.

EDITORIAL OVERVIEW

Kenneth B. Cummings

Trump provides a scholarly overview of the timing of androgen deprivation following PSA failure in patients who have undergone local therapy. He aptly points out early in the chapter that there are no randomized clinical trials from which data are available to address this issue. He observes that lacking clinical trials data, one is forced to address this issue by examining the natural history of PSA failure following local therapy and drawing inferences from studies in related situations. Unfortunately, upon review of a large series from institutions in which significant numbers of patients have been treated, the inconsistency in pattern of care with variable use of androgen deprivation has made observations on the natural history of PSA failure after prostatectomy almost impossible.

He cites data from the Hopkins series reported by Pound et al. [1] in which 304 men who underwent anatomic radical prostatectomy had no systemic or local therapy until the discovery of metastatic disease. From this, factors predictive of clinical evident metastasis following prostatectomy include the short interval from surgery to PSA detection (less than 2 years), PSA doubling time (less than 10 months), Gleason Score 7 or more. There are limitations to these data, the follow-up is relatively short, with only 36% of patients having been followed for more than 10 years, and the number of men with metastasis is small (103). 43% of these men died of prostate cancer, and no man who had developed metastatic disease died of other causes. Median survival after recognition of metastasis was slightly less than 5 years, with the only variable predictive of survival being the interval between the surgery and detectable metastatic disease. An interval of 1–3 years was associated with a median survival of slightly less than 5 years, while the median survival has not yet been reached for those men whose metastasis were detected more than 8 years following prostatectomy.

These data are pure in that they do reflect the natural history of a population with prostate cancer following radical prostatectomy and prognostic factors related to the timing of metastatic disease, but do not contribute any insight into the appropriate timing or androgen deprivation to alter a pattern of survival or which subgroup would benefit from such treatment. He cites the initial work of Huggins and Hodges, who received the Nobel Prize for their work in demonstrating that androgen deprivation therapy for prostate cancer is very good treatment for advanced disease [2].

He cites several animal studies where early androgen deprivation appears to be beneficial with respect to tumor progression [3–5].

Trump further examines the 1967 Veteran's Affairs Collaborative Urologic Research Group (VACURG) and examines their conclusions as well as the subsequent subset analysis, which are conflicting because of flaws in subset design [6]. Walsh and colleagues have reassessed the VACURG studies, focusing on comparisons of orchiectomy and placebo patients, and, in this subset analysis, find no indication of improved survival in patients undergoing orchiectomy, albeit the results support the concept that earlier androgen deprivation therapy (ADT) is not useful, but are confounded by the fact that the analysis relies on subgroup results of rather small group sizes [7].

Trump further reviews contemporary studies addressing the role of early vs. delayed androgen deprivation therapy in prostate cancer in a randomized fashion, and is unable, because of study design, to come to a firm conclusion on whether there is a distinct advantage to early vs. delayed therapy [8–10].

When I requested that he write the lead chapter for this text, he had recently contributed as senior author to the ECOG study comparing immediate androgen deprivation in node-positive radical prostatectomy patients vs. observation in which a survival advantage was demonstrated for the androgen deprived patient group [11]. He aptly points retrospectively to the demonstrated flaws in this study and turns his attention to the risks of androgen deprivation therapy (diminished potency, loss of libido, weight gain, loss of muscle strength, breast tenderness and swelling, hot flashes, osteoporosis) and notes that the magnitude and importance of these side effects is uncertain.

Somewhat to my surprise, his conclusion is that until adequate data are available, he does not believe in adjuvant androgen deprivation and believes that ADT should be delayed until the PSA reaches 15–20 ng/mL and would further individualize on a case-by-case basis. He further observes that Wasson et al. surveyed urologists and found that 66% recommended ADT for "PSA-only failure" following prostatectomy—even though most did not believe ADT would increase survival [12].

Crawford, addressing the same subject, while in agreement with most of Dr. Trump's conclusion and affirming the need for appropriate clinical trials as well as the need to weigh treatment with side effects, has a much earlier threshold than 15–20 ng/mL PSA, and, in fact, chooses a PSA of 2 ng/mL. He believes that this should give time to evaluate PSA velocity, but raises a question as to how long treatment should be given; should it be life long or for a period of years? He cites that, at the present time, we only have data on the previously discussed trials, which vary from 3 years to lifelong, and, indeed, the question remains unanswered.

Eisenberger offers a very scholarly review of the subject and, interestingly, raises the same questions regarding the emergence of androgen independence as a herald event to death in the absence of effective chemotherapy. While his position is similar to that of Trump's in that while he favors use of experimental agents while the PSA is rising as part of clinical trials, he prefers to withhold ADT until there is succinct progression.

Messing, who was the lead author on the ECOG Study randomizing node-positive prostatectomy patients to ADT vs. observation [11], as reported by Trump in his article, provides follow-up at 10 years in the ECOG study. Despite the flaws acknowledged by the study that the overall disease burden was considered to be minuscule when treatment was given, those patients who received immediate treatment enjoy a 72.3% survival at 10 years compared to the deferred group with a 49% survival (p = 0.025) and immediate treatment with a 87.2% and deferred at 56.9% (p = 0.001) for disease-specific survival. He further highlights that roughly 80% of patients in both arms had undetectable PSAs after surgery at the time of randomization. This represents a succinctly different group of patients from the studies referred to by Trump in the existing clinical trials, which were reviewed.

Messing further describes alternative means of androgen ablation to those already discussed: (a) High dose antiandrogens [13] or (b) intermittent hormone therapy. The latter, while first advocated by Herr [14] was primarily targeted to improve quality of life, particularly sexual function, than has been examined by others as well [15]. He further points out that neither treatment has been deemed as effective as the standard castrative approach in terms of arresting tumor. Further analysis of the economics of such therapies, which include antiandrogens alone, are currently not approved by the FDA or paid for by commercial insurance, would be a significant economic impact on the roughly 30,000 men each year that Trump correctly indicates are PSA-only failures after prostatectomy.

Despite the forgone discussion by Messing, he, in essence, finds the arguments by Trump agreeable and, in essence, follows a similar approach in patient management.

REFERENCES

1. Pound CR, Partin AW, Eisenberger MA, Chan DW, Pearson JD, Walsh PC. Natural history of progression after PSA elevation following prostatectomy. J Amer Med Assoc 1999; 281(17):1591–1597.

2. Huggins C, Hodges CV. Studies on prostate cancer: effect of castration, of estrogen and of androgen injection on serum phosphatases in metastatic carcinoma of the prostate. Cancer Res 1941; 1:293–297.

3. Nonomura N, Nakamura N, Uchida N, Noguchi S, Sato B, Sonoda T, Matsumoto K. Growth-stimulatory effect androgen-induced autocrine growth factors(s) secreted from Shionogi carcinoma 115 cells on androgen-unresponsive cancer cells in a paracrine mechanism. Cancer Res 1988; 48(17):4904–4908.

4. Isaacs JT. The timing on androgen ablation therapy and/or chemotherapy in the treatment of prostatic cancer. Prostate 1984; 5(1):1–17.

5. Henry JM, Isaacs JT. Relationship between tumor size and the curability of metastatic prostatic cancer by surgery alone or in combination with adjuvant chemotherapy. J Urol 1988; 139(5):1119–1123.

6. The Veterans Adminstration Cooperative Urological Research Group. Treatment and survival of patients with cancer of the prostate. Surg Gynecol Obstet 1967; 124(5): 1011–1017.

7. Walsh PC, Deweese TL, Eisenberger M. A structured debate: Immediate vs. deferred androgen suppression in prostate cancer—evidence for deferred treatment. J Urol 2001; 166:508–516.

8. The Medical Research Council—Prostate Cancer Working Party Investigators Group. Immediate vs. deferred treatment for advanced prostatic cancer: initial results of the Medical Research Council Trial. Br J Urol 1997; 79(2):235–246.

9. Kirk D. Immediate vs deferred hormone treatment for prostate cancer. How safe is androgen deprivation? Medical Research Council—Prostate Working Party Investigators Group. Br J Urol 2000; 86(suppl):220 (abstr).

10. Bolla M, Gonzalex D, Warde P, Dubois JB, Mirimanoff RO, Storme G, Bernier J, Kuten A, Sternberg C, Gil T, Collette L, Pierart M. Improved survival in patients with locally advanced prostate cancer treated with radiotherapy and goserelin. N Engl J Med 1997; 337(5):295–300.

11. Messing EM, Manola J, Sarosdy M, Wilding G, Crawford ED, Trump D. Immediate hormonal therapy compared with observation after radical prostatectomy and pelvic lymphadenectomy in men with node-positive prostate cancer. N Engl J Med 1999; 341(24):1781.

12. Wasson JH, Fowler FJ, Barry MJ. Androgen deprivation therapy for asymptomatic advanced prostate cancer in the prostate specific antigen era: a national survey of urologist beliefs and practices. J Urol 1998; 159:693–696.

13. Iversen P, Tyrrell C, Karisary A, Anderson JB, Baert L, Tammela T, Chamberlain M, Carroll K, Gotting-Smith K, Blackledge GR. Casodex (bicalutamide) 150 mg monotherapy compared with castration in patients with previously untreated nonmetastatic prostate cancer: results from two multicenter randomized trials at a median follow-up of 4 years. Urology 1998(51):389.

14. Herr H. Intermittent hormone therapy for advance prostate cancer. J Urol 1987(137): 255A (abstract).

15. Akukura K, Bruchovsky N, Goldenberg SL, Tenniswood M, Fox K. Effects of intermittent androgen suppression on androgen-dependent tumors: apoptosis and serum prostate-specific antigen. Cancer 1993; 71:2782–2790.

11

Novel Therapies for PSA Progression in the Absence of Imagable Disease Following Local Therapy

Robert S. DiPaola

Associate Professor of Medicine, The Robert Wood Johnson Medical School, University of Medicine and Dentistry of New Jersey, The Cancer Institute of New Jersey, New Brunswick, New Jersey, USA

Prostate cancer is only temporarily controlled with androgen ablation (AA) therapy and subsequent chemotherapy, secondary to the development of molecular mechanisms of resistance [1]. Additionally, molecular mechanisms of tumor resistance are increased in metastatic disease compared to primary tumors [1–7]. Potential mechanisms of resistance to therapy recently have been identified, including the overexpression of bcl-2, p53 mutations, and the multidrug resistance protein MRP [2–9]. For example, the development of androgen-independent disease is associated with an increase in the overexpression of the antiapoptotic protein bcl-2 [1,2]. McDonnell et al. demonstrated increased overexpression of bcl-2 in tumors obtained from patients with hormone-refractory prostate cancer (HRPC) in comparison to tumors from patients with hormone-naive disease [1]. Recent studies also demonstrated that the overexpression of bcl-2 is associated with resistance to chemotherapy [9]. In prostate cancer, mutations in p53 are more common in metastatic disease compared to primary tumors [3,4]. Mutated

"

p53 is found in 25% of advanced hormone refractory disease, but in less than 10% in earlier disease [3]. Although it is clear that more effective systemic therapies are needed in the treatment of prostate cancer, these data suggest that targeting such therapies before AA, with minimal disease, before the development of molecular mechanisms of therapy resistance, may further improve antitumor activity. This chapter reviews the data on the use of both systemic standard therapies (AA or the early use of chemotherapy) and novel therapies that might be considered or studied in patients with PSA progression and no imagable disease after local therapy. The use of local salvage radiation therapy will be considered elsewhere, and is not covered in this chapter.

TIMING OF ANDROGEN ABLATION THERAPY

It is indisputable that AA, as standard therapy, is temporarily effective in reducing PSA in most patients with PSA progression after local therapy; however, controversy exists on the timing of such therapy [10]. Given the potentially long period with absence of imagable disease, many opportunities for other interventions exist prior to the use of AA therapy. If AA therapy can be postponed without altering survival, opportunities for novel therapies in clinical trials should be offered.

Multiple studies have been conducted to determine if AA therapy is beneficial if administered early in the course of prostate cancer. For example, the medical research council (MRC) studied 934 patients with advanced or metastatic disease who were treated with either observation or AA [11]. In this study, 328 patients died with immediate AA compared to 361 in the delayed group (p = 0.02). 203 patients died from prostate cancer in the immediate AA group compared with 257 in the delayed group (p = 0.001). Despite these positive results, a significance for these differences did not occur in the group with metastasis. Additionally, patients were not followed closely in this study, as evidenced by the fact that 29 patients in the delayed group never received AA therapy; if these patients were removed, the difference in survival would not be significant. Current followup for most patients may be much more rigorous than in the MRC study, making this study less applicable for most patients. Therefore, one conclusion may be that this study demonstrated differences in survival with delays in AA if patients are not followed carefully, which may not apply to most patients seen today. More importantly, and relevant to this chapter, the MRC study, which enrolled patients with more advanced disease, did not address the timing of AA therapy in earlier disease.

The use of AA therapy in earlier disease is addressed in studies of AA therapy adjuvant to surgery or radiation therapy. For example, Soloway et al. completed a randomized trial with 303 patients treated with either 3 months of AA followed by surgery or surgery alone [12]. Although the percentage of patients with positive surgical margins (18% versus 48%, p <.001) and capsular penetration (53% versus 22%, p<.001) improved in the study, no difference in morbidity or overall survival was noted. Messing et al. enrolled 98 men with node-positive disease after radical prostatectomy to goserelin or orchiectomy versus observation [13]. At a median of 7.1 years, survival was improved in patients treated with AA therapy; 7 patients died (3 from prostate cancer) out of 47 treated, and 18 patients died (16 from prostate cancer) out of 51 observed (p = .02). Although the study was a positive study, multiple criticisms of the study include the lack of central pathology review, fewer enrolled patients than planned, more patients with Gleason scores 8–10 in the observed group (22 versus 14), and the survival rate in the observation group was less than expected historically.

Trials with AA along with radiation therapy have also not conclusively demonstrated a role for immediate AA therapy for most patients. For example, Bolla et al. completed a randomized trial with 198 patients treated with AA therapy for 3 years starting with radiation therapy compared to radiation therapy alone [14]. Most patients had more advanced disease (clinical stage T3 and T4). Patients treated with AA therapy had disease-free survival (DFS) and overall survival (OS) significantly improved over patients with radiation alone (DFS at 5 years of 85% versus 48%, and OS 79% versus 62%). The RTOG 86–31 trial randomized patients to AA therapy starting the last week of radiation (n = 477) versus radiation alone (n = 468) with AA at relapse. Although a statistically significant difference in DFS occurred at 8 years (36% versus 25%), no OS difference was noted in the initial report of this study [15]. However, when the subset of patients with Gleason scores 8–10 was considered, OS was significantly improved with AA therapy (35% versus 25%). RTOG 86–10 randomized 226 patients to 2 months of AA prior to radiation and combined with radiation compared to 230 patients treated with radiation alone [16]. At 8 years, only DFS was significantly improved in the group (33% versus 21%). However, in the subgroup of patients with Gleason scores 2–6, OS was significantly improved (70% versus 52%). Taken together, these data suggest that AA therapy may improve survival in patients with advanced disease who receive radiation therapy. However, the only studies discussed with an overall survival benefit in the entire study group was the study by Bolla et al. in which therapy was administered for 3 years and recent reports of RTOG 86–31 both in a group of patients with mostly advanced disease. A subsequent report of this study with longer followup did demonstrate an improvement in overall survival.

Overall, the data on the timing of AA therapy in prostate cancer is inadequate to define a standard approach that will alter survival; however, a few conclusions can be made [17]. First, AA can probably be delayed in patients with advanced disease only if patients are followed closely to avoid spinal cord compression problems or urological difficulties, although this point has not been proven. Second, AA does not improve survival as adjuvant therapy to radical prostatectomy, though one small study demonstrated a survival advantage for patients found with D1 disease. Third, AA therapy may improve survival in patients with T3 and T4 tumors to radiation therapy when added for 3 years or longer. Fourth, there is no data to support the early use of AA therapy in patients with PSA progression and absent imagable disease after local therapy, making the consideration of novel approaches in this group reasonable.

CHEMOTHERAPY IN PATIENTS WITH PSA PROGRESSION?

Given the development of mechanisms of tumor resistance in prostate cancer after the use of AA or in metastatic disease, one hypothesis that can be considered is that the early use of chemotherapy in the progression of prostate cancer will improve clinical results. Multiple studies have assessed the use of chemotherapy as early therapy in prostate cancer. For example, we recently completed a trial using mitoxantrone in patients with PSA progression [18]. Twenty-three hormone-naive patients with PSA progression after prostatectomy or radiation therapy were registered, and 22 treated with 10 mg/m^2 of mitoxantrone initially, followed by 12 mg/m^2 every three weeks for a maximum of 8 cycles, with a total of 131 cycles of therapy. Therapy was well tolerated, as expected; three patients had transient grade 3 or 4 neutropenia without fever. Ten of 22 patients demonstrated a decrease in PSA without an associated decrease in testosterone. The mean PSA decrease was 29% at three months and 43% at six months; overall 4 out of 22 patients had a decrease in PSA of $\geq$50%. Immunohistochemistry was performed to determine if any molecular markers of resistance correlated with this response. PSA decreased in 3 out of 7 patients whose cancer overexpressed MRP and in 3 out of 7 patients that overexpressed bcl-2. No patient with overexpression of topoisomerase II alpha (n = 4) had a decrease in PSA during the study but this was only assessed in a small number of patients. We concluded that mitoxantrone was safe and biochemically active, with a response rate that did not appear superior to prior studies in HRPC. In fact, prior studies using mitoxantrone in HRPC demonstrated a PSA response rate of 19% to 33% [19,20]. For example, Tannock et al. treated 111 patients with HRPC with a combination of 12mg/m^2 mitoxantrone every 3 weeks and 10 prednisone each day, or prednisone alone and found improved quality of life (29% treated with the combination compared to 12% treated with prednisone alone). Although serum PSA decreased by 50% or more in 33% of patients treated with mitoxantrone and prednisone, it was not statistically different from the serum PSA decrease in 22% of patients treated with prednisone alone [19]. Kantoff et al. treated 242 patients with HRPC with 14mg/m^2 mitoxantrone every 3 weeks combined with hydrocortisone or hydrocortisone alone [20]. Again, the difference in PSA decrease between arms was not significant; serum PSA decreased by 50% or more in 19% of patients treated with the combination compared to 14% treated with hydrocortosone alone.

Taken together, these data suggest that mitoxantone administered after PSA progression with hormone-naive disease may not be better than waiting for HRPC, although more studies would be needed to confirm this hypothesis. Other investigators have also studied the use of mitoxantrone as adjuvant therapy before PSA progression. Halford et al. treated 96 patients in a randomized trial with an LHRH agonist and flutamide with and without adjuvant mitoxantrone [21]. Patients enrolled had advanced disease, including 88 patients with T3 or T4 tumors and 55 patients with metastasis. Median survival was better in the group of patients with localized disease with adjuvant mitoxantrone (80 versus 36 months, p = 0.04). In contrast to the group of patients with localized disease (n = 38), there was no significant benefit of treatment with adjuvant mitoxantrone in the group of patients with metastatic disease (n = 55). Although this study suggested a benefit of adjuvant mitoxantrone to patients with localized disease, this benefit was in only a small subset of patients within the trial and is not definitive. Other prior studies of adjuvant therapy in prostate cancer have also had limitations [22–24]. Schmidt et al. reported the results of a study of 437 patients with localized prostate cancer treated with local therapy followed by estramustine or cyclophosphamide or no treatment, and found a progression-free survival benefit but no overall survival benefit [23]. Kuriyama et al. treated patients with AA with orchiectomy and DES with and without UFT for 1 year. Although the group with UFT had a longer progression-free survival, overall survival was not significantly improved with adjuvant chemotherapy [24]. Other investigators have also studied the use of chemotherapy prior to local therapy. For example, Oh et al. completed a trial using taxotere prior to surgery in patients with localized disease [25]. These studies are therefore not definitive, but support phase III studies of adjuvant chemotherapy, which are ongoing.

The use of chemotherapy in patients with PSA progression may represent a different population than patients at the point of local therapy, since the completed studies suggest that response rate for patients with hormone-naive PSA progression is similar to patients with HRPC. Therefore, molecular mechanisms of chemotherapy resistance may already be present, requiring further study of chemotherapy earlier in the course of disease, such as adjuvant therapy. Prior studies of adjuvant chemotherapy or neoadjuvant chemotherapy are, in fact interesting, but not definitive at this point, and further study is warranted. Phase III studies such as SWOG 9921, RTOG P0014, and ECOG 1899 are important. SWOG 9921 tests the role of adjavant mitoxantrone. P0014 test the role of chemotherapy in hormone sensitive PSA progression. ECOG 1899 test the role of chemotherapy in hormone refractory PSA progression. Accural to therapy should be encouraged. Additionally the study of novel agents with more targeted mechanisms of action are appropriate for patients with PSA progression after local therapy.

NEW APPROACHES TO THERAPY OF PSA PROGRESSION

Novel approaches to the treatment of prostate cancer include the use of more targeted therapies to pathways critical to tumor cells. Although some approaches

TABLE 1 Targeted Therapies Under Investigation for the Treatment of Prostate Cancer

Catagory	Examples of agents under investigation	References
Pharmacology/cytotoxins	Epothilone, PSA-activated cytotoxic agents, novel taxanes	27–29
Growth factors, cytokines, and signal transduction	EGF inhibitors, Gleevec (STI-571), Endothelin-1 inhibitors, Estrogens	64–73
Molecular mechanisms of tumor growth and death	Bcl-2 inhibitors, BH3 peptides, Akt inhibitors	51, 52, 53–56, 60–62, 82, 83, 77, 78
Angiogenesis	Antibodies to vascular endothelial growth factor (VEGF), TNP-470	
Immunology	Monoclonal antibodies and vaccines	49, 87, 88

are currently being investigated against more advanced disease, further study in patients with PSA progression and unimagable disease is warranted. Current approaches include the study of novel cytotoxins, the manipulation of molecular mechanisms of tumor cell growth and death by targeting the apoptotic pathway, the study of growth factor and cytokine pathway inhibitors, the study of vaccines and antibody approaches, and the study of angiogenesis (Table 1).

Novel Cytotoxic Agents

Current agents used in the treatment of HRPC are limited by a short median duration of response; the earlier use of these agents in patients with PSA progression and no imagable disease is ongoing, as discussed earlier, but current results in this group of patients suggest the need for newer approaches (19,20,26). The development of better cytotxic agents is ongoing and may improve these results. One example is the development of agents that are selectively activated by prostate tumor cells through PSA. As a serine protease, PSA is responsible for liquefaction of semen through cleavage of proteins at specific amino acid sequences. We studied a novel agent that is dependent on enzymatically functional PSA for activity L-377202 [28]. This agent is a conjugate consisting of the peptide covalently linked to the aminoglycoside portion of doxorubicin (Dox), which is cleaved by PSA to produce the biologically active forms leucine-doxorubicin (Leu-Dox) and Dox. We treated 19 patients in a phase I trial with advanced

HRPC with 71 cycles of L-377202 at escalating dose levels of 20 mg/m^2 (n = 1), 40 mg/m^2 (n = 3), 80 mg/m^2 (n = 4), 160mg/m^2 (n = 3), 225mg/m^2 (n = 6), and 315 mg/m^2 (n = 2) once every 3 weeks. Toxicity, response, and PK of L-377202 were assessed. Therapy was well tolerated, and the recommended dosage for efficacy studies was determined. At 225 mg/m^2 and 315 mg/m^2, 5 patients completed at least 3 cycles of therapy; 2 patients had a >75% decrease in PSA; and 1 patient had a stabilized PSA. Further studies of this or similar agents are warranted in advanced and earlier disease. A second example of promising agents includes the study of epothilone, a taxane-like agent that induces polymerization of tubulin dimers into stable-microtubules that are cytotoxic to Taxol-sensitive and Taxol resistant cells [29]. Phase I trials have now been complete, and phase II trials in prostate cancer are ongoing. It will be critical to develop novel cytotoxic agents to improve on the limited results of current chemotherapy in HRPC and to give candidate agents for earlier testing in patients with PSA progression.

Targeting Molecular Mechanisms of Tumor Growth and Death

Multiple mechanisms of tumor resistance appear to increase during the progression of prostate cancer or during the development of resistance to AA. For example, the antiapoptotic protein bcl-2 is overexpressed in most prostate cancers and is associated with resistance to AA [1]. The bcl-2 protein family plays a critical role in the positive and negative regulation of apoptosis. An understanding of these proteins first came from the study of the nematode *Caenorhabditis elegans*, in which the *ced-9* gene that represses cell death is a structural and functional homologue of bcl-2 [30]. Bcl-2 expression in human cells can protect from various stimuli, including chemotherapy and radiation [31]. Bcl-2 belongs to a family of regulating proteins that have antiapoptotic effects such as bcl-2, bcl-XL, bcl-w, Bfl-1, Brag-1, Mcl-1, A1, and NR-13, and proapoptotic effects such as Bax, Bak, Bcl-Xs, Bad, Bid, Bik, Hrk, and Bim [32,57–63]. Bcl-2 family proteins exert their effect at the mitochondria [33]. The release of cytochrome c from the mitochondria is a critical event in the pathway of apoptosis [34]. The release of cytochrome c from the mitochondria is dependent on Bax [34]. Bax forms a heterodimer with bcl-2, which inhibits the antiapoptotic effect of bcl-2 and enhances cell death. Multiple proteins regulate cytochrome-c release including Bcl-2 and Bcl-XL, which act to regulate pore opening, and Bax, which mediates release of cytochrome c. Bid and Bad antagonize the antiapoptotic effect of Bcl-2 and Bcl-XL. Additionally, Bad is rapidly phosphorylated in response to a growth factor, which results in its binding to 14–3–3 and sequestration in the cytosol. This process makes Bad incapable of binding and antagonizing the antiapoptotic protein Bcl-XL. This process of growth factor regulation of apoptosis through

Bad phosphorylation and sequestration may also be an important pathway that links growth regulators to apoptosis.

Since bcl-2 expression appears to increase during AA therapy, the study of agents that alter bcl-2 expression might be studied along or before the use of AA. McDonnell et al. detected bcl-2 by immunohistochemistry in only 6 out of 19 patients (30%) with hormone-sensitive tumors, whereas bcl-2 was detected with intense staining in 10 out of 13 patients (77%) with hormone-resistant tumors [1]. Other investigators found that bcl-2 immunostaining is greater in tumors from patients with resistance to AA [35]. McDonnell et al. also demonstrated increased bcl-2 expression in the ventral prostate tissue of a rat within 5 days of castration, consistent with the hypothesis that bcl-2 expression results from AA [1]. Direct evidence that bcl-2 expression is associated with the development of hormone-independence was reported by Raffo et al. who transfected prostate cancer cell lines that were initially sensitive to AA (LNCaP) with a cDNA encoding human *bcl-2* [31]. Tumors grown in male nude mice from the bcl-2 transfected cells were resistant to the antitumor effects of castration. In contrast, the growth of tumors formed from the nontransfected cells was inhibited by castration. Overexpression of bcl-2 is also associated with resistance to chemotherapy in prostate cancer [9]. Tu et al. transfected Dunning-G rat prostate cancer cells with a *bcl-2* expression vector and found that the transfectants were significantly resistant to the cytotoxic effects of doxorubicin compared to controls (cells transfected with the empty vector). This finding appeared to be due to the resistance of *bcl-2* transfectants to apoptosis.

The modulation of apoptotic targets such as bcl-2, therefore, may improve therapy for patients with prostate cancer. In fact, commonly used antimicrotubule agents may target bcl-2 function; antimicrotubular agents induce bcl-2 phosphorylation, which may abrogate bcl-2 antiapoptotic activity. Halder et al. demonstrated that multiple antimicrotubule agents such as paclitaxel, vinblastine, and taxotere could induce apoptosis in bcl-2 expressing PC-3 prostate cancer cells associated with the phosphorylation of bcl-2 [36–38]. Bcl-2 phosphorylation may be a mechanisms of apoptosis, since bcl-2 protects cells from apoptosis by dimerizing with Bax, and phosphorylation of bcl-2 interferes with dimerization [37]. Blagosklonny et al. demonstrated that paclitaxel could induce phosphorylation of bcl-2 in association with activation of Raf-1, a mitogen-stimulated protein serine/threonine kinase [36]. These data raise the possibility that use of antimicrotubular agents may bypass bcl-2 resistance in prostate cancer, and that this modulation of resistance is associated with the phosphorylation of bcl-2.

The study of novel agents that reduce bcl-2 expression have promise to induce or potentiate the apoptotic effect of known cytotoxic drugs [39,40]. As one example, preclinical and clinical studies of retinoids demonstrated antitumor activity and associated reduction in the expression of bcl-2 [40–43]. Investigators demonstrated antitumor activity of retinoids against both hormone-resistant and hormone sensitive prostate tumor cell lines that overexpress bcl-2 [42,43]. Studies that combined interferon (IFN) with 13 cis retinoic acid (CRA) demonstrated increased antitumor effects of CRA/IFN compared to either one alone in both laboratory and clinical studies [45–47]. For example, Majewski et al. found that the combination of CRA with IFN produced significant inhibition of angiogenesis as compared to the effects of the drugs given alone *in vivo* [45–46]. Lippman et al. demonstrated clinical activity of the combination of CRA/IFN in patients with advanced cervical carcinoma and the activity of CRA/IFN alone and combined with platinum against squamous cell carcinoma [47–48]. Zhang et al. demonstrated that CRA/IFN decreased cell viability in a highly resistant transformed rat kidney cell line transfected to overexpress bcl-2 and significantly enhanced the effect of paclitaxel (TAX) chemotherapy, as well a decreased the expression of bcl-2 in a hormone refractory prostate tumor cell line [50].

CRA/IFN has been studied further in the clinic to determine if chemotherapy resistance in tumor cells can be abrogated. For example, a pilot trial of CRA/IFN alone in patients with early recurrence of prostate cancer defined by rising prostate-specific antigen (PSA) after local therapy with unimagable disease demonstrated the safety of the regimen and clinical activity [51]. In a group of 30 patients, 38% had a decrease of PSA with a mean decrease of 20% (2% to 55%) at 3 months. Plasma TGF-beta1 levels increased with CRA/IFN therapy and correlated with a decrease in PSA. A phase I trial with CRA/IFN combined with TAX enrolled 22 patients with prostate cancer (n = 10) or other advanced malignancies [52]. Therapy was well tolerated, with a partial response noted in patients and stable disease in 5 patients. CRA/IFN decreased bcl-2 in peripheral blood mononuclear cells. Further studies of CRA/IFN and taxane therapy are ongoing.

Bcl-2 antisense oligonucleotides have also been studied in the clinic to determine if bcl-2–induced chemotherapy resistance can be abrogated. The antisense oligonucleotides studied were stretches of single-stranded DNA with a phosphorothioate backbone complementary to RNA regions of *bcl-2* [53]. Jansen et al. demonstrated that bcl-2 antisense improved chemosensitivity in melanoma cells grown in SCID mice and decreased bcl-2 in tumors by western analysis [54–55]. Pretreatment with antisense bcl-2 prior to dacarbazine chemotherapy resulted in decreased tumor size compared to sense and mismatched controls. Phase I clinical trials were completed in patients with non-Hodgkin's lymphoma and demonstrated clinical responses [53]. Jansen et al. studied the effect of bcl-2 antisense in combination with dacarbazine in patients with melanoma [54–55]. Seventeen patients with melanoma were treated with bcl-2 antisense combined with dacarbazine (antisense doses from 0.6 to 6.5 mg/kg/d). Therapy was well tolerated and induced a response in 3 out of 14-evaluable patients (1CR, 2PR, along with decreased bcl-2 expression in tumors. More recently, the study of bcl-2 antisense in prostate cancer was initiated. Scher et al. studied bcl-2 antisense alone and in combination with taxane in patients with hormone-refractory prostate cancer (n = 23) and other advanced malignancies (n = 12) [56]. Therapy was well tolerated and resulted in decreased bcl-2 in PBMCs in some patients. A study with bcl-2 antisense combined with docelareel demonstrated activity and additional studies are ongoing [64]. The study of these well-tolerated agents alone and in combination in early disease is also warranted.

Other efforts to target the apoptotic pathway include the study of natural apoptotic pathway inhibitors or promotors. Many proapoptotic bcl-2 family members such as Bad, Bax, Bik, and Bak, have bcl-2 homology 3 (BH3) domains that participate in apoptosis and inhibit the antiapoptotic members of the bcl-2 family [57,58]. For example, Bad promotes apoptosis by forming inactivating dimmers with death suppressors such as Bcl-XL through its BH3 domain [59]. Studies of synthetic peptides corresponding to the BH3 domain are ongoing [59]. One example has been published by Holinger et al., with the study of synthetic peptides corresponding to the BH3 domain of Bak [57]. Inhibitor of apoptosis proteins (IAP) are also promising drug targets. These proteins contain a conserved amino acid domain capable of suppressing apoptosis through the inhibition of caspases [60–62]. In contrast to the study of apoptotic inhibitors, the study of Bax adenoviral vectors exploit the enhancement of proapoptotic protein effects. For example, Tai et al. studied the effect of replication deficient adenoviral vectors containing Bax under the control of the DF3 promoter, which is expressed in ovarian cancers but not in normal peritoneal mesothelial cells [63]. Therapy was capable of selective cytotoxicity in ovarian cancer cells **in vitro** and nude mice.

Growth Factors, Cytokines, and signal transduction

Prostate cancer growth is regulated by several growth mediators independent of androgen, creating novel opportunities to control tumor growth independent of AA. These identified growth factors include epidermal growth factor (EGF), transforming growth factor (TGF), insulin like growth factor (IGF), fibroblast growth factor (FGF), platelet-derived growth factor (PDGF) and endothelin-1 [65–66]. For example, EGF, which is highly concentrated in the prostate, acts through the EGF receptor (EGFR) to activate intracellular tyrosine kinase activity [63]. Both androgen-sensitive and androgen-insensitive prostate tumors are stimulated by EGF, and agents that inhibit this pathway are under investigation. Selective inhibitors of EGFR tyrosine kinase activity are under study multiple malignancies. Endothelin-1, produced by endothelial and epithelial cells, binds to receptors in the prostate, increasing tumor cell proliferation [67]. Selective inhibitors of the Endothelin-1 receptor have been studied in prostate cancer with initial promising results, and further studies are underway [65].

The (PDGF) pathway may be a novel specific area to target in the treatment of prostate cancer. PDGF is a ubiquitous growth factor that drives cell proliferation during normal development and in malignancy [66]. Dysregulation of

PDGFR signaling in tumors can lead to autocrine- or paracrine-stimulation of cell growth [66]. Studies of prostate cancer have demonstrated both the expression of PDGFR and production of ligand (67,68). Fudge et al. found that alpha and beta receptor PDGF antibodies labeled adenocarcinoma with greater intensity in low Gleason-grade tumors [67]. Sitaras et al. demonstated that DU-145 and PC-3 prostate tumor cells express both platelet-derived growth factor-1 and PDGF-S/sis genes [68]. Vlahos et al. demonstrated that PDGF was mitogenic to human cells derived for patients with prostatic hyperplasia [69]. Taken together, these data support the study of agents that interrupt the PDGF pathway in prostate tumor. In fact, clinical studies of inhibitors of PDGFR in prostate cancer have already been reported in HRPC. Ko et al. tested a PDGFR, inhibitor (SU101) in patients with HRPC and found that 3 out of 39 had a decrease of PSA of >50% and 9 out of 39 with pain improvement, suggesting some antitumor activity [70]. The authors concluded that studies of other PDGFR inhibitors may be warranted.

Gleevec is a potent and clinically more active protein-tyrosine kinase inhibitor, which inhibits the Abl tyrosine kinase, PDGFR and receptor for stem cell factor, c-Kit [71–73]. Druker et al. demonstrated that Gleevec had impressive clinical activity against CMI and Ph-positive ALL [71]. In this study, 58 patients were treated with doses of Gleevec ranging from 300mg to 1000mg daily with minimal toxicity. Carroll et al. demonstrated that Gleevec also inhibits PDGFR kinase [72]. Gilbert et al. demonstrated that Gleevec reduced PDGF–stimulated mesangial cell proliferation in a dose-dependent manner, with complete abrogation at 0.4 uM [73]. Gleevec strongly inhibited the growth of v-sis-transformed BALB/c 3T3 mouse fibroblasts, which respond to autocrine PDGF production (Novartis investigators brochure, 4th edition). Despite these hypothesis generating data, a recent study with Gleevec in patients with PSA progression without metastasis had no detectable clinical activity in a study recently concluded at our institution [27].

Although growth factors have been shown to impact prostate tumor cell growth, these mediators also have molecular effects directly on the apoptotic pathway. In fact, exposure to various cell-growth stimuli maintain cell proliferation and decrease the apoptotic signal through a pathway involving the kinase Akt, which is upstream of Bad [74–78]. The kinase activity of Akt is induced by IGF-1, EGF, and PDGF in a phosphatidylinositide 3'-OH kinase (PI3K) dependent manner. One mechanism of activation is through the direct binding of PI3K generated phospholipids to Akt, which causes Akt to translocate from the cytoplasm to the inner surface of the plasma membrane, where regulatory kinases phosphorylate and activate Akt. Subsequently, active Akt phosphorylates Bad, a proapoptotic protein that normally interferes with the antiapoptotic protein Bcl-XL [75]. Phosphorylation of Bad at Ser-112 and Ser-136 results in the dissociation of Bad from Bcl-XL and the association of with cytoplasmic 14–3–3 protein, which sequesters Bad away from its targets at the mitochondria and increases the antiapoptotic signal. Therefore, the discovery of agents that are capable of abrogation of various growth-factor–induced events may be expected to effect both proliferation and apoptosis. Agents with the potential to inhibit individual growth factor pathways and multiple pathways, including the inhibition of Akt, are underway.

NF-kB also interacts with the apoptotic machinery and is another target for novel agents under investigation. NF-kB is a transcription factor that forms dimers with the Rel family of proteins [79]. NF-kB regulates the expression of multiple antiapoptotic genes via cytokine stimulation (i.e., IL-1 and TNF). Normally, NF-kB is found in the cytoplasm bound to IkB proteins. Upon cytokine stimulation, a cascade of events leads to IkB degradation and releases NF-kB. Functional IkB kinase phosphorylates IkB resulting in its degradation, which then allows NF-kB to disassociate from IkB and translocate to the nucleus where it upregulates suppressors of caspase activation [80]. Therefore, cytokine stimulation can result in an antiapoptotic signal through release of NF-kB and subsequent upregulation of other antiapoptotic proteins. The study of agents that may alter this pathway are ongoing. For example, proteosome inhibitors are a unique class of drugs that inhibit the proteosome, which is a multisubunit protease complex capable of degrading several proteins involved in cell-cycle regulation and survival including Ik-B/NF-kB [81–86].

The list of these potential targets continues to grow with the number of agents available to study growing rapidly, leading to great hope of future clinical outcomes. These more targeted therapies have the promise to potentially increase efficacy with reduced toxicity, making them attractive for study in earlier disease, such as in patients with only PSA progression.

Immunology

Immunotherapy offers an alternative approach to current therapy for prostate cancer, including AA therapy and chemotherapy. Although covered in detail elsewhere in this text, a brief overview of some of the efforts in patients with PSA progression will be summarized here.

Based on the work done previously with CEA, other antigens have been identified and selected for use in vaccine protocols in prostate cancer. Prostate epithelial cells lining the prostatic acini and ducts produce the glandular kallikrein-like protease PSA, which becomes markedly elevated when adenocarcinoma of the prostate occurs [49]. Because PSA is relatively tissue-specific, and because many patients have little or no remaining prostate tissue after local therapy, PSA is one logical target for vaccine strategies. Identification of HLA-A2-restricted, PSA-specific epitopes has now been reported by several authors [87–88]. More recently, a vaccinia virus expressing human PSA was constructed and tested in a rhesus monkey model, which minimal toxicity and increased anti-PSA IgM antibody titers after vaccination [49]. Studies have been published demonstrating the safety and potential efficacy of vaccination with PSA in man using various approaches [87,88]. Meidenbauer et al. [87] studied the JBT 1001 vaccine, which consists of recombinant PSA with lipid A formulated in liposomes in patients with prostate cancer. They demonstrated that after vaccination, 8 of 10 patients had measurable PSA-reactive T-cell frequencies when measured in peripheral blood mononuclear cells using in vitro sensitization, suggesting that vaccination induced T cell responses in most patients. Eder et al. recently completed a phase I trial using a recombinant vaccinia virus expressing PSA in patients with advanced prostate cancer [88]. The vaccine was administered in 3 monthly doses at increasing dose levels. Ten patients at the higher dose level also received GM-CSF as an immunostimulatory adjuvant. The vaccine was well tolerated. Immunologic studies demonstrated a T cell response, and 9 of 33 patients remained with stable PSA for 11 to 25 months. The combination of vaccinia and fowlpox virus with the PSA gene was recently studied in a pilot trial in patients with PSA progression and no imagable disease [49]. Therapy was safe, and further studies are planned with PSA and other antigens to determine if a vaccine approach will improve clinical outcomes.

In addition to efforts to induce an immune response, multiple studies have utilized monoclonal antibodies to alter prostate cancer progression. For example, McDevitt et al. studied a novel alpha-particle emitting monoclonal antibody targeting the external domain of PSMA in vitro and in vivo. This antibody improved tumor-free survival in mice and reduced PSA [89]. Smith-Jones studied 131I radiolabeled monoclonal antibodies which bind to the extracellular domain of PSMA [90]. Clinical trials using monoclonal antibodies to target PSMA are now ongoing and include patients with PSA progression and the absence of imagable disease [91].

FUTURE EFFORTS

The treatment of patients with PSA progression in the absence of imagable disease requires extensive thought and discussion. Patient options include close follow-up without therapy until needed for metastatic or symptomatic disease. Since data does not exist to demonstrate any survival advantage to early induction of AA in this patient group, other novel options can be considered. Studies of chemotherapy in patients with PSA progression before imagable disease develops have not yet been conclusive. Further study of these agents, and more novel cytoxic agents, are warranted. Accrual should be encouraged to the large national studies of chemotherapy in early prostate cancer. Even more intriguing are studies of novel, be targeted therapies with the potential of greater efficacy and less toxicity. The study of drugs that target the apoptotic pathway, growth factor, and cytokine pathways; the study of vaccines and antibody approaches; and the study of angiogenesis are the hope for the future of these patients with minimal yet progressive disease.

REFERENCES

1. McDonnell TJ, Troncoso P, Brisbay SM, et al. Expression of the proto-oncogene bcl-2 in the prostate and its association with emergence of androgen-independent prostate cancer. Cancer Research 1992; 52(24):6940.

2. Chiou S-K, Rao S-K, White E. Bcl-2 blocks p53-dependent apoptosis. Mol Cell Biol 1994; 14:2556–2563.

3. Bookstein R, MacGrogan D, Hilsenback SG, et al. P53 is mutated in a subset of advanced-stage prostate cancers. Cancer Res 1993; 53:3369–3373.

4. Aas T, Borresen A-L, Geisler S, et al. Specific p53 mutations are associated with de novo resistance to doxorubicin in breast cancer patients. Nature Med 1996; 2: 811–814.

5. Cole SP, Bharkwaj G, Gerlach JH, Mackie JE, Grant CE, Almquist KC, Stewart AJ, Kurz EU, Duncan AM, Deeley RG. Overexpression of a transporter gene in a multidrug-resistant human lung cancer cell line. Science 1992; 258:1650–1654.

6. Cole SP, Sparks KE, Fraser K, Loe DW, Grant CE, Wilson GM, Deely RG. Pharmacological characterization of multidrug resistant MRP-transfected human tumor cells. Cancer Res 1994; 54:5902–5910.

7. Futscher BW, Abbaszadegan MR, Domann F, Dalton WS. Analysis of MRP mRNA in mitoxantrone-selected, multidrug-resistant human tumor cells. Biochem Pharmacol 1994; 47:1601–1606.

8. Sullivan GF, Amenta PS, Villanueva JD, Alvarez CJ, Yang JM, Hait WN. The expression of drug resistance gene products during the progression of human prostate cancer. Clin. Cancer Res. 1998; 4:1393.

9. Tu S, McConnell K, Marin MC, et al. Combination adriamycin and suramin induces apoptosis in bcl-2 expressing prostate carcinoma cells. Cancer Letters 1995; 93: 147.

10. Pound CR, Partin AW, Eisenberger MA, Chan DW, Pearson JD, Walsh PC. JAMA 1999; 281:1591–1597.

11. Medical Research Council. Immediate vs. deferred treatment of advanced prostatic cancer: initial results of the MRC trial. BJU 1997; 79:235–246.

12. Soloway MS, Sharkfi R, Wajsman Z, et al. Randomized prospective study comparing radical prostatectomy alone vs. radical prostatectomy preceded by androgen blockade in clinical stage B2 prostate cancer. J Urol 1995; 154:424.

13. Messing et al. Z, et al. Immediate hormonal therapy compared with observation after radical prostatectomy and pelvic lymphadenectomy in men with node-positive prostate cancer. NEJM 1999; 341:1781.

14. Bolla et al. Z, et al. Improved survival in patients with locally advanced prostate cancer treated with radiotherapy and goserelin. NEJM 1997; 337:295.

15. Lawton et al. Z, et al. Updated results of the phase II radiation therapy oncology group trial 85–31 evaluating the potential benefit of androgen suppression following standard radiation therapy for unfavorable prognosis carcinoma of the prostate. IJROBP 2001; 49:937–946.

16. Pilepich et al. Z, et al. Phase III radiation therapy oncology group trial 86–10 of androgen deprivation adjuvant to definitive radiotherapy in locally advanced carcinoma of the prostate. IJROBP 2001; 50:1243–1252.

17. DiPaola RS. Approaches to the treatment of patients with hormone sensitive prostate cancer. Seminars of Oncology 1999; 26:24–27.

18. DiPaola RS, Chenven ES, Shih WJ, Lin Y, Amenta P, Goodin S, Shumate A, Rafi MM, Capanna T, Cardiella M, Cummings KB, Aisner J, Todd M. Mitoxantrone in patients with prostate specific antigen progression after local therapy for prostate cancer. Cancer 2001; 92:2065–71.

19. Tannock IF, Osoba D, Stockler MR, Ernst DS, Neville AJ, Moore MJ, Armitage GR, Wilson JJ, Venner PM, Coppin CM, Murphy KC. Chemotherapy with mitoxantrone plus prednisone or prednisone alone for symptomatic hormone-resistant prostate cancer: a Canadian randomized trial with palliative end points. J Clin Oncol 1996; 14:1756.

20. Kantoff PW, Halabi S, Conaway M, Picus J, Dirshner J, Hars V, Trump D, Winer EP, Vogelzang NJ. Hydrocortisone with and without mitoxantrone in men with hormone-refractory prostate cancer: Results of the cancer and leukemia Group B. J Clin Oncol 1999; 17:2506–2513.

21. Wang J, Halford S, Rigg A et al. Adjuvant mitozantrone chemotherapy in advanced prostate cancer. BJU international 2000; 86:675–680.

22. Murphy GP, Beckley S, Brady MF, et al. Treatment of newly diagnosed metastatic prostate cancer patients with chemotherapy agents in combination with hormones vs. hormones alone. Cancer 1983; 51:1264–1272.

23. Schmidt JD, Gibbons RP, Murphy GP, et al. Adjuvant therapy for localized prostate cancer 1993; 71:1005–1013.

24. Kuriyama et al. GP, et al. Prospective and randomized comparison of combined androgen blockade vs. combination with oral UFT as an initial treatment for prostate cancer. Jpn J Clin Oncol 2001; 31:18–24.

25. Oh WK. The evolving role of chemotherapy and other therapy for managing localized prostate cancer. J Urol 2003; 170:528–530.

26. Petrylak et al. SWOG 99–16: Randomized phase III trial of docataxel/estramustine vs. mithoxantrane/prednisone in men with AIPCA. PASCO 22:3, 2004.

27. Rao K et al. A phase II study of ematinib in patients with PSA progression after local therapy for prostate cancer. The Prostate (In Press 2004).

28. DiPaola RS, Rinehart J, Nemunaiti J, Effinghaus S, Rubin E, Capanna T, Ciardella M, Fontaine M, Adams N, Williams A, Schwartz M, Winchell G, Wickersham K, Deutsch P, Yao S. Characterization of a novel prostate-specific antigen activated peptide-doxorubicin conjugate in patients with prostate cancer. Journal of Clinical Oncology 2002):(In Press.

29. Goodin S, Kane MP, Ruben EM. Epothilones: Mechanism of action and biologic activity. J Clin Oncology 15: 2015, 2004.

30. Tsujimoto Y, Croce CM. Analysis of the structure, transcripts and protein products of bcl-2, the gene involved in human follicular lymphoma. Proc Natl Acad Sci USA 1986; 83:5214–5218.

31. Raffo AJ, Perlman H, Chen M, Day ML, Streitman JS, Buttyan R. Overexpression of bcl-2 protects prostate cancer cells from apoptosis in vitro and confers resistance to androgen depletion in vivo. Cancer Res 1995; 55:4438.

32. Korsmeyer SJ. Bcl-2 gene family and the regulation of Programmed Cell Death. Cancer Res 1999; 59:1693–1700.

33. Heiden MG, Thompson CB. Bcl-2 proteins: Regulators of apoptosis or of mitochondrial homeostasis?. Nature Cell Biology 1999; 1:209–216.

34. Reed JC. Bcl-2 family proteins: Regulators of Apoptosis and Chemoresistance in Hematologic Malignancies. Seminars in Hematology 1997; 34:9–19.

35. Colombel M, Symmans F, Gil S, et al. Detection of the apoptosis-suppressing oncoprotein bcl-2 in hormone-refractory human prostate cancers. Am J Pathol 1993; 143:390–400.

36. Blagosklonny MV, Schulte T, Nguyen Pet al. Taxol-induced Apoptosis and Phosphorylation of bcl-2 protein involves c-Raf-1 and represents a novel c-Raf-1 signal Tansduction Pathway. Cancer Res 1996; 56:1851–1854.

37. Hadlar S, Chintapalli J, Croce CM. Taxol induces *bcl-2* Phosphorylation and death of Prostate Cancer Cells. Cancer Res 1996; 56:1253.

38. Hadlar S, Jena N, Croce CM. Inactivation of bcl-2 by phosphorylation. Proc Natl Acad Sci USA 1995; 92:4507–4511.

39. Hu ZB, Minden MD, McCulloch EA. Regulation of the synthesis of bcl-2 protein by growth factors. Leukemia 1996; 10:1925–1929.

40. Smith MA, Parkinson DR, Cheson BD, et al. Retinoids in Cancer Therapy. J of Clin Onc 1992; 10(5):839–864.

41. Calmon G, Chabot GG, Valeriote F, et al. Phase I study and pharmacokinetics of weekly high-dose 13-cis-Retinoic acid. Cancer Res 1985; 45:1874–1878.

42. Kerr IG, Lippman ME, Jenkins Jet al. Pharmacology of 13-cis-retinoic acid in humans. Cancer Res 1982; 42:2069–2073.

43. Dahiya R, Park HD, Cusick J, et al. Inhibition of tumorigenic potential and prostate-specific antigen expression in LNCaP human prostate cancer cell line by 13-cis-retinoic acid. Int J of Can 1994; 59(1):126–32.

44. Hwang MS, Thompson KL. Independent induction of p21waf1 and apoptosis by all-trans-retinoic acid and 9-cis-retinoic acid in human prostate cancer cell lines. Amer Assoc for Cancer Res 1995; 36.

45. Majewski S, Szmurlo A, Marczak M, et al. Synergistic effect of retinoids and interferon alpha on tumor-induced angiogenesis: anti-angiogenic effect on HPV-harboring tumo-cell lines. Int J Cancer 1994; 57:81–85.

46. Slovin SF, Scher HI, Divgi CR, et al. Interferon-gamma and monoclonal antibody 131I-labeled CC49: Outcomes in patients with androgen-independent prostate cancer. Clin Cancer Res 1998; 4(3):643–651.

47. Lippman SM, Kavanagh JJ, Paredes-Espinoza M, et al. 13-cis-retinoic acid plus interferon-2alpha: highly active systemic therapy for squamous cell carcinoma of the cervix. J of the Nat Cancer Inst 1992; 84:4.

48. Lippman SM, Parkinson DR, Itri LM, et al. 13-cis-Retinoic Acid and interferon - 2a: Effective combination therapy for advanced squamous cell carcinoma of the skin. J of the Nat Cancer Inst 1992; 84(4):235–240.

49. Kaufman ML et al. Phase II randomized study of vaccine treatment of advanced prostate cancer (E7897): a trial of the Eastern Cooperative Oncology Group. J Clin Oncol 22:2122–2132, 2000.

50. Zhang C, DiPaola R, White E, Hait W. Restoration of taxol sensitivity in a p53 mutant, Bcl-2 overexpressing cell line by interferon-alpha and Retinoic acid. Am Asso for Cancer Res 1997:3563.

51. DiPaola RS, Weiss RE, Cummings KB, Kong FM, Jirtle R, Anscher M, Gallo J, Goodin S, Thompson S, Rasheed Z, Aisner J, Todd M. Effect of 13-cis Retinoic acid and alpha interferon on transforming growth factor Betal in patients with rising prostate specific antigen. Clin Cancer Research 1997; 3:1999–2004.

52. DiPaola RS, Rafi M, Vyas V, Gupta E, Toppmeyer D, Rubin E, Patel G, Goodin S, Medina P, Zamek R, Zhang C, White E, Hait WN. Phase I clinical and pharmaco-logic study of 13-cis retinoic acid, alpha interferon and paclitaxel in patients with prostate cancer and other advanced malignancies. J Clin Oncol 1999; 17: 2213–2218.

53. Webb A, Cunningham D, Cotter F, et al. BCL-2 antisense therapy in patients with non-Hodgkin lymphoma. Lancet 1997; 349(9059):1137–1141.

54. Jansen B, Wacheck V-, Ress E. Systemic treatment with bcl-2 antisense down-regulates tumor content of bcl-2 protein and induces major antitumor responses in patients with melanoma when combined with dacarbazine. Proceedings of the American Association of Cancer Research 2000:LB23.

55. Jansen B-, Wadl H, Brown BD, et al. Bcl-2 antisense therapy chemosensitizes human melanoma in SCID mice. Nature Medicine 1998; 4:232.

56. Scher HI, Morris MJ, Tong WP, et al. A phase I trial of G3139, a bcl-2 anti-sense drug, by continuous infusion as a single agent and with weekly taxol. Proceedings of the American Society of Clinical Oncology 2000; 19:774.

57. Holinger EP, Chittenden T, Lutz RJ. Bak BH3 peptides antagonize BCL-XL func-tion and induce apoptosis through cytochrome-c independent activation of caspases. J Bio Chem 1999; 274:13298–13304.

58. Krajewski M, Krafewski S, Epstein JIet al. Immunohistochemical analysis of bcl-2, bax, bcl-X, and mcl-1 expression in prostate cancers. Am J Pathol 1996; 148: 1567–1576.

59. Wang J, Zhang Z, Choksi S, et al. Cell permeable bcl-2 binding peptides: A chemical approach to apoptosis induction in tumor cells. Cancer Res 2000; 60:1498–1502.

60. Deveraux Q, Reed JC. IAP family proteins-suppressors of apoptosis. Genes Dev 1998; 13:239–252.

61. Deveraux QL, Leo E, Stennicke HR, et al. Cleavage of human inhibitor of apoptosis protein XIAP results in fragments with distinct specificities for caspases. EMBO J 1999; 18(19):5242–5251.

62. Deveraux QL, Takahashi R, Salvesen GSet al. X-linked IAP is a direct inhibitor of cell death proteases. Nature 1997; 388(6639):300–324.

63. Tai YT, Strobel T, Kufe D, et al. In vivo cytotoxicity of ovarian cancer cells through tumor-selective expression of the BAX gene. Cancer Res 1999; 59(9):2121–2126.

64. Chi KN, Gleave MD. Antisense approaches in prostate cancer. Expert Opin Biol Ther 2004; 4:927–936.

65. Carducci et al. Effect of endothelin-A receptor blockade with atrasentan on tumor progression in men with hormone refactory prostate cancer: a randomized Phase II, placebo-controlled trial. J Clin Oncol 2003; 21:679–689.

66. Kim HE, Han SJ, Kasza T, Han R, Choi HS, Palmer KC, Kim HR. Platelet derived growth factor signaling mediates radiation induced apoptosis in human prostate cancer cells with loss of p53 function. Int J Radiat Oncol Biol Phys 1997; 39: 731–736.

67. Fudge K, Wang CY, Stearns ME. Immunohistochemistry analysis of PDGF A and B chains and PDGF alpha and beta receptor expression in benign prostate hyperplasias and Gleason graded human prostate adenocarcinomas. Mod Pathol 1994; 7: 549–554.

68. Sitaras NM, Sariban E, Bravo M, Pantazis P, Antoniades HN. Constitutive production of PDGF-like proteins by human prostate adenocarcinoma cell lines. Cancer Res 1988; 48:1930–1935.

69. Vlahos CJ, Kriauciunas TD, Gleason PE, Jones JA, Eble JN, Salvas D, Falcone JF, Hirsch KS. PDGF induces proliferation of hyperplastic human prostatic stormal cells. J Cell Biochem 1993; 52:404–413.

70. Ko YJ, Small EJ, Kabbinavar F, Chachoua A, Taneja S, Reese D, DePaoli A, Hannah A, Balk SP, Bubley GJ. A multi-institutional phase II study of SU101, a platelet-derived growth factor receptor inhibitor, for patients with HRPC. Clin Cancer Res 2001; 7:800–805.

71. Druker BJ, Sawyers CL, Kantarjian H, Resta DJ, Reese SF, Ford JM, Capdeville R, Talpaz M. Activity of a specific inhibitor of the BCR-Abl tyrosine kinase in the blast crisis of chronic myeloid leukemia and acute lymphoblastic leukemia with the Philadelphia chromosome. NEJM 2001; 344:1038.

72. Carroll M-, Jones S, Tamura S, Buchdunger E, Zimmermann J, Lydon ND, Gilliland DG, Druker BJ. CGP 57148, a tyrosine kinase inhibitor, inhibits the growth of cells expressing BCR-ABL, TEL-ABL, and TEL-PDGFR fusion proteins. Blood 1997; 90:4947–4952.

73. Gilbert RE, Kelly KJ, McKay T, Chadban S, Hill PA, Cooper ME, Atkins RC-, Paterson DJ. PDGF signal transduction inhibition ameliorates experimental mesnagial proliferative glomerulonephritis. Kidney Int 2001; 59:1324–1332.

74. Cairns P, Okami K, Halachmi S, et al. Frequent inactivation of PTEN/MMAC1 in primary prostate cancer. Cancer Res Nov 15 1997; 57(22):4997–5000.

75. Whang YE, Wu X, Suzuki H et al. Inactivation of the tumor suppressor PTEN/MMAC1 in advanced human prostate cancer through loss of expression. Proc Natl Acad Sci USA Apr 28 1998; 95(9):5246–5250.

76. Wu X, Senechal K, Neshat MS, et al. The PTEN/MMAC1 tumor suppressor phosphatase functions as a negative regulator of the phosphoinositide 3-kinase/Akt pathway. Proc Natl Acad Sci USA Dec 22 1998; 95(26):15587–15591.

77. Datta SR, Brunet A, Greenberg ME. Cellular survival: A play in three Akts. Genes and Development 1999; 13:2905–2927.

78. Teng D, Hu R, Lin H. MMAC1/PTEN mutations in primary tumor specimens and tumor cell lines. Cancer Research 1997; 57:5221–5225.

79. Ozes ON, Mayo LD, Gustin JA, et al. NFk-B activation by tumour necrosis factor requires the Akt serine-threonine kinase. Nature 1999; 401:82–85.

80. Wang CY, Mayo MW, Korneluk RG, et al. NF-kB antiapoptosis: induction of TRAF-1 and TRAF-2 and cIAP1 and cIAP2 to suppress caspase-8 activation. Science 1998; 281:1680–1683.

81. King RW, Deshaies RJ, Peters JM, et al. How proteolysis drives the cell cycle. Science 1996; 274(5293):1652–1659.

82. Loda M, Cukor B, Tam S, et al. Increased proteasome-dependent degradation of the cycl independent kinase inhibitor p27 in aggressive colorectal carcinomas. Nature Medicine 1997; 3:231–4.

83. Papandreou CN, Pagliaro L, Millikan R, et al. Phase I study of PS-341, a novel proteasome inhibitor, in patients with advanced malignancies [abstract 6]. In Proceedings of the 1999 AACR-NCI-EORTC International Conference on Molecular Targets and Cancer Therapeutics. Washington. DC, 1999.

84. Rao L, Perez D, White E. Lamin proteolysis facilitates nuclear events during apoptosis. J Cell Biol 1996; 135:1441–1445.

85. Scheffner M, Huibregtse JM, Viersta RD, et al. The HPV-16 and E6-AP complex functions as a ubiquitin-protein ligase in the ubiquitination of p53. Cell 1993; 57(3): 495–505.

86. Zong WX, Edelstein LC, Chen C, et al. The prosurvival BCL-2 homolog Bfl-1/A1 is a direct transcriptional target of NF-kappaB that blocks TNF-Alpha induced apoptosis. Genes Dev 1999; 13:382–387.

87. Mandenbauer N. et al. Generation of PSA-reactive of test cells after vaccination with a PSA-based vaccine in patients with prostate cancer. Prostate 43:88–100, 2000.

88. Eder JP. et al. A phase I trial of a recombinant vaccinia virus expressing prostate-specific antigen in advanced prostate cancer. Clin Cancer Res 6:1632–1638, 2000.

89. McDevitt et al. C, et al. An alpha-particle emitting antibody for radioimmunotherapy of prostate cancer. Cancer Res 2000; 60:6095–6100.

90. Smith-Jones PM, et al. In vitro characterization of radiolabeled monoclonal antibodies specific for the extracellular domain of prostate-specific membrane antigen. Cancer Res 2000; 15:5237–5243.

91. Gong et al. PM, et al. Prostate-specific membrane antigen specific monoclonal antibodies in the treatment of prostate and other cancers. Cancer Metastasis Rev 1999; 18:483–490.

EDITORIAL COMMENTARY

Neil H. Bander

Bernard & Josephine Chaus Professor, Weill Medical College of Cornell University, Attending Surgeon, Brady Urology New York-Presbyterian Hospital-Cornell University Medical Center, New York, NY, USA

DiPaola addresses a problem of substantial significance. Despite the fact that we can now, in the "PSA era" diagnose prostate cancer far earlier than previously, in most cases while the patient still has a palpably normal gland, there is still a high failure rate after local therapy. Estimates of failure after surgery or radiotherapy range from 25–50% in cases. Some 75,000–100,000 new patients fall into this category of "biochemical (PSA) failure" or "D0" disease each year. According to the Hopkins data [1], the median time from PSA failure to imagable, metastatic disease is 8 years, followed by a median of 5 years until death. As there is no current adequate systemic therapy beyond palliative hormonal therapy, all of these patients have an inexorable course that ultimately leads to death from prostate cancer unless they die of another cause first. It is an unfortunate reality that the only thing keeping prostate cancer from being the largest cancer killer is the fact that a large proportion of these patients suffer from co-morbidities to which they succumb prior to death from prostate cancer. During this long period of progressing cancer, even in the absence of symptoms, patients are stressed by the sense that the Sword of Damocles is inching ever closer. Clearly, this is an unacceptable situation and we need to do better.

DiPaola makes a persuasive case for the study of novel therapies in patients with PSA failure prior to the development of imagable disease. He points out that earlier treatment may be more successful if instituted prior to years of hormone therapy and the acquisition of multiple mutations that lead to ever increasing treatment resistance. He similarly points out the additional benefit that disease burden is low in this setting. He appropriately indicates that there is little persuasive evidence that early hormone therapy provides any *meaningful* survival benefit to patients and, therefore, offering patients options of novel therapies prior to hormonal therapy is not likely to compromise their eventual survival.

Rather than discuss the specific therapeutic options presented by DiPaola, I will provide my basic approach for deriving recommendations for patients in this setting. My own preference for selecting novel therapies to recommend to patients is, first, therapies that have shown some benefit in patients with more advanced prostate cancer. Absent such options, a second choice of options would be therapies that may not yet have demonstrated benefit but do have some scientific rationale compelling one to put them to the test. Recognizing that these trials will provide real benefit to few participating patients, I also prefer therapies that have little or no significant side effects, as one does not want to compromise the quality of life of these patients who are a long way from being symptomatic from their underlying disease.

In conclusion, I strongly support DiPaolo's well-explained position that D0 patients be offered novel therapies as an option to early hormone-therapy. The latter provides patients with little meaningful benefit in quantity of life and clearly causes significant, albeit insidious, side effects. It is imperative that we develop improved systemic therapies, as adjuncts to local treatments, for this large and growing group of patients.

REFERENCE

1. Pound CR, Partin AW, Eisenberger MA, Chan DW, Pearson JD, Walsh PC. Natural
    history of progression after PSA elevation following radical prostatectomy. JAMA
    1999; 281:1591–1597.

EDITORIAL COMMENTARY

Susan F. Slovin

Genitourinary Oncology Service, Memorial Sloan-Kettering Cancer Center, New
York, NY, USA

There has been a transformation in the tableau that once defined the prostate
cancer population; in the 1980s, prostate cancer patients were usually older with
larger tumor burdens at presentation with multiple medical comorbidities, and
often there was a delay in the actual time to diagnosis. Within the last decade,
we are clearly seeing a different trend in the prostate cancer patient who presents
to the clinic, i.e., a younger man with often a more aggressive and clinically
localized tumor compared with those patients who presented for treatment over
a decade ago. In addition, we are seeing the emergence of a unique subpopulation
of men who are living longer and have, as the only manifestation of disease
recurrence following primary therapy, a rising biomarker, prostate-specific antigen (PSA), in the absence of radiographic progression of disease. There is no
doubt that the treatments needed for the patient with biochemically relapsed prostate cancer should be distinct from those with more advanced disease; however,
there is evidence to suggest that the age-old treatment algorithms which favor
specific and distinctive treatments for use at a particular stage in the disease are
no longer tenable, and that hormones, chemotherapy and biologic agents, may
be interspersed at any time along the treatment pathway.

RISK PROGNOSTICATION IN THE TREATMENT DECISION

Both urologists and oncologists are now basing their treatment decisions on risk
prognostication. Risk of disease recurrence has always been a key factor in the
discussion by the physician with any patient who either has early clinically localized disease or disease relapse. The odds that a treatment will work and the
percent response rate that will delay disease recurrence is what often sways a
patient toward a particular treatment option. However, the data presented by
Pound et al. [1] crystallized how we, as urologists and medical oncologists, should
really evaluate a patient either in the throes of initial diagnosis or beyond. Based
on a single urologist's collective experience of 1,997 patients, it was determined
that the initial Gleason grade, baseline PSA, and PSA doubling time contributed

to disease outcome. The authors were then able to stratify based on an algorithm constructed to predict metastatic progression, those who would have a biochemical failure within 2, 5, or 10 years postsurgery. Patients at low and high risk were identified. Patients with Gleason tumor scores of between 8 and 10, for example, had a probability of metastatic progression of 37%, 60%, and 71% at 3, 5, and 7 years, respectively. Combining a high-grade histology and time to recurrence of PSA, the proportion of patients with metastases at 3, 5, and 7 years was 23%, 40%, and 53%. In addition, those patients who had evidence of PSA relapse within two years of surgery, with PSA doubling times of less than ten months, often did worse prognostically compared with patients whose PSAs relapsed after five or ten years. Though this single study of patients was followed expectantly postprostatectomy, and although there are considerably larger data bases which exist in the radiation oncology literature (2–4), it, nevertheless, set the stage for practitioners to at least examine how risk may play a role in treatment decision and development. Scher et al. [5] and Logothetis [6] offered alternative views as to how medical oncologists should approach the development of disease progression and showed that, by defining the biologic and clinical risk factors which contribute to disease evolution, one could then develop appropriate treatment strategies. In the "clinical states model" by Scher and Heller [5], the model included a depiction of both the natural and treated history of the disease and provided a framework to assess and reassess prognosis over a timeline. Based on the understanding that cancer and its evolution is a dynamic process, this model offered a statistical probability paradigm which could predict the likelihood of disease progression. As many models now do, this model tries to take into consideration both the biologic behavior of the tumor as well as its clinical presentation within the patient. Logothetis [6] has concentrated on understanding the biologic and molecular factors which govern metastatic tumors and has developed several models by which the risk of these molecular events can occur.

TREATMENT BASED ON UNDERSTANDING PATIENT'S UNIQUE TUMOR BIOLOGY

The idea of trying to understand the biology of the tumor's behavior and its impact on the clinical manifestation of disease is not new. What is more problematic, however, is trying to reconcile the vagaries between tumor behavior and factors which define behavior and the real clinical adaptation of the tumor as manifested within the patient. These include evaluation of the prostatic biopsy cores at diagnosis to determine the number of cores and extent of tumor involvement within each [7]; presence of high grade Gleason score [8]; presence of p27 or p53 mutations [9–11]; ploidy [12] and microvascular density [13]; expression of E-cadherin [14]; and the isolation and characterization of prostate cancer cells from the circulation [15]. While many of these elements can assist in characterizing the behavior of the tumor to a small extent, there remains a considerable distance to be traversed before these variables impact on decision making.

TARGETED THERAPIES IN THE MINIMAL AND METASTATIC DISEASE STATES

As can be gleaned by DiPaolo's comprehensive review, biologic agents are clearly making their way into the treatment roster based on the presence of multiple cytoplasmic and nuclear targets. The impact of many of these treatments also depends on the clinical stage at which the treatment is given, the number of pretreatments, including hormone and chemotherapeutic agents, and the extent of tumor burden. Many oncologists would agree that the greater the number of prior treatments, the lower the probability that many investigational treatments will work. This may be due in part to extensive bone marrow compromise by the tumor lending to a "burned out" marrow, which may contribute to myelosuppression during treatment. Patients treated with multiple radiations in a "band-aid"–like approach also run the risk of having marrows that will not support even the mildest of biologic agents. Yet many of the clinical trials target just that population; those who have failed conventional modalities have no other recourse but to be treated in a phase I or II setting. This had led many oncologists to try to treat patients with biologic agents earlier in the disease with minimal tumor burden such as those in the setting of a rising PSA alone following primary treatment or those who have failed hormone treatments and are now in the castrate state in the absence of radiographic disease. One of the great controversies in prostate cancer management is whether patients will be amenable to such therapies. Clearly, the patient who has responded well to hormones in the past and has a rising PSA may favor a second- or third-line hormone in an attempt to not "rock the boat." On the other hand, a patient whose PSA is rising following definitive radiation therapy or surgery and has a slow biochemical relapse (Gleason grade 7 or less, PSA doubling time > 6 months) may opt to undergo expectant monitoring compared with a similar patient who has a history of a Gleason 8 or greater tumor and PSA doubling time of less than six months. Because there is no standard of care for these patients and because many who have failed hormones may do so without evidence of radiographic disease, the options for treatment, once quite limited, have grown enormously. To date, no cytotoxic approach in the phase III setting has shown to improve survival significantly although recent data suggest that taxane-based regimens may contribute to improving survival marginally. Unfortunately, there have been an overall paucity of phase III trials in prostate cancer; phase I and phase II trials using biologic agents have not shown significant efficacy. This may be due to the fact that many of the earlier trials were not designed with appropriate clinical trial endpoints in mind. It may well be that using variables associated with risk prognostication may be helpful in defining a more uniform population for clinical trial entry, limiting those patients to the trial who most require it and for whom a more rapid clinical response may be determined.

HOW SHOULD SPECIFIC PATIENT POPULATIONS OR STATES PROCEED WITH TREATMENT?

So how does one proceed with treatment recommendations given the patient populations which are now presenting in the new millennium? Once again, it is advisable to use either a disease-state model or some other means of evaluating the type of patient for whom a treatment is to be considered. If it is a patient in the rising PSA population (noncastrate with biochemical relapse after initial therapy), expectant monitoring or biologic approaches are indeed reasonable. Given the varied and abundant expression of many altered "self" antigens on prostate cell surfaces, such as PSA, PSMA acid phosphatase, glycoproteins such as mucins or glycolipids such as Globo H, GM2, and Lewis y, immunologic strategies have been developed in the form of conjugate carbohydrate vaccines [16], dendritic cell vaccines [17,18] and DNA vaccines [19], all of which are currently in clinical trials. It should be stressed that the biggest detriment to biologic trials performed in the setting of a rising PSA in the minimal disease state, is the lack of appropriate target endpoints. At present, the FDA will not accept changes in PSA slope, as the impact of slope changes either by per cent or log slope as observed in many trials, has not as yet been validated. All clinical trials must have a "time to disease progression" as a trial endpoint with progression of disease in bone as a final determinant of disease progression. A consensus conference as part of a consortium with the Prostate Cancer Foundation (formerly CaP CURE), the NIH, the Food and Drug Administration (FDA), and multiple academic institutions within the country, are currently putting together recommendations for treatment options for these patients and how to best evaluate the clinical endpoint.

Molecular targeting is another important treatment approach that has been relegated to trials for more advanced patients. It may be naive of investigators to assume that the biologic behavior of the disease remains the same throughout its natural history. Assuming that is the case, the biology of the cancer that fails one particular treatment is a different cancer behaviorally and molecularly compared to when it fails another therapy, so it should be easy to develop reasonable agents to deal with the treatment failure. Unfortunately, the mechanism by which failure occurs with each treatment remains unknown. This is why biologic agents, when given alone and show no effect, are often given adjunctively with a chemotherapy agent that may, in fact, act synergistically with the biologic agent at a different level of function, for example, as seen in trials using bcl-2 alone and then in concert with a taxane.

Novel nuclear targets, including the androgen receptor, RXR superfamily, and even PPAR-α, as well as signal transduction pathways, have been targeted by a variety of compounds that interfere with nuclear or cellular signaling, respectively [20]. Despite the elucidation of these target–drug interactions, there remains a dichotomy between the success seen in preclinical models and the success seen in vivo in man. This has led to widespread disappointment in the general public who want a "cure," and has disappointed scientists whose rationale for these targets are often logical and substantiated by their preclinical work. What is especially promising now is the fact that novel targets do exist and that, with time and better designed clinical trials based on risk prognostication and biological characteristics of the tumor, there is a greater likelihood that an impact on biologic behavior and clinical outcome will be achieved.

REFERENCES

1. Pound CR, Partin AW, Eisenberger MA, Chan DW, Pearson JD, Walsh PC. Natural history of progression after PSA elevation following radical prostatectomy. JAMA 1999; 281:1591–1597.
2. Roach MR, Lu J, Pilepich MV, Asbell SO, Mohiuddin M, Grignon D. Four prognostic groups predict long-term survival from prostate cancer following radiotherapy alone on Radiation Therapy Oncology Group clinical trials. Int J Radiat Oncol Biol Phys 2000; 47:609–615.
3. Roach M, Weinberg V, McLaughlin P, et al:. Death due to prostate cancer following radiotherapy alone: Defining candidates for early "salvage" trials. Proc J Clin Oncol 2001; 20:176a.
4. D'Amico A. Combined-modality staging for localized adenocarcinoma of the prostate. Oncology 2001; 15:1049–1059.
5. Scher HI, Heller G. Clinical states in prostate cancer: toward a dynamic model of disease progression. Urology 2000; 55:323–327.
6. Logothetis CJ. Introduction: a therapeutically relevant framework for the classification of human prostate cancer. Sem Onc 1999; 26:369–374.
7. Stamey TA. Making the most out of six systematic sextant biopsies. Urology 1995; 95:2–12.
8. Stamey TA, McNeal JE, Yemoto CM, Sigal BM, Johnstone IM. Biological determinants of cancer progression in men with prostate cancer. JAMA 1999; 281:1395–1400.
9. Yang RM, Naitoh J, Murphy M, Wang HJ, Phillipson J, deKernion JB, Loda B, Reiter RE. Low p27 expression predicts poor disease-free survival in patients with prostate cancer. J Urol 1998; 159:941–945.
10. Cordon-Cardo C, Koff A, Drobnjak M, Capodieci P, Osman I, Millard SS, Gaudin PB, Fazzari M, Zhang ZF, Massgue J, Scher HI. Distinct altered patterns of p27kip1 expression in benign prostatic hyperplasia and prostatic carcinoma. J Natl Cancer Inst 1998; 90:1284–1291.

11. Bookstein R, Bova GS, MacGrogan D, Levy A, Isaacs WB. Tumour-suppressor genes in prostatic oncogenesis: a positional approach. Br J Urol 1997; 79(Suppl 1): 28–36.

12. Lieber M. DNA ploidy in prostate cancer: potential measurement as a surrogate endpoint biomarker. J Cell Biochem 1994; 19:246–248.

13. Brawer MJ. Quantitative microvessel density: a staging and prognostic marker for human prostatic cancer. Cancer 1996; 78:345–349.

14. Umbas R, Isaacs WB, Bringuier PP, et al:. Decreased-E-cadherin expression is associated with poor prognosis in patients with prostate cancer. Cancer Res 1994; 54: 1284–1291.

15. Slovin SF, Scher HI. Detectable tumor cells in the blood and bone marrow: smoke or fire?. Cancer 1998; 83:394–398.

16. Slovin SF. Vaccines as treatment strategies for relapsed prostate cancer: approaches for induction of immunity. Hematol Oncol Clin North Am 2001; 15:477–496.

17. Small EJ, Fratesi P, Reese DM, Strang G, Laus R, Peshwa MV, Valone FH. Immunotherapy of hormone-refractory prostate cancer with antigen-loaded dendritic cells. J Clin Oncol. 2000; 18:3894–3903.

18. Simons JW, Mikhak B, Chang JF, DeMarzo AM, Carducci MA, Lim M, Weber CE, Baccala AA, Goemann MA, Clift SM, Ando DG, Levitsky HI, Cohen LK, Sanda MG, Mulligan RC, Partin AW, Carter HB, Piantadosi S, Marshall FF, Nelson WG. Induction of immunity to prostate cancer antigens: results of a clinical trial of vaccination with irradiated autologous prostate tumor cells engineered to secrete granulocyte-macrophage colony-stimulating factor using ex vivo gene transfer. Cancer Res 1999; 59:5160–5168.

19. Wolchok JD, Livingston PO. Vaccines for melanoma: translating basic immunology into new therapies. Lancet Oncol 2001; 2:205–211.

20. Smith MR, Manola J, Kaufman D, George D, Mueller E, Bittman L, Kazanis M, Slovin S, Spiegelman B, Small E, and Kantoff PW. Rosiglitazone versus placebo for men with prostate cancer and a rising serum prostate specific antigen after radical prostatectomy and/or radiation therapy. Cancer, in press.

EDITORIAL OVERVIEW

Kenneth B. Cummings

DiPaola observes that, overall, the data on the timing of androgen ablation therapy in prostate cancer is inadequate to define the standard approach that will alter survival. However, a few conclusions can be made: (a) androgen ablation probably can be delayed in patients with advanced disease only if patients are followed closely to avoid problems with spinal cord compression or urologic difficulties, (b) androgen ablation does not improve survival as adjuvant therapy to radical prostatectomy, (c) androgen ablation therapy may improve survival when added for 3 years to radiation therapy in patients with advanced T3 and T4 tumors, and (d) there is no data to support the early use of androgen ablation therapy in patients with PSA progression in absence of imageable disease after local therapy making the considerations of novel approaches in this group reasonable [1].

The availability of PSA, in addition to employment in the diagnosis, with associated "lead time" bias, has been a valuable tool in following patients after local therapy and is a surrogate to response to novel therapies. The ability to randomize patients with PSA progression to clinical trials rests heavily on the investigator's integrity to persuade the patient that we have no compelling data to exhibit that eliminating a PSA value when it first manifests after local therapy has documented impact on disease-specific survival. The opportunity to exploit this marker in a patient population who have, albeit, slow but progressive disease manifested by PSA progression, and who likely can be safely deferred androgen deprivation until a value of 15–20 ng/mL is reached, offers an unusual opportunity to "drug discover."

DiPaola provides a scholarly approach to drug-resistance mechanisms as well as an understanding of emerging concepts employing drug discovery to known mechanisms of tumor cell resistance. He has illustrated in his Table 1 the category of mechanisms that can be targeted and examples of agents that are under investigation, which are most appropriately referenced.

Bander supports DiPaola's efforts in that he concurs that there is little persuasive evidence to support that early hormone therapy provides any meaningful survival benefit to patients, and, therefore, offering patients options of novel therapies prior to hormone therapy is unlikely to compromise survival.

Slovin is in accord with DiPaola's search for novel therapies in the population of patients with PSA progression only and cites that, to date, no cytotoxic approach in Phase III setting has shown to improve survival significantly. She makes a strong argument for the use of biologics and vaccines given the varied expression of many altered self-antigens on prostate cell surfaces. Slovin states that immunologic strategies have been developed in the form of conjugate carbohydrates vaccines [2], dendritic cell vaccines [3,4], and DNA vaccines [5], all of which are currently in clinical trials. She stresses that the biggest detriment to biologic trials performed in a setting of rising PSA in minimal disease state is a lack of appropriate target endpoints. At present, the FDA will not accept changes in PSA slope, as the impact of slope changes either by percent or log slope as observed in many trials, has not as yet been validated. All clinical trials must have a "time-to-disease progression" as a trial endpoint, with progression of disease in bone as a final determinant of disease progression.

The observation that many patients with PSA progression only, depending on their original tumor characteristics, may, in fact, have a significant disease-free interval and a survival of up to 10 years has made application of clinical trials with significant toxicity unattractive. In contrast to germ cell tumors, where the availability of serum markers allowed the definition of cytotoxic chemotherapy, which, albeit, could be life threatening, has, in fact, led to a cure of the disease, does not have a similar paradigm in prostate cancer.

It may be necessary to consider that the earlier use of cytotoxic agents, which are novel but not associated with life-threatening toxicity, with application for select patients could alter the current paradigm of ineffective chemotherapy when the disease is advanced and hormone refractory. It seems likely that employment of a combination of agents with activity and potential to be mechanically synergistic could, with justification, be employed. It would be necessary to identify a subset of PSA-progression only patients with unfavorable tumor characteristics. Certainly, the timing of such intervention should be early prior to the acquisition of major drug-resistance mechanisms.

In a disease where a marker "PSA" is available and where androgen deprivation has, since its discovery, not been curative [6] as man's life expectancy has been extended, novel albeit toxic chemotherapy may be appropriate and necessary to cure those who will "benefit from cure."

To expand on the now famous quote from Whitmore, who died of prostate cancer while still in his intellectual prime "age 78," "curative treatment is possible for whom it is unnecessary, but impossible for whom it is necessary." Man's advancing life expectancy should force us to reexamine our therapy in a disease for whom a cure is necessary but historically has not been possible.

REFERENCES

1. DiPaola RS. Approaches to the treatment of patients with hormone sensitive prostate cancer. Seminars of Oncology 1999; 26:24–27.
2. Slovin SF. Vaccines as treatment strategies for relapsed prostate cancer: approaches for induction of immunity. Hematol Oncol Clin North Am 2001; 15:477–496.
3. Small EJ, Fratesi P, Reese DM, Strang G, Laus R, Peshwa MV, Valone FH. Immunotherapy of hormone-refractory prostate cancer with antigen-loaded dendritic cells. J Clin Oncol 2000; 18:3894–3903.
4. Simons JW, Mikhak B, Chang JF, DeMarzo AM, Carducci MA, Lim M, Weber CE, Baccala AA, Goemann MA, Clift SM, Andro DG, Levitsky HI, Cohen LK, Sanda MG, Mulligan RC, Partin AW, Carter HB, Piantadosi S, Marshall FF, Nelson WG. Induction of immunity to prostate cancer antigens: results of a clinical trial of vaccination with irradiated autologous prostate tumor cells engineered to secrete granulocyte-macrophage colony-stimulating factor using ex vivo gene transfer. Cancer Res 1999; 59:5160–5168.
5. Wolchok JD, Livingston PO. Vaccines for melanoma: translating basic immunology into new therapies. Lancet Oncol 2001; 2:205–211.
6. Huggins C, Hodges CV. Studies on prostate cancer: effect of castration, of estrogen and of androgen injection on serum phosphatases in metastatic carcinoma of the prostate. Cancer Res 1941; 1:292–297.

12

Future Perspectives: Immunotherapy and Vaccines in Prostate Cancer

Johannes Vieweg and Jens Dannull

Division of Urology, Duke University Medical Center, Durham,
North Carolina, USA

INTRODUCTION

According to data from the Surveillance, Epidemiology and End Results (SEER) Program Registries, approximately 185,000 men present with prostate cancer every year in the United States [1]. Almost one-third of these newly diagnosed patients have locally advanced or metastatic disease. Further, standard therapies for presumed organ-confined prostate cancer produce failure rates of 30–50% [2]. Recurrent or metastatic disease is initially treated with hormone deprivation, which temporarily achieves disease stabilization or tumor regression in approximately 80% of patients. However, despite primary or secondary hormonal manipulations, androgen-refractory disease will eventually develop and is ultimately fatal. The median survival for the hormone-refractory group of patients is approximately one year. Even with the administration of second- or third-line chemotherapy, no improvement in survival is achieved. Therefore, experimental therapies conducted in peer-reviewed clinical trials should be recommended to all subjects with metastatic prostate cancer. As these epidemiologic figures clearly illustrate, prostate cancer has a marked impact upon our society with major socioeconomic implications. It is evident, then, that current standard therapies are inadequate and new treatment approaches are warranted. Accordingly, any new strategy that improves the outcome for prostate cancer patients has the potential to exert profound benefit for the individual patient as well as for our society as a whole.

THE RATIONALE FOR IMMUNOLOGIC TREATMENT OF PROSTATE CANCER

New cancer therapy approaches seek to employ "targeted therapies" to selectively eradicate tumors or disrupt mechanisms essential for tumor and metastatic growth and metastasis. Therefore, there is a renewed enthusiasm for the use of cancer immunotherapy since immune-based approaches are highly specific, exploiting biologic differences between malignant and normal cells, thereby exacting tumor cell death in a highly targeted manner.

Historically, immune interventions have been largely unsuccessful in impacting tumor growth and disease progression in prostate cancer settings. Therefore, the prostate was regarded as an immuno-privileged site in which tumors can arise without interference from the immune system [3]. However, over the last decade, this view has changed profoundly since many studies demonstrated that inflammatory responses against prostate tumors exist and that T effector cells can naturally infiltrate prostate cancers [4]. Furthermore, many novel tumor-associated antigens (TAA) have now been identified that are prostate or prostate cancer specific, thus providing highly authentic and relevant targets for prostate cancer immunotherapy [5]. One major milestone that has advanced the field of cancer immunotherapy in general is the unveiling of mechanisms that regulate the interactions between professional antigen-presenting cells (APC) and T effector cells. Dendritic cells (DC) are professional APC that play a key role in the initiation of cellular and humoral immune responses by capturing, processing and presenting antigen to naive T cells [6,7]. Circulating DC can naturally be found in trace numbers throughout the human body, but are predominantly present at sites of potential antigen encounter, such as skin, lung and gastrointestinal (GI) tract. They reside in these tissues mainly as immature, antigen-capturing cells. Following antigen exposure and uptake, however, DC migrate to the secondary lymphoid organs where they mature and become able to select and activate naive antigen-specific T-cells, thereby inducing immune responses. Effective T cell priming necessitates appropriate costimulatory signals, such as CD40 or B7 during DC-T cell engagement, in order to prime a vigorous and antigen-specific immune response [8].

The immune system is equipped with two different effector arms against tumors, each of which involves different lymphocytes subsets and different mechanisms of attack. The effector cells generated by active immunotherapy strategies, such as cancer vaccines, are cytotoxic T cells (CD8$^+$), which are capable of killing tumor cells in an antigen-specific manner. Accumulating evidence suggests that

CD4$^+$ T cell responses also play a key role in antitumor immunity. The Th1 subset of CD4$^+$ T cells is essential for the induction and persistence of CD8$^+$ cytotoxic T lymphocytes (CTL). In addition, by secretion of effector cytokines, CD4$^+$ T cells stimulate antibody secreting B cells and sensitize tumor cells to CTL lysis via up-regulation of major histo-compatibility complex (MHC) class I molecules and other components of the endogenous presentation pathway [9]. Emerging evidence suggests that an optimal antitumor immune response will most likely require the concomitant activation of a sustained CD4$^+$ and CD8$^+$ T-cell response with the CD4$^+$ T cells playing a more important role than previously thought [10].

The B-cell effector arm can contribute to an antitumor effect through antibodies which bind noncovalently to cell surface-based antigens via specific receptors in their Fab region (Fig. 1). Antibodies mediate tumor cell lysis by a variety of mechanisms including (1) antibody dependent cellular cytotoxicity (ADCC), (2) complement dependent cytotoxicity (CDC), (3) interference with ligand-receptor interactions, and (4) opsonization of tumor cells that stimulate innate immune responses from phagocytes, NK cells, and other components of innate immunity.

Another key component required for the stimulation of antitumor responses is the presence of molecules through which cancer cells can be distinguished from normal cells. Such molecules, termed tumor-associated antigens (TAA), can be divided into two main categories: (1) Patient-specific mutated self antigens

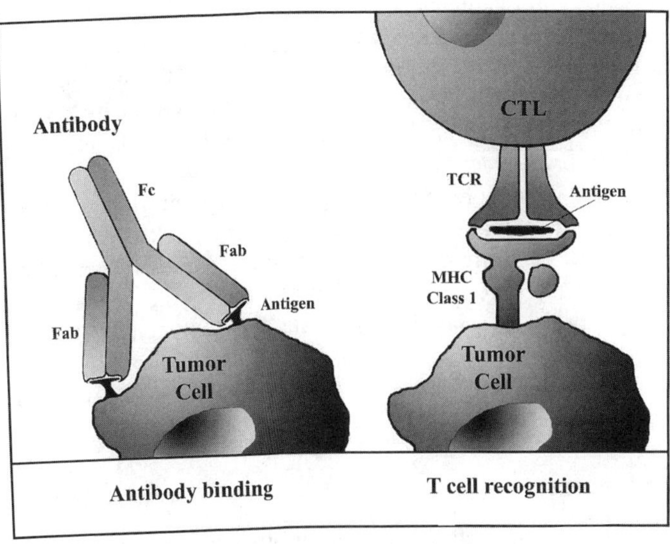

FIGURE 1

and (2) shared non-mutated self antigens (discussed in reference) [11]. Mutated self antigens result from somatic mutations of normal gene products reflecting the genetic instability of tumor cells [12]. Such mutations have arisen in a random fashion and are incidental to the oncogenic process. Shared antigens (with a few notable exceptions) frequently correspond to normal gene products overexpressed by cancer cells or to fetal gene products re-expressed in immunoprivileged sites. While whole-cell vaccines have generated much enthusiasm in the past, antigen-specific targeting of cancers has marked the beginning of the next generation of cancer immunotherapy by circumventing the need to immunize with unfractionated, tumor cell-derived preparations, making the vaccine more practical, especially for tumors that are difficult to access [13].

Unlike in many other tumor systems, many prostate or prostate cancer-specific antigens have been identified that can be recognized by the cellular or humoral arm of the immune system. The discovery of these antigens has facilitated the development of highly promising strategies that will likely augment, and may even supplant, the conventional therapies currently used for cancer treatment. This review will discuss these antigenic targets and will describe their application in context with modern monoclonal antibody drugs and cancer vaccine strategies

PROSTATE CANCER ANTIGENS

Immune-based cancer therapies attempt to take advantage of the unique and exquisitely specific mechanisms by which the body distinguishes and defends itself from foreign pathogens and malignant tumors. Antigens expressed by prostate cancer cells have attracted scientific interest due to their potential capacity to serve as targets for immune attack. Continued identification of the novel markers and therapeutic targets in prostate cancer, especially in advanced disease, is critical for improving diagnosis and therapy, including immunotherapy. Considerable efforts in antigen discovery are ongoing and it is reasonable to expect that in the age of modern genomics, even more relevant targets will be identified in the near future. Table 1 depicts the most relevant prostate tumor antigens identified to date that are under current investigation as targets for the humoral (monoclonal antibodies) or cellular arm (cancer vaccines) of the immune system. These antigens can be categorized as (1) "classical" prostate tissue antigens, (2) targets that regulate prostate cancer growth, (3) targets that are altered or overexpressed during oncogenesis, and (4) stromal targets involved in angiogenesis or tumor-stromal interactions.

Monoclonal Antibodies

In recent years, monoclonal antibody therapy has greatly benefited from the discovery of highly relevant TAA, thereby transforming this technology into an

TABLE 1 Target Antigens for Prostate Cancer Immunotherapy

	Location	Function	Clinical application
Prostate Tissue Specific Antigens			
Prostate-Specific Antigen (PSA)	Secretory protein produced by prostatic epithelial and ductal cells	Serine protease (involved in liquefaction of semen)	**Diagnostic:** mAB (serum marker for disease progression, PCA screening, immunohistochemistry) **Therapeutic:** mAB, Cancer vaccines
Prostate-Specific Membrane Antigen (PSMA)	Membrane-bound protein with both intra- and extracelullar epitopes	Acidic dipeptidase	**Diagnostic:** mAB (Prostascint Scan™) **Therapeutic:** mAB, Cancer vaccines
Prostatic Acid Phosphatase (PAP)	Secretory protein produced by prostatic epithelial and ductal cells	Acid phosphatase	**Diagnostic:** mAB (serum marker of disease progression) **Therapeutic:** mAB, Cancer vaccines
Prostate Stem Cell Antigen (PSCA)	Cell-surface protein	Unknown	**Diagnostic:** mAB (immunohistochemistry) **Therapeutic:** mAB, Cancer vaccines
Genes Regulating Prostate Growth			
Epidermal Growth Factor Receptor (EGFR)	Cell-surface receptor with kinase activity	Activation promotes malignant cell proliferation	**Therapeutic:** mAB (ERBITUX™, ABX-EGF™, EMD72000™)
HER2/neu	Transmembrane protein with tyrosine kinase activity	Promotes oncogenic transformation through dysregulated intracellular signaling	**Therapeutic:** mAB (Herceptin™, Omnitarg™, MDX-H210™)

(continued)

TABLE 1 *continued*

	Location	Function	Clinical application
Genes Altered or Overexpressed During Oncogenesis			
Epithelial Mucins and Glycolipids Antigens	Cell-surface glycoproteins/ glycolipids	Involved in cell-to-cell interaction and signaling	**Therapeutic:** Cancer vaccines (glycolipids, mucin-core structures, blood group-related AGs)
Human Telomerase Reverse Transcriptase (hTERT)	Cell nucleus	Reconstitutes telomere length and promotes unregulated tumor cell proliferation	**Therapeutic:** Cancer vaccines (peptides, DC-based)
Antiangiogenic Targets			
Vascular epithelial growth Factor (VEGF)	Tumor/Tumor stroma	Initiation of blood vessel formation	**Therapeutic:** mAB (Bevacizumab™) **Experimental:** Cancer vaccines **Developmental:** Preclinical studies only
Basic Fibroblast Growth Factor (bFGF)	Tumor/Tumor stroma	Induction of blood vessel formation early in tumorigenes	
Matrix Metalloproteinases (MMP)	Tumor/Tumor stroma	Involved in extracellular matrix interaction, metastasis, angiogenesis	**Therapeutic:** Small molecule inhibitors **Experimental:** Cancer vaccines

important tool for prostate cancer diagnosis and therapy. Antibodies are molecules normally produced by activated B lymphocytes that can be used to target cellular antigens. With the advent of cell engineering, hybridoma technology [14] and methods of "humanization," many approaches now exist that engineer antibodies conjugated to radionuclides, cytotoxic- or immunostimulatory-molecules, capable of initiating either local tumor cell destruction or stimulating a systemic antitumor response. Monoclonal antibody therapy is the only immunological approach to date that has demonstrated proven activity against cancer, as exemplified by the introduction of anti-CD20 (Rituximab™) in B-cell lymphoma and anti-HER-2 (Herceptin™) in breast cancer. Despite this progress, the development of monoclonal antibody drugs with clinical activity against prostate cancer is not yet as advanced as in breast and hematopoietic cancers. However, monoclonal antibodies remain an important vehicle for the staging and diagnosis of recurrent or metastatic disease. Antibodies directed against prostate-specific membrane antigen (PSMA) are currently used to detect prostate cancer metastases [15] and are also being evaluated for prostate cancer treatment [16]. Furthermore, new molecular approaches to antibody design have led to the development of multivalent constructs, which can recognize more than one antigen, thereby potentially improving clinical efficacy. Thus, new antibody-based strategies are emerging that, when applied as monotherapy or in combination with cytotoxic drugs, have shown activity in hormone-refractory prostate cancer (HRPC).

Cancer Vaccines

Active immunotherapy via cancer vaccines has now evolved from first generation tumor cell-based preparations into more advanced approaches that employ defined tumor-associated antigens in context with activated professional antigen presenting cells, such as dendritic cells. Cancer vaccines focus on stimulating the cellular arm of the immune system by de novo induction of antigen-specific T cells in the tumor-bearing host. While antibodies bind noncovalently to a particular antigen via Fab fragments, T-cell recognition is more complex since it involves processing of antigens through the MHC class I or class II pathway (Fig. 1). Each T-cell receptor binds only to its cognate MHC/antigen complex. This strict recognition ensures that T cells are able to recognize subtle changes in the repertoire of antigens expressed by most somatic cells, thus improving specificity. Mechanisms that facilitate efficient T-cell recognition and function rely on (1) effective antigen presentation, (2) MHC class I and II expression by tumor cells, and (3) costimulation during DC T-cell interaction in lymphatic organs. Finally, the pattern of antigen expression influences the processing pathway to T cells. It is known that endogenously synthesized antigens (cytoplasmatic proteins) are presented on MHC class I, but not on MHC class II, molecules, while exogenous proteins (secretory and some membrane proteins) that are internalized by fluid phase absorption or receptor-mediated endocytosis are presented mainly in context with MHC class II, and, to a lesser extent, with MHC class I molecules.

PROSTATE TISSUE-SPECIFIC ANTIGENS

Prostate-Specific Antigen (PSA)

The most widely recognized and consistently expressed prostate cancer-associated antigen is prostate-specific antigen (PSA). PSA is a 34-kD glycoprotein and is a member of the serine protease family with trypsin- or chymotrypsin-like protease activity. Since PSA expression is almost exclusively restricted to prostatic epithelial or ductal cells, and is retained in the majority of androgen-refractory cancer cells, much research has focused on whether or not PSA could represent a relevant target for prostate cancer immunotherapy. The ability to generate T cell-mediated immune responses against PSA in normal men and prostate cancer patients has been well documented by many investigators. Correale and co-workers have shown that cytotoxic T cell lines can be generated by stimulation with HLA-A0201-restricted PSA peptides (PSA-1, PSA-3) and that these CTL are capable of lysing PSA-expressing, HLA-A0201$^+$ prostate cancer cells in vitro [17]. In a subsequent study, this group of investigators demonstrated that in vitro stimulation with a 30-mer oligopeptide spanning the PSA-1 and PSA-3 epitopes can induce a polyvalent, PSA-specific CTL response cytotoxic for prostate tumor cells [18]. Recently, Heiser et al. demonstrated that a vaccine consisting of PSA RNA-transfected DC is capable of stimulating a PSA-specific T-cell response in vitro [19]. The major advantage with this approach, when compared to the peptide strategy, lies in the fact that the vaccine-induced T-cell response was directed against multiple epitopes on the PSA molecule and that could be generated from patients with different HLA backgrounds. The same group of investigators recently reported the results a phase I clinical study in which 13 patients with metastatic prostate cancer were vaccinated using PSA RNA-transfected DC. There was no evidence of dose-limiting toxicity or adverse effects [20]. Induction of PSA-specific T-cell responses was consistently detected in all patients, suggesting in vivo bioactivity of the vaccine. Vaccination was further associated with a significant decrease in the log PSA slope (PSA velocity) and with molecular clearance of circulating tumor cells after vaccination.

Other investigators have focused on activating a cytotoxic T-cell response against PSA through recombinant gene technologies that incorporate genes encoding PSA into viral delivery vectors. Investigators at the NCI and their industry collaborators have developed a recombinant, PSA-expressing vaccinia virus cassette (PROSTVAC) that has been validated in preclinical models, as well as used in several clinical trials [21]. Three phase I clinical trials performed with this recombinant vaccinia PSA vaccine (two with GM-CSF used as adjuvant) have demonstrated only minimal toxicity, except for low grade fever and local erythema at the inoculation site [22–24]. One major drawback of this particular strategy is that vaccinia viruses are highly immunogenic after previous exposure (vaccination), thus leading to the generation of neutralizing antibodies and T-cell responses against viral proteins expressed by previously infected cells. In order to circumvent this problem, prime-boost strategies using alternate viral vectors have been developed that have been shown to enhance antitumor immunity [25,26]. For example, the combination of a PROSTVAC (for priming) and a non-replicating fowlpox virus (boosting) is now being studied in clinical trials and may represent one way to enhance anti-PSA immunity. Other concepts to enhance T-cell activation against PSA include (1) delivery of PSA antigens via recombinant poxviral vectors, (2) the use of multiple T-cell costimulatory molecules [27], and (3) cytokines as biological adjuvants. Clinical trials designed to evaluate these concepts in different stages of disease and through different routes of administration are being performed to define the optimal strategy and schedule for PSA vaccines in patients with prostate cancer, or for those at high risk for disease recurrence.

Prostate-Specific Membrane Antigen (PSMA)

Another potential immune target is prostate-specific membrane antigen (PSMA), a 100-kD transmembrane glycoprotein highly homologous with the human N-acetylated-α-linked acidic dipeptidase. Although PSMA is highly expressed by prostate cells, PSMA is not as organ-specific as originally thought, since PSMA is also expressed by other tissues or neoplasms, such as brain, salivary glands, and intestine, as well as on the surface of new blood vessels induced by neoplastic growth [16]. PSMA is recognized by the murine 7E11-C5 monoclonal antibody, generated against membrane preparations of the human LNCaP prostate adenocarcinoma cell line [28]. This antibody recognizes an intracellular epitope (N-terminus) of the PSMA molecule and is currently used clinically for the diagnosing, localization, and staging of recurrent and metastatic prostate cancer via the ProstaScint™ scan. The ProstaScint™ scan has shown a 44% overall sensitivity and 86% specificity to detect soft tissue nodal disease [29] and, further, can provide valuable staging information when local adjuvant radiation therapy is considered in men with biochemical cancer recurrence following radical prostatectomy [30].

Despite the undisputed diagnostic benefits of using this imaging modality, there are several drawbacks to this technique: adverse reactions to the murine antibody (HAMA formation) have been reported in 4% to 5% of patients upon initial and repeated injection of the antibody. Secondly, a false-positive accumulation of antibodies can occur in secondary tumors or nontumor tissue with high blood content, such as bowel and vascular structures. To minimize false-positive interpretations of the scan, repeat studies are performed 72 to 120 hours following initial injection of radio-labeled antibodies to allow clearance of the isotopes from the vascular and intestinal structures. Finally, the 7E11-C5 antibody targets the intracellular domain of the PSMA molecule, thus necessitating cellular penetration of the antibody to bind to its cognate epitope. Recently, humanized antibodies that bind to the extracellular domain of PSMA have been developed that can be linked to tracer molecules or radioisotopes [16,31]. These antibodies are currently undergoing evaluation for their use in diagnostic and therapeutic applications and may aid in the development of novel methods for delivering toxins, drugs, or short-range radioisotopes to prostate cancer cells.

Recognizing the immunogenicity of PSMA, investigators have identified antigenic peptides within the PSMA protein that serve as epitopes restricted to the HLA-A201 molecule, a common MHC-I molecule found in over 50% of the Caucasian and the African American population. In an initial phase I trial, PSMA peptide-loaded DC were used as a vaccine in 51 patients with metastatic prostate cancer. Administration of autologous DC loaded with two HLA-0201-restricted peptides, derived from PSMA (PSM-P1 and PSM-P2) was well tolerated except for mild to moderate infusion-related side-effects [32]. In a subsequent phase II trial, serum PSA responses were seen in 25%–30% of the patients [33]. However, it was unclear whether or not these PSA reductions could, in fact, be attributed to an immunologic response against the PSMA epitopes since PSA responses were also obtained in patients who lacked the restriction element for the PSMA peptides.

Prostatic Acid Phosphatase

Human prostatic acid phosphatase (PAP) was the first urological tumor marker used for staging and monitoring prostate cancer patients. PAP, a glycoprotein with histidine phosphatase activity, is synthesized by prostatic epithelial cells and secreted into seminal fluid. Like PSA, PAP serum levels increase progressively with advancing stage [34]. However, similar to PSA, the expression of PAP is reduced in neoplastic cells of poorly differentiated tumors, when compared with normal prostatic tissue and well-differentiated adenocarcinomas. The immunogenicity of PAP was previously demonstrated in several studies. First, it was shown that immunization with mouse, but not rat PAP protein resulted in significant T cell-mediated autoimmune prostatitis in Copenhagen rats [35]. Second, DC loaded with PAP-specific peptides have proven effective in stimulating antigen-specific T-cell responses in vitro [36]. Third, PAP-specific antibodies have demonstrated their ability to target and inhibit the growth of established LNCaP tumors [37,38].

The clinical application of PAP-targeting prostate cancer vaccines was recently presented by Small and coworkers, who used APC preparations that were loaded with a recombinant fusion protein consisting of PAP and GM-CSF [39]. In a phase I/II study that enrolled patients with HRPC and, in some cases, chemotherapy refractory metastatic prostate cancer, 3 of 20 subjects had a more than 50% decline in serum PSA levels, and another three demonstrated a partial biochemical response (25–49% serum PSA reduction). Notably, in 40% of the patients, PAP was immunologically recognized as a foreign target. Based on these data, a phase III, placebo-controlled study in 127 patients with HRPC was performed. Although no overall survival benefit was achieved by DC-PAP-based vaccination over placebo, subset analysis revealed that patients with a Gleason score of 7 or below may have benefited from therapy; therefore, additional trials are currently planned.

In a separate trial reported by Fong and colleagues, DC pulsed with recombinant murine PAP were administered as a tumor vaccine to patients with metastatic prostate cancer [40]. Twenty-one patients received monthly vaccinations of xenoantigen-loaded DC with minimal treatment-associated side effects. All patients developed T-cell immunity to murine PAP following immunization. Eleven of the 21 patients also developed T-cell proliferative responses to the homologous PAP antigen. These responses were associated with antigen-specific Interferon-γ and tumor necrosis factor-α (TNF-α) secretion, but not with IL-4 or IL-10 expression, consistent with a Th1-type immune response. Finally, 6 of 21 patients experienced clinical stabilization of their previously progressing prostate cancer. All 6 of these patients developed T-cell immunity to human PAP following vaccination. Together, these results demonstrate that (1) PAP is a potential cancer vaccine candidate and (2) xenoantigen immunization is able to break tolerance against the self antigen PAP in humans and can result in a clinically significant antitumor effect.

Prostate Stem Cell Antigen (PSCA)

Prostate stem cell antigen (PSCA) was discovered in the LAPC-4 xenograft model of human prostate cancer using polymerase chain reaction (PCR)-based representational difference analysis as a gene product that was up-regulated in tumor xenografts when compared to normal prostate tissues [41]. PSCA is a glycosyl-phosphatidylinositol-anchored cell surface antigen that is expressed by both androgen-dependent and independent prostate tumors. It also has been found in transitional cell carcinomas of the bladder and pancreatic carcinomas. PSCA is a unique glycoprotein that shares only some structural homology with stem cell antigen 2. Studies have shown a correlation between the level of PSCA protein expression with later pathological stages of prostate cancer or increasing Gleason score [42]. The cell surface expression of PSCA, coupled with its restricted pattern of expression, makes it a promising target for cancer immunotherapy. Dannull et al. have demonstrated that in vitro stimulation with HLA-A201-binding PSCA peptides can induce a tumor-specific CTL response [43]. These PSCA-specific CTL recognized peptide-pulsed target cells as well as three prostate cancer cell lines in cytotoxicity assays. Saffran and colleagues reported that polyclonal antibodies directed against PSCA can inhibit tumor growth and metastasis formation in mice [44]. Although the exact mechanisms by which tumor growth is inhibited are under current investigation, the above results underscore the therapeutic and diagnostic potential for anti-PSCA immunotherapy in treating advanced and metastatic prostate cancer.

TARGETS THAT REGULATE PROSTATE CANCER GROWTH

Epidermal Growth Factor Receptor

A particularly promising antibody-based strategy entails the targeting of mechanisms essential for tumor cell proliferation and tumor survival, such as those that regulate autocrine growth or angiogenesis. One such target for antibody-based therapy is the epidermal growth factor receptor (EGF). Studies have shown that many tumors have mutations and deletions in the extracellular or the intracellular domain of EGF, some of which promote constitutive kinase activity in the absence of ligands. Furthermore, constitutive activation of EGF, associated with autocrine loops of its ligands, namely EGF, transforming growth factor-α (TGF-α), and amphiregulin, is often observed in human tumors, leading to stimulation of cancer growth, cellular proliferation, tissue invasion, angiogenesis, and metastasis [45]. EGFR is activated by trans-phosphorylation, which, in turn, results in signal transduction that stimulates the cellular mechanisms promoting tumor cell proliferation and survival. EGFR is aberrantly expressed in approximately 80% of prostate cancers and appears to be associated with de-differentiation and the development of androgen-independent disease. Several humanized, EGFR-specific antibodies, including cetuximab (ERBITUX™), ABX-EGF™, and EMD72000™, are now available and are currently undergoing active clinical investigation for the treatment of advanced cancers, including prostate and renal cancers refractory to conventional therapies [46]. An initial clinical trial combining cetuximab with doxorubicin has shown promising results in the form of disease stabilization in 38% of patients [47]. ABX-EGF™, a human monoclonal antibody directed against the human EGFR is currently undergoing evaluation in the setting of a phase II clinical trial in patients with metastatic RCC and HRPC [48]. Although the overall toxicity profiles of antibodies directed against EGFR are favorable, particularly at lower doses, skin toxicities in the form of flushing, seborrhoic dermatitis, and acneiform follicular skin rash have been identified as the major and characteristic side-effect of this particular approach [49]. The rash commonly presents on the head, neck, and trunk and resolves without scarring once the treatment has been discontinued [50].

HER2/neu

The HER-2/neu protein is overexpressed in approximately 63% of primary breast cancers and in 40–60% of metastatic prostate cancers, dependent on the clinical stage of the patient [51]. The proto-oncogene HER2/neu (c-erbB-2) encodes a 185 kD transmembrane protein with intrinsic tyrosine kinase activity (reviewed in [52]). Oncogenic Neu (NeuT), the rat homologue of HER2 that was first isolated from tumors developed in carcinogen-treated rats, was found to have an activating point mutation in its transmembrane region. HER2 shares homology with the rat gene neu, hence the name HER2/neu. The transforming capacity of HER2/neu is solely associated with its overexpression resulting from gene amplification. Since no direct ligand for HER2/neu has been identified, it is believed that high levels of HER2 promote spontaneous dimerization, thus causing constitutive HER2/neu activation and signaling. In addition, heterodimerization between HER2/neu and the other EGFRs (EGFR1, 3, and 4) leads to enhanced ligand affinity along with a decelerated rate of ligand dissociation, which, in turn, results in prolonged signaling by EGFR ligands. In normal cells, up to 20,000 to 50,000 copies of the HER2 receptor are present on the plasma membrane in a tissue-specific manner. However, tumor cells that overexpress HER2 may have up to 2 million copies of the receptor on their cell surface, making the receptor an attractive target for immune-based therapies. The structure of HER2 in malignant cells is the same as that seen in normal cells, therefore, no mutated forms of HER2 have been identified in human prostate cancer. Trastuzumab, also known as Herceptin™, is a humanized monoclonal antibody that binds to the HER2 receptor. In 1998, the U.S. Food & Drug Administration (FDA) approved trastuzumab for the treatment of HER2 protein overexpressing metastatic breast cancers in combination with paclitaxel as a first line therapy and as a single agent for second- and third-line therapy. The usefulness of targeting HER2 in metastatic prostate cancers has been widely debated, since HER2 positivity in prostate cancer is usually weak in intensity and focal in distribution. Accordingly, trastuzumab was not found to be an effective single agent for prostate cancer. However, in combination with docetaxel and estramustin, anti-HER therapy has demonstrated clinical activity in patients with androgen-refractory disease [53]. More contemporary experimental studies have highlighted the important role of HER2/neu signaling and its direct involvement in the progression of prostate cancer to a hormone-refractory state by activation of the androgen receptor pathway, even in the absence of ligand. Thus, rather than simply being a marker that identifies a malignant cell, it is believed that HER2 overexpression contributes to oncogenic transformation through dysregulated intracellular signaling cascades. Therefore, there is continued interest in HER2 and its downstream signaling pathway molecules as potential treatment targets for human prostate carcinoma. Pertuzumab (Omnitarg™) is a humanized HER2-targeted antibody that binds to a cell surface-based epitope distinct from trastuzumab. Pertuzumab acts by blocking ligand-associated heterodimerization of HER2 with other HER-kinase family members (HER1 [EGFR], HER3, and HER4), thereby inhibiting intracellular signaling through MAP and PI3 kinases. The inhibition of mitogenic signaling has shown to arrest cancer-cell growth and to affect cell death. A phase II multicenter trial is currently ongoing to evaluate the efficacy and safety of pertuzumab in subjects with HRPC. The bispecific MDX-H210, has recently been developed and is directed against HER2 as well as the CD64 receptor. CD64, the high affinity receptor for IgG (FcγRI), is expressed by NK cells, monocytes, and macrophages, and is attracting these cells to (HER-2 expressing) tumor sites [54]. In a phase II trial in patients with metastatic prostate cancer, MDX-H210 administered in conjunction with GM-CSF demonstrated a 50% reduction of PSA serum levels in 35% of patients, and a decrease in PSA velocity in 83% of patients [55].

TARGETS ALTERED OR OVEREXPRESSED DURING ONCOGENESIS

Epithelial Mucins and Oligosaccharide Antigens

Among the many structural and functional transformations that occur during oncogenesis, altered expression of cell-surface glycoproteins, such as mucins, has now been recognized as an opportunity for the development of vaccine strategies. Epithelial mucins are high molecular weight glycoproteins that provide a protective layer on epithelial and glandular cell surfaces and are involved in cell-to-cell interactions and signaling [56]. In recent years, several human mucins (MUC1–MUC8) have been identified, at least one of which (MUC-1) shows cell-surface expression on prostate cancer cells. MUC-1 consists of a large, highly glycosylated core region comprising 30–100 tandem repeats of a 20–amino acid sequence. Oligosaccharide structures make up 50% to 90% (by weight) of all mucin molecules. Mucin overexpression and altered glycosylation (hypoglycosylation) in malignant cells result in the exposure of the core protein of the tandem repeats on the cell surface, which can trigger both cytotoxic and humoral immune responses. For example, it is well established that MUC-1 peptides can be processed and presented in conjunction with MHC complex to the immune system for recognition [57] and that cytotoxic T lymphocytes bearing specificity for MUC proteins can arise de novo in patients with cancer, highlighting the potential importance of this antigen in the development of immunotherapeutics.

Several clinical trials using MUC-1 antigens have demonstrated safety in and an increased antibody response after vaccination, the latter of which was associated with a reduction of PSA velocities in some responders (reviewed by [58]). Active immunization with carbohydrate tumor antigens is also being explored as a possible therapeutic modality for prostate cancer since the appearance of unusual, glycolipid or glycoprotein-derived oligosaccharide motifs on the cell surface has shown to correlate with more advanced cancer or hormone-refractory disease. A number of carbohydrate-based cancer vaccines that target the gangliosides GM2, GD2, GD3, and FucM1 [59], mucin-core structures such as TF, Tn, and S-Tn [60], and blood group-related antigens, including globoH and Le^Y [61], have been investigated in a vaccine setting. While measurable antibody responses were achieved, clinical efficacy remains to be demonstrated. Newer strategies seek to enhance the immunogenicity of glycoprotein or carbohydrate vaccines by conjugation with keyhole limpet hemocyanin (KLH) and by coadministration of immunological adjuvants such as the saponin derivatives QS-21 or GP-0100. In a recently completed phase I clinical trial, 20 patients with relapsed prostate cancer received 5 subcutaneous injections (over 26 weeks) of a globoH-KLH conjugate in combination with the adjuvant QS21 [62]. Humoral (IgM and IgG) responses were obtained in all patients and treatment effects occurred 3 months after completion of vaccine therapy. Treatment effects manifested as a decline of serum PSA velocities in 5 patients for more than 2 years. These encouraging results provide a rationale for pursuing immunotherapy trials with tumor-derived oligosaccharide motifs as targets for active immunotherapy.

Telomerase Reverse Transcriptase

The ongoing search for broadly expressed (''universal'') tumor antigens has intensified following the identification of human telomerase reverse transcriptase (hTERT) as a potential antigenic target expressed in the majority of cancer patients. hTERT is a protein essential for maintaining the proliferative capacity and survival of tumor cells. Most somatic tissues and primary cultured cells demonstrate low to undetectable hTERT activity, leading to a steady decline in telomere length with continued cell proliferation in vivo or with passage in culture. Telomerase activity is dramatically up-regulated in virtually all tumors of murine and human origin, including prostate cancers. Telomerase activity is, however, transiently expressed in proliferating tissues such as activated T and B cells, hematopoietic progenitors, germ cells, and cells within intestinal tissues and skin. Because of this differential expression, hTERT has been investigated as a potential target for immunotherapy. Vonderheide and colleagues have shown that hTERT is processed for class I presentation in a broad range of human tumors [1]. In this study, an HLA-A0201 binding hTERT peptide was used to generate a CTL line which lysed HLA-A0201$^+$, but not HLA-A0201$^-$, hTERT positive human tumors [63]. Minev et al. have confirmed and extended these observations by demonstrating that hTERT-specific CTL can be stimulated from the PBMC of healthy individuals as well as of patients with prostate cancer [64]; however, in a recent publication hTERT peptide-specific CTL clones failed to recognize hTERT- and HLA A-201 expressing tumors cells due to inadequate antigen processing by the proteasome [65]. Finally, Nair and colleagues have shown that hTERT-specific CTL can be stimulated from the PBMC of prostate and renal cancer patients by using hTERT-RNA-transfected DC, and that these CTL can recognize and kill autologous prostate and renal cell tumor targets [66]. Cumulatively, these studies provided evidence that hTERT could function as a tumor antigen in a broad range of cancers, including prostate carcinoma. At Duke University, clinical trials are ongoing to test the immunogenicity of hTERT RNA-transfected DC in patients with metastatic prostate cancer. Preliminary data suggest vaccine safety and the induction of hTERT-specific T cells in all subjects enrolled. If such studies demonstrate encouraging results, hTERT will ultimately become an important target for immunotherapy given its wide expression in many tumors.

TARGETING THE TUMOR STROMA

Vascular Epithelial Growth Factor and Matrix Metalloproteinases

The notion of targeting the tumor stroma, especially the angiogenic process, is not new. It has long been known that all tumors beyond a minimal size (2–3 mm) require blood supply and depend on intratumoral neoangiogenesis [67]. Particularly in prostate cancer, stromal-epithelial interactions have shown to play a major role in tumorigenesis and the development of androgen-refractory disease by providing a constant feedback circuit that promotes tumor growth. The tumor stroma offers a broad range of potential molecular therapeutic targets such as vascular epithelial growth factor (VEGF) and its receptors, or basic fibroblast growth factor (bFGF), both of which are proteins involved in endothelial cell differentiation, vessel assembly, and metastatic behavior [68].

Other stromal targets include the matrix metalloproteinases (MMP), key molecules involved in tumor/extracellular matrix interactions, tumor invasion, metastasis, and angiogenesis [69]. Preclinical studies using a synthetic, selective MMP inhibitor, (Prinomastat^{TM}), have demonstrated encouraging results in human prostate cancer xenograft models (as reviewed in reference [70]). Therefore, several of the MMP inhibitors, such as Marimastat and Prinomastat, are currently being clinically investigated in HRPC and other cancers. Although no convincing evidence of antitumor activity has been demonstrated in controlled trials thus far, studies are continuing in order to gain insight as to the role of these agents in the management of prostate cancer [70]. The concepts derived from small molecule-based inhibition studies of MMPs have recently been translated into the field of immunotherapy, since CTL or antibodies may represent an alternative approach for targeting stromal antigens. Support for this novel concept was recently provided by the demonstration in which a vaccine based on chicken MMP-2 as a model antigen could induce both protective and therapeutic antitumor immunity. In addition, angiogenesis was effectively inhibited within the tumor following vaccine treatment [71].

In addition to MMP blockade, natural angiogenesis inhibitors, such as endostatin, angiostatin, and other receptor inhibitors, have been shown to interfere with tumor progression and metastatic development [67]. Consequently, many antiangiogenic compounds are under active clinical investigation in a prostate cancer setting. Previous trials have included therapy with Suramin, Carboxyamido-triazole, Endostatin, SU5416, SU6668, 2-methoxyestradiol (Panzem), TNP-470, and thalidomide [72]. The National Cancer Institute (NCI) has performed a phase II trial of thalidomide in patients with HRPC [73]. Therapy with thalidomide was associated with reduced serum PSA and clinical improvement in selected subjects. Based on these data, a phase III national trial of thalidomide versus placebo in patients with rising PSA is currently ongoing. Two antibody-based approaches that target angiogenic products are being clinically pursued in a metastatic prostate cancer setting. First, Small and colleagues treated 15 patients with HRPC using a humanized antibody that binds to VEGF (Bevacizumab) [72]. Since only 4 patients demonstrated attenuated serum PSA levels after treatment, the investigators concluded that single agent VEGF antibody therapy, at the dose level and frequency administered in this trial, did not produce an objective response in HRPC. In a subsequent study, the same group is now investigating the therapeutic efficacy of Bevacizumab in combination with PAP-loaded antigen-presenting cells in patients with progressive prostate cancer after primary therapy. Second, the investigational antibody Vitaxin™ (MEDI-522) has recently been shown to inhibit neovascularization by binding to $\alpha_V\beta_{III}$ integrin, a molecule present on the surface of endothelial cells [74]. Phase I pharmacokinetic studies have been conducted in patients with mixed solid tumors and Phase II clinical trials in metastatic prostate cancer are planned. Regarding the development of antiangiogenic tumor vaccines, several studies have now established a new ''proof of concept'' that stromal or angiogenic proteins can also be effectively targeted by T cells. This was demonstrated in recent studies in which mice were immunized with (1) paraformaldehyde-fixed xenogeneic endothelial cells [75], (2) VEGFR-2 protein loaded dendritic (DC) [76], (3) VEGFR-2 cDNA-encoding Salmonella based vectors [77], or with (4) DC transfected with VEGR-2, Tie-2 or VEGF mRNA [78]. In all studies, tumor growth was significantly inhibited without induction of detectable autoimmune pathology. The conceptual advantage of these vaccine-based approaches is that their action profile is expected to be lytic rather than cytostatic, the latter of which is the case with small, molecule-based inhibitors that require repeated re-administration to maintain antitumor efficacy [79]. Furthermore, it is anticipated that the antibody- or T cell-mediated antiangiogenic and antitumoral effects can be further improved by combining them with other potentially synergistic strategies such as (1) metronomic therapy via low dose continuous chemotherapy to inhibit proliferation of endothelial cells [80], (2) the use of pleiotropic inhibitors of MMPs such as Neovastat™ (AE-941), (3) treatment with "standard" angiogenesis inhibitors (mechanisms not yet defined) such as thalidomide [81] and TNP-470, and (4) administration of endogenous inhibitors of angiogenesis, such as endostatin (a collagen XVIII fragment) or angiostatin (a plasminogen fragment) [82,83].

ANTIGEN DISCOVERY

Although the previously described antigens have shown promise as therapeutic targets in the treatment of prostate cancer, many potential limitations exist. First, it has long been recognized that prostate tumors are comprised of a diverse population of malignant cells. Correspondingly, the expression of antigenic targets by prostate cancers is also heterogeneous, thus potentially limiting the therapeutic effectiveness of therapies for prostate cancer that target a single or limited repertoire of tumor cell antigens. Secondly, even when target antigens are expressed, prostate malignancies often employ mechanisms to escape identification and destruction by immune surveillance, i.e., through down-regulation of MHC antigens [84]. Nonetheless, although cytotoxic T cells cannot recognize malignant cells that completely lack MHC class 1 expression, antibody-mediated therapies are not necessarily compromised by loss of MHC class I. Finally, antigen-specific vaccinations direct the immune response to a narrow range of single epitopes, which may lead to "antigen escape" by tumor cells [85]. Given these limitations, both the detection and treatment of prostate cancer would be greatly improved by the identification of new targets that can overcome the obstacles associated with single-antigen vaccination. Numerous methods for antigen discovery are now available, and considerable efforts are underway in academic and industry settings to identify new therapeutic targets such as:

1. *cDNA libraries:* T cell antigens can be identified using CTL clones that selectively recognize and kill specific target cells. To allow T cell recognition, target cells are transferred with cDNA libraries prepared from prostate tumor tissues.
2. *Reverse immunology:* This approach takes advantage of computer-assisted prediction models to identify antigenic peptides that fulfill the established criteria for binding to a MHC class I molecule. Once identified, these peptides can be synthesized and their clinical relevance can

be determined by measuring the frequency of T cells in patient blood that reacts with a given peptide epitope [86].

3. *SEREX analysis:* The SEREX approach (serological analysis of autologous tumor antigens by recombinant expression cloning) entails serologic analysis of tumors CDNA used in combination with molecular cloning techniques [87]. It is a promising means of identifying novel antigens that allows an unbiased search for an antibody response and the direct molecular identification of immunogenic tumor proteins based on their reactivity with autologous patient sera. SEREX analyses have led to identification of a variety of novel antigens, the clinical potential of which is currently under investigation.

4. *Surface Epitope Masking (SEM):* This procedure is based on selective blocking of antigens expressed by a genetically modified target cell (tester) using polyclonal antibodies produced against the same unmodified cell line (driver). Antigen-blocked target cells are used to vaccinate mice and, subsequently, to generate hybridomas that can be characterized for antigen specificity. The SEM approach has been successfully used to identify antibodies specific for cell surface-based molecules, both with known and unknown function [88].

5. *Molecular-based approaches:* Many other approaches for antigen discovery have been developed that utilize molecular techniques that identify differential expression patterns between normal versus cancerous tissues. These approaches include: (a) differential display or representational difference analysis [89], (b) subtractive cDNA libraries, (c) use of microarrays (gene chips), or (d) database mining of expressed sequence tag libraries followed by rapid amplification of cDNA ends (RACE) [90].

Using these techniques, several new prostate or prostate cancer-specific genes or gene products have been identified, including Part-1 [91], STEAP [92] DD3 [89], PAGE-4 [93], and PCTA-1 [88], all of which have yet to be explored for their therapeutic and diagnostic potential. In the age of modern genomics, it is expected that newer and more powerful screening techniques will be forthcoming that will provide an overwhelming choice of potential targets for further exploration and development.

CONCLUSION

An improved understanding of the molecular changes associated with the onset and progression of prostate cancer is providing a rational basis for the development of new diagnostic and prognostic tools, as well as novel targets for therapy. Numerous methods for antigen discovery are now available, and considerable efforts are underway in academic and industrial settings to further identify even more relevant prostate cancer targets. The continued identification and characterization of these highly specific targets will be instrumental in the development of more effective treatment modalities, including immunotherapy. Immune-based strategies have emerged as a promising form of targeted therapy that can induce an antitumor response in a highly specific fashion, thus reducing toxic side effects. It is only a matter of time before powerful tools for antigen discovery, combined with modern genomic technologies, will expand our repertoire of treatment options to include tumor vaccines and antibody therapies for prostate cancer patients.

REFERENCES

1. Ries LAG EM, Kosary CL, Hankey BF, et al. (eds.). SEER Cancer Statistics Review; 1975–2000. Bethesda, MD 2003.
2. Badalament RA, Miller MC, Peller PA, et al. An algorithm for predicting nonorgan-confined prostate cancer using the results obtained from sextant core biopsies with prostate specific antigen level. J Urol 1996; 156:1375–1380.
3. Abubakr YA, Redman BG. The role of immunotherapy in urologic malignancies. Cancer Treat Res 1996; 88:235–248.
4. Vesalainen S, Lipponen P, Talja M, et al. Histological grade, perineural infiltration, tumor infiltrating lymphocytes and apoptosis as determinants of long-term prognosis in prostate adenocarcinoma. Eur J Cancer 1994; 12:1797–1803.
5. Saffran DC, Reiter RE, Jacobovits A, et al. Target antigens for prostate cancer immunotherapy. Cancer and Metastasis Reviews 1999; 18:437–449.
6. Steinman RM. The dendritic cell system and its role in immunogenicity. Annu Rev Immunol 1991; 9:271.
7. Steinman RM. Dendritic cells and immune-based therapies. Exp Hematol 1996; 24: 859–862.
8. Banchereau J, Steinman RM. Dendritic cells and the control of immunity. Nature 1998; 392:245–252.
9. Qin Z, Blankenstein T. CD4 + T cell–mediated tumor rejection involves inhibition of angiogenesis that is dependent on IFN gamma receptor expression by nonhematopoietic cells. Immunity 2000; 12:677–686.
10. Toes REM, Ossendorp F, Offringa R, et al. CD4 T cells and their role in antitumor immune responses. Journal of Experimental Medicine 1999; 189:753–756.
11. Gilboa E. The makings of a tumor-rejection antigen. Immunity 1999; 56:223–229.
12. Lengauer C, Kinzler KW. Vogelstein B. Genetic instabilities in human cancers. Nature 1998; 396:643–649.
13. Rosenberg SA. A new era for cancer immunotherapy based on the genes that encode cancer antigens. Immunity 1999; 10:281–287.
14. Kohler G, Milstein C. Continuous cultures of fused cells secreting antibody of predefined specificity. Nature 1975; 256:495–497.
15. Lange PH. PROSTASCINT scan for staging prostate cancer. Urology 2001; 57: 402–406.

16. Liu H, Moy P, Kim S, et al. Monoclonal antibodies to the extracellular domain of prostate-specific membrane antigen also react with tumor vascular endothelium. Cancer Res 1997; 57:3629–3634.

17. Correale P, Walmsley K, Nieroda C, et al. In vitro generation of human cytotoxic T lymphocytes specific for peptides derived from prostate-specific antigen [see comments]. Journal of the National Cancer Institute 1997; 89:293–300.

18. Correale P, Walmsley K, Zaremba S, et al. Generation of human cytolytic T lymphocyte lines directed against prostate-specific antigen (PSA) employing a PSA oligoepitope peptide. Immunology 1998; 161:3186–3194.

19. Heiser A, Dahm P, Yancey D, et al. Human dendritic cells transfected with RNA encoding prostate specific antigen stimulate prostate specific CTL responses in vitro. J Immunol 2000; 164:5508–5514.

20. Heiser A, Coleman DM, Dannull J, et al. Dendritic cells transfected with prostate-specific antigen RNA induces PSA specific T cell responses in metastatic prostate cancers. J Clin Invest 2002; 159.

21. Hodge JW, Schlom J, Donohue SJ, et al. A recombinant vaccinia virus expressing human prostate-specific antigen (PSA): safety and immunogenicity in a non-human primate. International Journal of Cancer 1995; 63:231–237.

22. Sanda MG, Smith DC, Charles LG, et al. Recombinant vaccinia-PSA (PROSTVAC) can induce a prostate-specific immune response in androgen-modulated human prostate cancer. Urology 1999; 53:260–266.

23. Eder JP, Kantoff PW, Roper K, et al. A phase I trial of a recombinant vaccinia virus expressing prostate-specific antigen in advanced prostate cancer. Clin Cancer Res 2000; 6:1632–1638.

24. Gulley J, Chen AP, Dahut W, et al. Phase I study of a vaccine using recombinant vaccinia virus expressing PSA (rV-PSA) in patients with metastatic androgen-independent prostate cancer. Prostate 2002; 53:109–117.

25. Irvine KR, Chamberlain RS, Shulman EP, et al. Enhancing efficacy of recombinant anticancer vaccines with prime/boost regimens that use two different vectors. J Natl Cancer Inst 1997; 89:1595–1601.

26. Hodge JW, McLaughlin JP, Kantor JA, et al. Diversified prime and boost protocols using recombinant vaccinia virus and recombinant non-replicating avian pox virus to enhance T cell immunity and antitumor responses. Vaccine 1997; 15:759–768.

27. Zhu M, Terasawa H, Gulley J, et al. Enhanced activation of human T cells via avipox vector-mediated hyperexpression of a triad of costimualtory molecules in human dendritic cells. Cancer Res 2001; 61:3725–3734.

28. Horoszewicz JS, Kawinski E, Murphy GP. Monoclonal antibodies to a new antigenic marker in epithelial prostatic cells and serum of prostatic cancer patients. Anticancer Res 1987; 7:927–935.

29. Babaian RJ, Sayer J, Podoloff DA, et al. Radioimmunoscintigraphy of pelvic lymph nodes with 111indium labeled monoclonal antibody CYT-356. J Urol 1994; 152: 1952–1955.

30. Kahn D, Williams RD, Haseman MK, et al. Radioimmunoscintigraphy with In-111-labeled capromab pendetide predicts prostate cancer response to salvage radiotherapy after failed radical prostatectomy. J Clin Oncol 1998; 16:284–289.

31. Smith-Jones PM, Vallabhajosula S, Navarro V, et al. Radiolabeled monoclonal antibodies specific to the extracellular domain of prostate-specific membrane antigen: preclinical studies in nude mice bearing LNCaP human prostate tumor. J Nucl Med 2003; 44:610–617.

32. Murphy G, Tjoa B, Ragde H, et al. Phase I clinical trial: T-cell therapy for prostate cancer using autologous dendritic cells pulsed with HLA-A0201-specific peptides from prostate-specific membrane antigen. Prostate 1996; 29:371–380.

33. Lodge PA, Jones LA, Bader RA, et al. Dendritic cell-based immunotherapy of prostate cancer: immune monitoring of a phase II clinical trial. Cancer Res 2000; 60: 829–833.

34. Jacobs EL, Haskell CM. Clinical use of tumor markers in oncology. Curr Probl Cancer 1991; 15:299–360.

35. Fong L, Ruegg CL, Brockstedt D, et al. Induction of tissue-specific autoimmune prostatitis with prostatic acid phosphatase immunization: implications for immunotherapy of prostate cancer. J Immunol 1997; 159:3113–3117.

36. Peshwa MV, Shi JD, Ruegg C, et al. Induction of prostate tumor-specific CD8+ cytotoxic T-lymphocytes in vitro using antigen-presenting cells pulsed with prostatic acid phosphatase peptide. Prostate 1998; 36:129–138.

37. Deguchi T, Chu TM, Leong SS, et al. Effect of methotrexate-monoclonal anti-prostatic acid phosphatase antibody conjugate on human prostate tumor. Cancer Res 1986; 46:3751–3755.

38. Deguchi T, Chu TM, Leong SS, et al. Potential therapeutic effect of adriamycin-monoclonal anti-prostatic acid phosphatase antibody conjugate on human prostate tumor. J Urol 1987; 137:353–358.

39. Small EJ, Fratesi P, Reese DM, et al. Immunotherapy of hormone-refractory prostate cancer with antigen-loaded dendritic cells [In Process Citation]. J Clin Oncol 2000; 18:3894–3903.

40. Fong L, Brockstedt D, Benike C, et al. Dendritic cell-based xenoantigen vaccination for prostate cancer immunotherapy. J Immunol 2001; 167:7150–7156.

41. Reiter RE, Gu Z, Watabe T, et al. Prostate stem cell antigen: a cell surface marker overexpressed in prostate cancer. Proceedings of the National Academy of Sciences of the United States of America 1998; 95:1735–1740.

42. Gu Z, Thomas G, Yamashiro J, et al. Prostate stem cell antigen (PSCA) expression increases with high gleason score, advanced stage and bone metastasis in prostate cancer. Oncogene 2000; 19:1288–1296.

43. Dannull J, Diener PA, Prikler L, et al. Prostate stem cell antigen is a promising candidate for immunotherapy of advanced prostate cancer. Cancer Res 2000; 60: 5522–5528.

44. Saffran DC, Raitano AB, Hubert RS, et al. Anti-PSCA mAbs inhibit tumor growth and metastasis formation and prolong the survival of mice bearing human prostate cancer xenografts. Proc Natl Acad Sci USA 2001; 98:2658–2663.

45. Blackledge G, Averbuch S, Kay A, et al. Anti-EGF receptor therapy. Prostate Cancer Prostatic Dis 2000; 3:296–302.

46. Mendelsohn J. Antibody-mediated EGF receptor blockade as an anticancer therapy: from the laboratory to the clinic. Cancer Immunol Immunother 2003; 52:342–346.

47. Ciardiello F, Tortora G. A novel approach in the treatment of cancer: targeting the epidermal growth factor receptor. Clin Cancer Res 2001; 7:2958–2970.

48. Kim HL, Pantuck AJ, Zomorodian N, et al. Monoclonal antibody (MAB) in patients with advanced cancer. Curr Urol Rep 2003; 4:11–12.

49. Bunn PA, Franklin W. Epidermal growth factor receptor expression, signal pathway, and inhibitors in non-small cell lung cancer. Semin Oncol 2002; 29:38–44.

50. Herbst RS, Madden TL, Tran HT, et al. Safety and pharmacokinetic effects of TNP-470, an angiogenesis inhibitor, combined with paclitaxel in patients with solid tumors: evidence for activity in non-small-cell lung cancer. J Clin Oncol 2002; 20:4440–4447.

51. Di Lorenzo G, Tortora G, D'Armiento FP, et al. Expression of epidermal growth factor receptor correlates with disease relapse and progression to androgen-independence in human prostate cancer. Clin Cancer Res 2002; 8:3438–3444.

52. Holbro T, Civenni G, Hynes NE. The ErbB receptors and their role in cancer progression. Exp Cell Res 2003; 284:99–110.

53. Small EJ, Bok R, Reese DM, et al. Docetaxel, estramustine, plus trastuzumab in patients with metastatic androgen-independent prostate cancer. Semin Oncol 2001; 28:71–76.

54. Lewis LD, Beelen AP, Cole BF, et al. The pharmacokinetics of the bispecific antibody MDX-H210 when combined with interferon gamma-1b in a multiple-dose phase I study in patients with advanced cancer. Cancer Chemother Pharmacol 2002; 49:375–384.

55. James ND, Atherton PJ, Jones J, et al. A phase II study of the bispecific antibody MDX-H210 (anti-HER2 × CD64) with GM-CSF in HER2+ advanced prostate cancer. Br J Cancer 2001; 85:152–156.

56. Parry S, Silverman HS, McDermott K, et al. Identification of MUC1 proteolytic cleavage sites in vivo. Biochem Biophys Res Commun 2001; 283:715–720.

57. Agrawal B, Reddish MA, Longenecker BM. In vitro induction of MUC-1 peptide-specific type 1 T lymphocyte and cytotoxic T lymphocyte responses from healthy multiparous donors. J Immunol 1996; 157:2089–2095.

58. Slovin SF, Livingston PO, Rosen N, et al. Targeted therapy for prostate cancer: the Memorial Sloan-Kettering Cancer Center approach. Semin Oncol 1996; 23:41–48.

59. Livingston PO, Natoli EJ, Calves MJ, et al. Vaccines containing purified GM2 ganglioside elicit GM2 antibodies in melanoma patients. Proc Natl Acad Sci USA 1987; 84:2911–2915.

60. Ragupathi G, Howard L, Cappello S, et al. Vaccines prepared with sialyl-Tn and sialyl-Tn trimers using the 4-(4-maleimidomethyl)cyclohexane-1-carboxyl hydrazide linker group result in optimal antibody titers against ovine submaxillary mucin and sialyl-Tn-positive tumor cells. Cancer Immunol Immunother 1999; 48:1–8.

61. Wang ZG, Williams LJ, Zhang XF, et al. Polyclonal antibodies from patients immunized with a globo H-keyhole limpet hemocyanin vaccine: isolation, quantification, and characterization of immune responses by using totally synthetic immobilized tumor antigens. Proc Natl Acad Sci U S A 2000; 97:2719–2724.

62. Slovin SF, Scher HI. Peptide and carbohydrate vaccines in relapsed prostate cancer: immunogenicity of synthetic vaccines in man—clinical trials at Memorial Sloan-Kettering Cancer Center. Semin Oncol 1999; 26:448–454.

63.	Vonderheide RH, Hahn WC, Schultze JL, et al. The telomerase catalytic subunit is a widely expressed tumor-associated antigen recognized by cytotoxic T lymphocytes. Immunity 1999; 10:673–679.

64.	Minev B, Hipp J, Firat H, et al. Cytotoxic T cell immunity against telomerase reverse transcriptase in humans. Proc Natl Acad Sci U S A 2000; 97:4796–4801.

65.	Ayyoub M, Migliaccio M, Guillaume P, et al. Lack of tumor recognition by hTERT peptide 540–548-specific CD8(+) T cells from melanoma patients reveals inefficient antigen processing. Eur J Immunol 2001; 31:2642–2651.

66.	Nair SK, Heiser A, Boczkowski D, et al. Induction of cytotoxic T cell responses and tumor immunity against unrelated tumors using telomerase reverse transcriptase RNA transfected dendritic cells. Nat Med 2000; 6:1011–1017.

67.	Folkman J. Angiogenesis in cancer, vascular, rheumatoid and other disease. Nat Med 1995; 1:27–31.

68.	Fong GH, Rossant J, Gertsenstein M, et al. Role of the Flt-1 receptor tyrosine kinase in regulating the assembly of vascular endothelium. Nature 1995; 376:66–70.

69.	Nelson AR, Fingleton B, Rothenberg ML, et al. Matrix metalloproteinases: biologic activity and clinical implications. J Clin Oncol 2000; 18:1135–1149.

70.	Scatena R. Prinomastat, a hydroxamate-based matrix metalloproteinase inhibitor. A novel pharmacological approach for tissue remodelling-related diseases. Expert Opin Investig Drugs 2000; 9:2159–2165.

71.	Su JM, Wei YQ, Tian L, et al. Active immunogene therapy of cancer with vaccine on the basis of chicken homologous matrix metalloproteinase-2. Cancer Res 2003; 63:600–607.

72.	Figg WD, Kruger EA, Price DK, et al. Inhibition of angiogenesis: treatment options for patients with metastatic prostate cancer. Invest New Drugs 2002; 20:183–194.

73.	Figg WD, Dahut W, Duray P, et al. A randomized phase II trial of thalidomide, an angiogenesis inhibitor, in patients with androgen-independent prostate cancer. Clin Cancer Res 2001; 7:1888–1893.

74.	Posey JA, Khazaeli MB, DelGrosso A, et al. A pilot trial of Vitaxin, a humanized anti-vitronectin receptor (anti alpha v beta 3) antibody in patients with metastatic cancer. Cancer Biother Radiopharm 2001; 16:125–132.

75.	Wei YQ, Wang QR, Zhao X, et al. Immunotherapy of tumors with xenogeneic endothelial cells as a vaccine. Nat Med 2000; 6:1160–1166.

76.	Li Y, Wang MN, Li H, et al. Active immunization against the vascular endothelial growth factor receptor flk1 inhibits tumor angiogenesis and metastasis. J Exp Med 2002; 195:1575–1584.

77.	Niethammer AG, Xiang R, Becker JC, et al. A DNA vaccine against VEGF receptor 2 prevents effective angiogenesis and inhibits tumor growth. Nat Med 2002; 8: 1369–1375.

78.	Nair S, Boczkowski D, Moeller B, et al. Synergy between tumor immunotherapy and antiangiogenic therapy. Blood 2003; 102:964–971.

79.	Sternberg CN. What's new in the treatment of advanced prostate cancer?. Eur J Cancer 2003; 39:136–146.

80.	Kerbel RS, Klement G, Pritchard KI, et al. Continuous low-dose antiangiogenic/ metronomic chemotherapy: from the research laboratory into the oncology clinic. Ann Oncol 2002; 13:12–15.

81. Amato RJ. Thalidomide therapy for renal cell carcinoma. Crit Rev Oncol Hematol 2003; 46(Suppl):59–65.
82. Eder J, Clark J, Supko J, et al. A phase I trial of recombinant human endostatin, ASCO. 2002.
83. Boehm T, Folkman J, Browder T, et al. Antiangiogenic therapy of experimental cancer does not induce acquired drug resistance. Nature 1997; 390:404–407.
84. Sanda MG, Restifo NP, Walsh JC, et al. Molecular characterization of defective antigen processing human prostate cancer. National Cancer Institute 1995; 87: 280–285.
85. Nestle FO, Alijagic S, Gilliet M, et al. Vaccination of melanoma patients with peptide- or tumor lysate-pulsed dendritic cells. Nature Medicine 1998; 4:328–332.
86. Maecker B, von B-B, Anderson KS, et al. Linking genomics to immunotherapy by reverse immunology—"immunomics" in the new millennium. Curr Mol Med 2001; 1:609–619.
87. Sahin U, Tureci O, Pfreundschuh M. Serological identification of human tumor antigens. Curr Opin Immunol 1997; 9:709–716.
88. Su Z, Lin J, Shen R, et al. Surface-epitope masking and expression cloning identifies the human prostate carcinoma antigen gene PTCA-1, a member of the galectin family. Proc Natl Acad Sci USA 1996; 93:7252–7257.
89. Bussemakers MJ, Bokhoven A, Verhaegh GW, et al. DD3: a new prostate-specific gene, highly overexpressed in prostate cancer. Cancer Res 1999; 59:5975–5979.
90. Vasmatzis G, Essand M, Brinkmann U, et al. Discovery of three genes specifically expressed in human prostate by expressed sequence tag database analysis. Proc Natl Acad Sci USA 1998; 95:300–304.
91. Lin B, White JT, Ferguson C, et al. PART-1: A novel human prostate-specific, androgen regulated gene that maps to chromosome 5q12. Cancer Res 2000; 60: 858–863.
92. Hubert RS, Vivanco I, Chen E, et al. STEAP: A prostate-specific cell-surface antigen highly expressed in human prostate tumors. Proc Natl Acad Sci USA 1999; 96: 14523–14528.
93. Brinkmann U, Vasmatzis G, Lee B, et al. Novel genes in the PAGE and GAGE family of tumor antigens found by homology walking in the dbEST database. Cancer Res 1999; 59:1445–1448.

EDITORIAL OVERVIEW

Kenneth B. Cummings

Vieweg reviews the historic background of immunotherapeutic approaches (e.g., monoclonal antibodies vs. highly targeted vaccines) and recent identification of many novel tumor-associated antigens (TAA), producing highly authentic and relevant targets for prostate cancer immunotherapy [1]. Improved understanding of the role of the dendritic cells (DC) as antigen-presenting cells (APC) in the interaction with T effector cells has advanced the field of immunotherapy [2–4].

The author's Table 1 depicts the most relevant prostate tumor antigens identified to date and currently under investigation as targets for the humoral (monoclonal antibodies) or the cellular arm (cancer vaccines) of the immune system. He further outlines their location, function, and current clinical application.

Despite ongoing research as outlined, there still exists significant limitations. It has long been recognized that prostate tumors represent a diverse population of malignant cells. Expression of antigenic targets by prostate cancers is also highly variable, limiting the therapeutic effectiveness of therapies for prostate cancer that target single or "limited" tumor cell antigens. Prostate cancer often employ mechanisms to escape identification and destruction, by immune surveillance, even when target antigens are expressed, by down-regulation of major histo-compatibility (MHC) antigens [5]. Although malignant cells completely lack MHC class I expression and cannot be recognized by cytotoxic T cells, antibody-mediated therapies may not be compromised.

Vieweg concludes that significant effort is underway employing powerful tools for antigen discovery combined with modern genomics. This will expand the identification of new genes and will overcome obstacles associated with single antigen vaccination. This should rapidly expand the treatment options with tumor vaccines and antibody therapies for prostate cancer patients.

REFERENCES

1. Saffran DC, Reiter RE, Jacobovits A, Witte O. Target antigens for prostate cancer immunotherapy. Cancer and Metastasis Reviews 1999; 18:437–449.
2. Steinman RM. The dendritic cell system and its role in immunogenicity. Annu Rev Immunol 1991(9):271.
3. Steinman RM. Dendritic cells and immune-based therapies. Exp Hematol 1996; 24: 859–862.
4. Banchereau J, Steinman RM. Dendritic cells and the control of immunity. Nature 1998; 392:245–252.
5. Sanda MG, Restifo NP, Walsh JC, Kawakama Y, Nelson WG, Pardoll DM, Simons JW. Molecular characterization of defective antigen processing human prostate cancer. National Cancer Institute 1995; 87:280–285.

Index

Page numbers followed by *f* indicate figures. Those followed by *t* indicate tables.

**